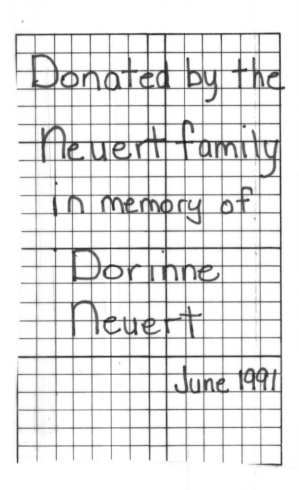

Donated by the
Neuert family
in memory of
Dorinne
Neuert
June 1991

NOTES ON SYMPTOM CONTROL IN HOSPICE & PALLIATIVE CARE

Notes on

SYMPTOM CONTROL

In Hospice & Palliative Care

PETER KAYE
MA, MB, MRCP, MRCGP, DRCOG

Consultant in Palliative Medicine
Oxford Regional Health Authority
&
Medical Director
Cynthia Spencer House
Northampton, England

Revised First Edition
USA Version

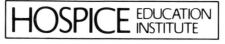

A NON-PROFIT ORGANIZATION
Essex, Connecticut, USA

For information please contact the publisher:

HOSPICE EDUCATION INSTITUTE
Five Essex Square
P.O. Box 713
Essex, Connecticut 06426, U.S.A.
(203) 767-1620
Fax: (203) 767-2746

Library of Congress Cataloging-in-Publication Data

Kaye, Peter.
   Notes on symptom control in hospice and palliative care / Peter
Kaye. -- Rev. 1st ed., USA version.

   Includes bibliographical references.
   Includes index.
   ISBN 0-9623438-1-1 (pbk.) : $24.95
   1. Cancer--Palliative treatment.   2. Symptomatology.   3. Hospice
care.   I. Hospice Education Institute.   II. Title.
   [DNLM: 1. Hospices.   2. Palliative Treatment.   3. Terminal Care-
psychology.   WB 310 K23n]
RC271.P33K39   1990
362.1'75--dc20
DNLM/DLC
for Library of Congress   90-4880
                                                                  CIP

To Karen

TABLE OF CONTENTS

Table of Contents

Table of Contents

Table of Contents

Table of Contents

Table of Contents

TABLE OF DRUGS
GENERIC/PROPRIETARY

This table is intended only for quick reference purposes. **Be sure to verify all information before prescribing.** Products listed may vary in availability of strengths and forms.

Generic Name	Representative U.S. Trade Name
Acetaminophen	TYLENOL
Acyclovir	ZOVIRAX
Adrenaline	ADRENALIN
Albuterol	VENTOLIN
Allopurinol	ZYLOPRIM
Aluminum Hydroxide	in MYLANTA
Amantadine	SYMMETREL
Amiloride	MIDAMOR
Aminoglutethimide	CYTADREN
Aminopropilidine Biphosphonate (*APD*)	nca
Aminophylline	AMINOPHYLLIN
Aminophylline Controlled-Release	PHYLLOCONTIN
Amitriptyline	ELAVIL
Aspirin	ASPIRIN
Atropine	ATROPINE
AZT-Azidothymidine	(see *Zidovudine*)
Baclofen	LIORESAL
Bisacodyl	DULCOLAX
Bleomycin	BLENOXANE
Bromocriptine	PARLODEL
Bumetanide	BUMEX
Bupivacaine	MARCAINE
Buprenorphine	BUPRENEX
Busulphan	MYLERAN
Calcitonin	CALCIMAR
Carbamazepine	TEGRETOL
Casanthrol + Docusate Sodium	PERI-COLACE
Chlorambucil	LEUKERAN
Chloramphenicol	CHLOROMYCETIN
Chlorhexidine Gluconate	PERIDEX ORAL RINSE
Chlorpromazine	THORAZINE
Cholestyramine	QUESTRAN
Choline Magnesium Trisalicylate	TRILISATE
Cimetidine	TAGAMET
Clonazepam	KLONOPIN
Clonidine	CATAPRES
Clotrimazole	MYCELEX
Codeine	CODEINE SULFATE
Crotamiton Cream	EURAX

Generic Name	Representative U.S. Trade Name
Cyclizine	MAREZINE
Cyproheptadine	PERIACTIN
Cyproterone Acetate (*Androcur*)	nca
Cytarabine	CYTOSAR-U
Demeclocycline	DECLOMYCIN
Desipramine	NORPRAMIN
Desmopressin	DDAVP
Dexamethasone	DECADRON
Dextroamphetamine	DEXEDRINE
Diamorphine	(see *Heroin*)
Diazepam	VALIUM
Diazepam Enema (*Stesolid*)	n/a
Dichloromethylene-Biphosphonate (*Clodronate*)	nca
Diclofenac	VOLTAREN
Diethylstilbestrol	DIETHYLSTILBESTROL
Digoxin	LANOXIN
Dihydrocodeine	in SYNALGOS-DC
Diphenoxylate	LOMOTIL
Dipipanone (*Diconal*)	n/a
Docusate Sodium	COLACE
Doxorubicin	ADRIAMYCIN
Erythromycin	ILOSONE
Ethinyl Estradiol	ESTINYL
Etidronate Disodium	DIDRONEL
Ferrous Sulfate Tablets	FEOSOL
Flecainide	TAMBOCOR
Fluorouracil	ADRUCIL
Flutamide	EULEXIN
Furosemide	LASIX
Haloperidol	HALDOL
Heparin	HEPARIN
Heroin	n/a
Hyaluronidase	WYDASE
Hydrocortisone	HYDROCORTONE
Hydrocortisone Foam	CORTIFOAM
Hydromorphone	DILAUDID
Hydroxyurea	HYDREA
Hyoscine	(see *Scopolamine*)
Ibuprofen	MOTRIN
Imipramine	TOFRANIL
Indomethacin	INDOCIN
Insulin	INSULIN (various)
Ketoconazole	NIZORAL

Generic Name	Representative U.S. Trade Name

Lactulose .... CHRONULAC
Lidocaine................................XYLOCAINE
Lidocaine Jelly ....XYLOCAINE 2% JELLY
Lidocaine Viscous ....XYLOCAINE 2% VISCOUS
Loperamide ....IMODIUM
Lorazepam ....ATIVAN

Magnesium Sulfate .... EPSOM SALTS
Medroxyprogesterone Acetate ....PROVERA
Megestrol Acetate .... MEGACE
Meperidine............................. DEMEROL
Methadone........................... DOLOPHINE
Methotrexate .... MEXATE
Methotrimeprazine ....LEVOPROME
Methylprednisolone .... MEDROL
Methyltestosterone .... ANDROID
Methysergide .... SANSERT
Metoclopramide .... REGLAN
Metolazone ....ZAROXOLYN
Metronidazole ....FLAGYL
Metronidazole Sterile Gel (*Topimet*).............. nca
Metyrapone ....METOPIRONE
Mexiletine............................. MEXITIL
Miconazole Lotion .... MONISTAT-DERM
Midazolam ....VERSED
Mitomycin .... MUTAMYCIN
Morphine Sulfate ....MSIR
Morphine Sulfate Controlled-Release ..... MS-CONTIN

Nabilone .... CESAMET
Nalbuphine................................ NUBAIN
Naloxone .... NARCAN
Naproxen .... NAPROSYN
Nifedipine............................PROCARDIA
Nortriptyline .... PAMELOR
Nystatin Suspension....................MYCOSTATIN

Orphenadrin ....DISIPAL
Oxybutynin...............................DITROPAN
Oxycodone .... ROXICODONE

Pancreatic Enzyme Replacement ....PANCREASE
Paracetamol (*see Acetaminophen*) .... n/a
Paraldehyde .... PARALDEHYDE
Pentazocine .... in TALWIN
Pentamidine PENTAM-300
Pentamidine Aerosol .... NEBUPENT
Phenazocine (*Narphen*) .... n/a

Generic Name	Representative U.S. Trade Name

Phenazopyridine .... PYRIDIUM
Phenobarbital .... PHENOBARBITAL
Phenoxybenzamine .... DIBENZYLENE
Phenytoin .... DILANTIN
Phosphate, Oral .... K-PHOS NEUTRAL
Phytonadione .... KONAKION
Piroxicam .... FELDENE
Potassium Citrate (*Urocit-K*) .... nca
Povidone-Iodine Solutions .... BETADINE
Prednisolone .... PREDNISOLONE
Prochlorperazine .... COMPAZINE
Procyclidine .... KEMADRIN
Promethazine .... PHENERGAN
Propanolol .... INDERAL
Protriptyline .... VIVACTIL

Quinacrine .... ATABRINE
Quinine Sulfate .... QUININE SULFATE

Ranitidine .... ZANTAC

Scopolamine .... SCOPOLAMINE
Scopolamine Trans-dermal Patch ... TRANSDERM-SCOP
Senna .... SENOKOT
Senna + Doscusate Sodium .... SENOKOT-S
Simethicone .... in MYLANTA
Sodium Bicarbonate .... SODIUM BICARBONATE
Spironolactone .... ALDACTONE
Streptokinase .... STREPTASE

Tamoxifen .... NOLVADEX
Temazepam .... RESTORIL
Terfenadine............................. SELDANE
Tetracycline...................... ACHROMYCIN V
Theophylline .... BRONKODYL
Theophylline Controlled-Release .... UNIPHYL
Thiethylperazine .... NORZINE
Thiotepa .... THIOTEPA
Thyroxine .... SYNTHROID
Tranexamic Acid.................... CYKLOKAPRON
Triamcinalone Acetonide
    Dental Paste .... KENALOG in ORABASE
Triamterene + Hydrochlorothiazide .... DYAZIDE
Triazolam............................. HALCION
Trihexyphenidyl .... ARTANE
Trimethoprim + Sulfamethoxasole .... BACTRIM
Trimipramine .... SURMONTIL

Generic Name	Representative U.S. Trade Name
Valproic Acid	DEPAKENE
Verapamil	CALAN
Vinblastine	VELBAN
Vitamin C	VITAMIN C
Warfarin	COUMADIN
Zidovudine	RETROVIR
Zinc Gluconate	ZE CAPS

n/a = Not available in the United States.
nca = Not commercially available in the United States, but may on occasion be obtained for compassionate or investigational use, or may be the subject of a new drug application pending with the FDA.

TABLE OF DRUGS
PROPRIETARY/GENERIC

This table is intended only for quick reference purposes. **Be sure to verify all information before prescribing.** Products listed may vary in availability of strengths and forms.

Representative U.S. Trade Name	Generic Name
Achromycin V	TETRACYCLINE
Adrenalin	ADRENALINE
Adriamycin	DOXORUBICIN
Adrucil	FLUOROURACIL
Aldactone	SPIRONOLACTONE
Aminophyllin	AMINOPHYLLINE
Android	METHYLTESTOSTERONE
Artane	TRIHEXYPHENIDYL
Aspirin	ASPIRIN
Atabrine	QUINACRINE
Ativan	LORAZEPAM
Atropine	ATROPINE
AZT	(see Retrovir)
Bactrim	TRIMETHOPRIM + SULFAMETHOXASOLE
Betadine	POVIDONE + IODINE
Blenoxane	BLEOMYCIN
Bronkodyl	THEOPHYLLINE
Bumex	BUMETANIDE
Buprenex	BUPRENORPHINE
Calan	VERAPAMIL
Calcimar	CALCITONIN
Catapres	CLONIDINE
Cesamet	NABILONE
Chloromycetin	CHLORAMPHENICOL
Chronulac	LACTULOSE
Codeine Sulfate	CODEINE
Colace	DOCUSATE SODIUM
Compazine	PROCHLORPERAZINE
Cortifoam	HYDROCORTISONE FOAM
Coumadin	WARFARIN
Cyklokapron	TRANEXAMIC ACID
Cytadren	AMINOGLUTETHIMIDE
Cytosar-U	CYTARABINE
DDAVP	DESMOPRESSIN
Declomycin	DEMECLOCYCLINE
Decadron	DEXAMETHASONE
Demerol	MEPERIDINE
Depakene	VALPROIC ACID

Dexedrine	DEXTROAMPHETAMINE
Dibenzylene	PHENOXYBENZAMINE
Didronel	ETIDRONATE DISODIUM
Diethylstilbestrol	DIETHYLSTILBESTROL
Dilantin	PHENYTOIN
Dilaudid	HYDROMORPHONE
Disipal	ORPHENADRIN
Ditropan	OXYBUTYNIN
Dolophine	METHADONE
Dulcolax	BISACODYL
Dyazide	TRIAMTERENE + HYDROCHLOROTHIAZIDE
Elavil	AMITRIPTYLINE
Epsom Salts	MAGNESIUM SULFATE
Estinyl	ETHINYL ESTRADIOL
Eulexin	FLUTAMIDE
Eurax	CROTAMITON CREAM
Feldene	PIROXICAM
Feosol	FERROUS SULFATE
Flagyl	METRONIDAZOLE
Halcion	TRIAZOLAM
Haldol	HALOPERIDOL
Heparin	HEPARIN
Hydrea	HYDROXYUREA
Hydrocortone	HYDROCORTISONE
Ilosone	ERYTHROMYCIN
Imodium	LOPERAMIDE
Inderal	PROPANOLOL
Indocin	INDOMETHACIN
Kemadrin	PROCYCLIDINE
Kenalog in Orabase	TRIAMCINALONE ACETONIDE DENTAL PASTE
Klonopin	CLONAZEPAM
Konakion	PHYTONADIONE
K-Phos Neutral	ORAL PHOSPHATE
Lanoxin	DIGOXIN
Lasix	FUROSEMIDE
Leukeran	CHLORAMBUCIL
Levoprome	METHOTRIMEPRAZINE
Lioresal	BACLOFEN
Lomotil	DIPHENOXYLATE
Marcaine	BUPIVACAINE
Marezine	CYCLIZINE
Medrol	METHYLPREDNISOLONE

Megace	MEGESTROL ACETATE
Metopirone	METYRAPONE
Mexate	METHOTREXATE
Mexitil	MEXILETINE
Midamor	AMILORIDE
Motrin	IBUPROFEN
Monistat-Derm	MICONAZOLE LOTION
MS-Contin	MORPHINE SULFATE CONTROLLED-RELEASE
MSIR	MORPHINE SULFATE
Mutamycin	MITOMYCIN
Mycelex	CLOTRIMAZOLE
Mycostatin	NYSTATIN SUSPENSION
Mylanta	contains ALUMINUM HYDROXIDE, SIMETHICONE
Myleran	BUSULPHAN
Naprosyn	NAPROXEN
Narcan	NALOXONE
Nebupent	PENTAMIDINE AEROSOL
Nizoral	KETOCONAZOLE
Nolvadex	TAMOXIFEN
Norpramin	DESIPRAMINE
Norzine	THIETHYLPERAZINE
Nubain	NALBUPHINE
Pamelor	NORTRIPTYLINE
Pancrease	PANCREATIC ENZYME REPLACEMENT
Paraldehyde	PARALDEHYDE
Parlodel	BROMOCRIPTINE
Pentam-300	PENTAMIDINE
Periactin	CYPROHEPTADINE
Peri-Colace	CASANTHROL + DOCUSATE SODIUM
Peridex Oral Rinse	CHLORHEXIDINE GLUCONATE
Phenergan	PROMETHAZINE
Phenobarbital	PHENOBARBITAL
Phyllocontin	AMINOPHYLLINE CONTROLLED-RELEASE
Prednisolone	PREDNISOLONE
Procardia	NIFEDIPINE
Provera	MEDROXYPROGESTERONE ACETATE
Pyridium	PHENAZOPYRIDINE
Questran	CHOLESTYRAMINE
Quinine Sulfate	QUININE SULFATE
Reglan	METOCLOPRAMIDE
Restoril	TEMAZEPAM

Representative U.S. Trade Name	Generic Name
Retrovir	ZIDOVUDINE (formerly AZT)
Roxicodone	OXYCODONE
Sansert	METHYSERGIDE
Scopolamine	SCOPOLAMINE
Seldane	TERFENADINE
Senokot	SENNA
Senokot-S	SENNA + DOCUSATE SODIUM
Sodium Bicarbonate	SODIUM BICARBONATE
Streptase	STREPTOKINASE
Surmontil	TRIMIPRAMINE
Symmetrel	AMANTADINE
Synalgos-DC	contains DIHYDROCODEINE
Synthroid	THYROXINE
Tagamet	CIMETIDINE
Talwin	contains PENTAZOCINE
Tambocor	FLECAINIDE
Tegretol	CARBAMAZEPINE
Thiotepa	THIOTEPA
Thorazine	CHLORPROMAZINE
Tofranil	IMIPRAMINE
Trilisate	CHOLINE MAGNESIUM TRISALICYLATE
Transderm-Scop	SCOPOLAMINE TRANS-DERMAL PATCH
Tylenol	ACETAMINOPHEN
Uniphyl	THEOPHYLLINE CONTROLLED-RELEASE
Valium	DIAZEPAM
Velban	VINBLASTINE
Ventolin	ALBUTEROL
Versed	MIDAZOLAM
Vitamin C	VITAMIN C
Vivactil	PROTRIPTYLINE
Voltaren	DICLOFENAC
Wydase	HYALURONIDASE
Xylocaine	LIDOCAINE
Xylocaine 2% Jelly	LIDOCAINE JELLY
Xylocaine 2% Viscous	LIDOCAINE VISCOUS
Zantac	RANITIDINE
Zaroxolyn	METOLAZONE
Zovirax	ACYCLOVIR
Zyloprim	ALLOPURINOL
ZE Caps	ZINC GLUCONATE

TABLE OF ABBREVIATIONS

ACTH . . . . Adrenocorticotropic Hormone
AIDS . . . . Acquired Immune Deficiency Syndrome
ADH . . . . Anti-diuretic Hormone
ALL . . . . Acute Lymphoblastic Leukemia
ALS . . . . Amyotrophic Lateral Sclerosis
AML . . . . .Acute Myeloid Leukemia
ANLL . . . . Acute Non-lymphoblastic Leukemia
A-P . . . . Abdomino-perineal
APD . . . . Aminopropilidine Biphosphonate
AZT . . . . Azidothymidine (Zidovudine)

C . . . . Centigrade
C1, C2, etc. . . . . .Cervical Vertebrae
cc . . . . Cubic Centimeter
cGy . . . . centi-Gray
CLL . . . . Chronic Lymphocytic Leukemia
cm . . . . Centimeter
CML . . . . Chronic Myelocytic Leukemia
CMV . . . . Cytomegalovirus
CNS . . . . Central Nervous System
CO_2 . . . . .Carbon Dioxide
COPD . . . . Chronic Obstructive Pulmonary Disease
CPB . . . . Celiac Plexus Block
CSF . . . . Cerebrospinal Fluid
CT . . . . Computerized Tomography
CTZ . . . . Chemoreceptor Trigger Zone

dl, dL . . . . Deciliter
DVT . . . . Deep Venous Thrombosis

ENT . . . . Ear, Nose & Throat
ERCP . . . . Endoscopic Retrograde
                                        Cholangiopancreatography
ESR . . . . Erythrocyte Sedimentation Rate

FDA . . . . U.S. Food & Drug Administration
Fr . . . . .French

g . . . . .Gram
GI . . . . Gastrointestinal

h . . . . Hour
H2 . . . . .Histamine Type 2
Hb . . . . .Hemoglobin
H2 . . . . .Histamine Type 2
Hb . . . . .Hemoglobin
Hg . . . . Mercury
HIV . . . . Human Immunodeficiency Virus

Table of Abbreviations

HPO . . . . Hypertrophic Pulmonary Osteoarthropathy
HSV2 . . . . Herpes Simplex Virus Type 2
Hz . . . . Hertz

ICP . . . . Intracranial Pressure
IgA . . . . Immunoglobulin A
IgG . . . . Immunoglobulin G
IgM . . . . Immunoglobulin M
IM . . . . Intramuscular
IV . . . . Intravenous
IVC . . . . Inferior Vena Cava

kg, Kg . . . . Kilogram
KS . . . . Kaposi's Sarcoma

l, L . . . . Liter
L1, L2, etc. . . . . Lumbar Vertebrae
lb, Lb . . . . Pound
LHRH . . . . Luteinizing Hormone-releasing Hormone

MAO . . . . Monoamine Oxidase Inhibitor
MCH . . . . Mean Corpuscular Hemoglobin
MCV . . . . Mean Corpuscular Volume
mEq . . . . Milliequivalent
mg . . . . Milligram
ml . . . . Milliliter
mm . . . . Millimeter
mmol . . . . Millimole
MMWR . . . . Morbidity and Mortality Weekly Report
mosmol . . . . Milliosmole
MRI . . . . Magnetic Resonance Imaging

Nd Yag . . . . Neodymium Yttrium Aluminum Garnet
NSAID(s) . . . . . . Non-Steroidal Anti-Inflammatory Drug(s)

PCC . . . . Percutaneous Cervical Cordotomy
pCO2 . . . . Carbon Dioxide Plasma Partial Pressure
PCP . . . . Pneumocystis Carinii Pneumonia
PRN . . . . As Needed (or, in hospice care,
Pain Relief Negligible)

SI . . . . International System Units
SVC . . . . Superior Vena Cava

T1, T2, etc. . . . . Thoracic Vertebrae
TENS . . . . Transcutaneous Electrical Nerve Stimulation

WBC . . . . White Blood Cells

5HT . . . . 5-Hydroxytryptamine (Serotonin)
μmol . . . . Micromole

NOTES

When referring to pharmaceuticals, we have used generic names whenever possible. Proprietary (product) names have been used when the length or complexity of the generic name would be unwieldy or potentially confusing. **Tables of generic and proprietary names appear directly after the Table of Contents.**

SI (International System) unit values are shown on occasion **in brackets and italics** following the listing of conventional unit values.

Throughout this book we have used the female gender for nurses, the male gender for doctors, and the male gender for patients of both sexes, unless specific examples require otherwise. This avoids the cumbersome use of both genders whenever nurses, doctors or patients are mentioned. We have chosen this usage because, in the United States at present, the majority of nurses are female, and the majority of doctors are male.

The author and publisher have taken precautions to ensure that the information in this book is error-free. However, readers must be guided by their own personal and professional standards of good practice in evaluating and applying recommendations made herein. The contents of this book represent the views and experience of the author, and not necessarily those of the publisher.

FOREWORD

Competent and compassionate care is not a privilege for the fortunate few who encounter hospice during their final illness. Competent and compassionate care is the absolute right of **every** patient, wherever he or she may be.

Skilled physical symptom control is the linchpin of good hospice and palliative care, around which revolve other key services to patient and family, and without which the many psychological, social and spiritual needs of patient and family cannot easily be met.

Over the past generation, hospices have developed and demonstrated the principles of good terminal care; among these the need for regular titrated analgesia, respect for the family as the unit of care, use of a multi-disciplinary team for problem-solving and support, emphasis on the quality of remaining life, and concern for those who are grieving.

The great challenge of the 1990s is to expand hospice principles and practices to the care of **all** patients and their families. This process is already underway through example, education, and consumer demand. The hospice movement must encourage and welcome responsible and innovative adaptation of existing principles and practices in varied settings and situations. Much more remains to be done, particularly in the areas of professional and public education.

The Hospice Education Institute is proud to publish this book by Dr. Peter Kaye. Dr. Kaye is among the growing number of health and caring professionals who combine strong scientific knowledge, broad clinical experience and active practical compassion in caring for patients and their families. These physicians, nurses, caring professionals and community volunteers are setting new and higher standards for the practice of hospice and palliative care, by demonstrating how patients with far advanced disease, and their families, can receive the best that modern home health care, day care and in-patient care can offer. This book explains what can be done, and encourages us all to do it well, wherever we are.

Michal Galazka
Executive Director
June, 1989   Hospice Education Institute

ACKNOWLEDGEMENTS

It was only possible to find the time to write this book because of the support of my wife, Karen, to whom the book is dedicated, with love.

I would like to warmly thank the whole team at Cynthia Spencer House for all their recent support and especially Ann Goodman, for her cheerful and efficient help with the manuscript. I am grateful to Yoshi Shimazu, who worked at Cynthia Spencer House as a volunteer, for some of the recorded comments from patients, which I use with permission.

Michal Galazka has played a very active part in the editing and production of the book, and I thank him for his sustained enthusiasm and encouragement.

I am very grateful to my colleague, Jill Stewart, for checking the sections on individual cancers.

Thanks to Ann Skinner and the staff at the Cripps Postgraduate Medical Centre Library, Northampton, England.

I would like to thank the following colleagues for their helpful comments: Lorna Allen, Sue Beresford, John Chapman, Pat Cooke, Brian Dowling, Alan Farnell, Charles Fox, Gillian Furguson, Rob George, Meg Green, Ken Lloyd, Maurice McClain, Barbara Malcomson, Evelyn Malloy, Leigh Moss, David Oliver, Jackie Phillips, Peter Robertson, Hamish Ross, Christine Russell and Liz Starmer.

Thanks to friends and colleagues in the U.S.A., including Ellen Laskarin at the Hospice Education Institute, Mary Pettit, Ruth Thayer and Eileen Torrenti at Visiting Nurses of the Lower Valley, Robert Delaney and Paul Schreiner at Doane's Pharmacy, Richard Beaser, George Bowers, Jr., Jeffrey Rabuffo, James A. Zibluk, over 300 hospice and palliative care professionals who made helpful suggestions and comments about the preliminary edition of this book, and Ed Ziobron and Diane Dugal at Illustrated Printing Company who coped competently and patiently with additions and corrections.

PREFACE

This book offers a problem-orientated approach to the physical and psycho-social aspects of advanced disease. It is intended for all who support adult patients (and their families) facing advanced illness in an in-patient hospice, a hospital, a nursing home, or at home.

This book attempts to convey straight-forward principles of care which can be applied in any setting, and which can make so much difference to patients and their families. While this book is mainly for doctors and nurses, other professionals and volunteers — especially those who work in hospice and palliative care teams — will find it useful.

The principles of good hospice care now seem like common sense, yet it has taken over twenty years for details of this team-based approach to evolve. Most of us now working in hospice and palliative care do not consider it to be a specialist subject, because the problems we encounter are so universal to all areas of health care.

The aim of this book is to be as useful and accurate as possible. If you have any comments, criticisms or suggestions I would be very grateful to receive them via the publishers, Hospice Education Institute.

Cynthia Spencer House   Peter Kaye
Northampton, England
June, 1989

DEFINITIONS

Palliative care is care of patients when cure is no longer possible, the aim being to control symptoms and prolong life (by means of surgery, radiotherapy, chemotherapy or hormone therapy). Palliative care is the aim at the outset of treatment for about 50% of cancer patients (since only about 50% at diagnosis have disease that is limited enough to realistically attempt cure).

Hospice care no longer hopes to prolong life, but emphasizes symptom control and quality of remaining life. It is characterized by a team approach, symptom control, rehabilitation of the whole person, good communication, psychological support, family counseling, awareness of spiritual needs, expert care of the dying person and bereavement follow-up.

These two areas of care overlap. Patients receiving palliative treatment benefit from a team approach to improve their quality of life. Patients receiving hospice care occasionally need to be referred for palliative treatments.

"A hospice is a team or community concerned with enhancing the quality of remaining life for a patient and family struggling with mortal illness." (Cicely Saunders)

"Here they treat me like a human being all the time, not just when they feel like it." (Jane Zorza, in *A Way to Die* by Rosemary and Victor Zorza)

INTRODUCTION

Symptom control is the foundation of good hospice care. It is impossible to address the problems of mental, social and spiritual anguish without first releasing a person from constant physical discomfort.

In general medicine symptoms have diagnostic usefulness, but in advanced disease symptoms become functionless. Good symptom control is important at all stages of care, but becomes particularly important when it is all we have to offer.

Symptom control is best achieved in the context of **team care**. A dying person has complex needs, and it takes a team of professionals (and volunteers) to help meet them all. The patient may not label his problems as physical, emotional or spiritual, but is often desperately seeking simultaneous help on all these fronts. In a good team, everyone is aware of the importance of physical comfort as the foundation of this work. For example, it may be the team's social worker who reports that when she saw the patient at home he still seemed to be in pain. The next step is an immediate reassessment of the patient by the doctor or nurse.

Team members include doctors, nurses, social workers or psychologists, clergy, and other professionals, often including physical, occupational and diversional therapists, dietitian, pharmacist, and if possible, art and music therapists. Well-trained volunteers are a very valuable part of any team, provided they are considered as full members, and have continuing liaison with, and supervision from, the professionals.

Since team care is so important to both patients and professionals, informal teams must be built where no formal structures exist for consultation and support. Teams must also identify and educate key health professionals whose help may occasionally be needed: a radiotherapist who understands palliative techniques, an orthopedic surgeon willing to operate promptly to fix fractured limbs, an anesthesiologist with a special interest in nerve blocks, a dentist, an optometrist, etc.

Supporting and educating family members is an essential part of symptom control. When a patient is at home, the family observe, witness and often cope with the physical symptoms. We often expect so much of carers, who apart from new roles, extra pressure of work, adjusting to loss (and physical exhaustion too very often) are usually expected to help with complicated regimes of medication. When caring family members are in partnership with the professionals, symptom control works very well in a home setting.

Patients with advanced cancer have many complex needs and can benefit from the expertise and support of a large number of professionals. It follows that team care by a team of professionals and volunteers is an effective model of care, provided it is **well coordinated**. However, good communication among busy professionals is often difficult to achieve. There is danger that a doctor in doing his best for a particular problem may not be acting in the patient's best interests, for example, admitting a terminally ill patient with jaundice for a biliary bypass procedure when the priority for the patient is to spend his last days at home.

In Britain, specialist nurses (often called Macmillan nurses) acting as key workers overcome many of these problems by coordinating care and improving communications and liaison among professionals. They also offer expertise in controlling symptoms, and in family counseling. In the United States, experienced hospice nurses, visiting nurses or oncology nurses can often serve the same important role.

It is nurses who have the most contact with the patient. One young man of 38 with advanced abdominal malignancy made the point to me when he said:

"The difference between being in St. Christopher's Hospice and being in the hospital is that when I was in the hospital, it would take ages for them to do anything if I got pain. They had to call a doctor, and it always took so long. But if I get pain here, the nurses deal with it right away."

In British hospices, the nurses are educated in the basic skills of prescribing, and are trusted to **increase** the dose of morphine when necessary. The dose is ordered by the doctor as a **range** — for example, "10mg to 20mg morphine every 4 hours" — meaning that the patient is on 10mg regularly, but the nurses have the option of increasing to 20mg. When the doctor is next contacted he will be asked to re-assess pain control, and if necessary change his order to "20mg to 30mg morphine every 4 hours". If this simple rule were adopted more widely, it would reduce unnecessary cancer pain considerably — but it depends upon investing time and energy to educate key nursing staff in the basic skills of using morphine, and then trusting them to teach and supervise other nurses.

Symptoms can usually be quickly controlled once a patient is admitted to an in-patient hospice. One reason for this is that the doctor on duty and the nurse in charge review all drug charts and patient orders together every day. For 20 in-patients this routine discussion usually only takes 20 to 30 minutes. It gives the doctor accurate feedback on whether medication is proving effective, whether it needs changing in dose, or whether another treatment needs to be considered. Again, if this simple procedure were adopted routinely, a good deal of unnecessary physical suffering would be avoided. In hospice home care, similar benefits would accrue if the home care nurse and the doctor **actually talked together daily**, however briefly.

Why are physical symptoms often managed so badly? Why is something so straightforward still often ignored, or done half-heartedly or ineffectively? One reason is because it is embarrassing and upsetting to talk to a patient if you feel, as a doctor or a nurse, that you have somehow failed.

What is the answer? Teaching young doctors and nurses (and older ones, too!) about symptom control empowers them again to be able to help these patients and dispels much of their sense of failure. It gives them some control over the situation and gives them expertise they can still offer. They then discover that patients are much more realistic (and often much more accepting of disability or death) than they are. They discover that patients will say "I realize you can't cure me, doctor, but if only you could get rid of this pain.". They discover that these patients are hoping for kindness not cure, and that relieving a person of physical discomfort brings genuine gratitude out of all proportion to the skills involved. And they discover that it is satisfying to care for terminally ill patients, that in fact there is a great deal that can be done to help them. They discover, to their surprise, that caring for patients can be just as rewarding as curing them.

PRINCIPLES OF SYMPTOM CONTROL

The important principles of symptom control are:

- Medical expertise
- High quality nursing care
- Full assessment
- Attention to detail
- Regular review
- Ability (and energy) to listen
- Communication skills

Many patients with advanced cancer continue to suffer unnecessary physical distress because many doctors and nurses remain unaware of what can be achieved.

★ **"Surely the most important principle of symptom control must be to get on and do it."** (Mary Baines)

Too often expressions like "We're waiting for the drugs to work " really mean "We don't know what else to do and can't be bothered to find out."

It is possible to significantly control the symptoms of pain, nausea, vomiting, dyspnea and dysphagia in **ALL** patients, and to abolish these unpleasant symptoms altogether in the great majority. It is almost always possible to control symptoms effectively in the patient's home, if there are willing carers and a competent home care team. It demands skillful medical care, skillful prescribing of drugs, and also skillful use of the doctor "as a drug" — using the skills of listening, reassurance and explanation to boost patient confidence and morale, and to reduce fear and insecurity. It demands high quality care from nurses who are committed to total care of patient and family, who are educated to identify and assess pain, who understand the use of analgesics, and who are willing, if necessary, to act as advocates for their patients. Visit regularly — at least daily if there are uncontrolled symptoms. Severe pain is a medical emergency. (*see Home Care*)

★ **Symptom control often enables rehabilitation.**

Once symptoms are controlled, the next step is to ask "Can this patient be helped to become more independent?" (*see Rehabilitation*)

Controlling physical symptoms is usually simple and straightforward (and often very rewarding for all con-

1

cerned). It demands proper assessment of each problem, including history and examination. Occasionally special tests such as x-rays, bone scans or blood tests are appropriate. It can seem more difficult to be methodical when a patient is very ill or very anxious, but it is still possible.

History — It is important first of all to **listen**. This builds trust, which improves compliance. The order in which problems are conveyed is in itself an important message.

Having listened, it is then important to **elicit symptoms**. (We usually talk of eliciting signs in general medicine.) There seems to be an unwritten rule in medicine that a patient is "allowed" only one problem at a time. The patient can be embarrassed to discuss more than two or three problems, when in fact there can be many more than this. It is possible to tackle a long list of problems at a first assessment only by knowing that there is a full team of people capable of absorbing some of the problems, and dealing with them.

Discover the **significance of symptoms**. Patients with cancer (and their families) often assume that new symptoms are due to the spread of the disease. Explanation reduces anxiety. (see *Explanation*)

Examination — Examination of the patient is an essential step in symptom control. It is in itself a **powerful, non-verbal message** saying, "I am interested in you, and this is how I am going to care for you." It is important to look for obvious physical signs of oral thrush, pressure areas, hepatomegaly, bony tenderness, impacted feces, ankle edema, etc.

It is also an important opportunity for the nurse or doctor to **make a positive comment** such as "You have lovely skin ", or "Your lungs sound completely healthy." These comments obviously need to be true, but it is usually possible to find something to be positive about. This can be a great boost to morale in the face of progressing disease.

Special tests — It is often unnecessary to subject people with advanced disease to special investigations, but occasionally it is essential.

For example:

- Chest x-ray, in the assessment of dyspnea
- X-rays or scans, in the assessment of metastases or possible pathological fractures
- Blood, to diagnose uremia or hypercalcemia (as causes of nausea, thirst, drowsiness, confusion)

★ **Routine measurements of temperature, pulse, respiration and blood pressure are not necessary in terminal illness.**

2

The symptoms listed below are those commonly seen on admission to St. Christopher's Hospice. The percentages are based on routine questioning of 6,677 patients admitted between 1975 and 1984. They give a useful overview of the frequency of particular problems, but they give no indication of the severity of symptoms or of the changing nature of symptoms.

For example, mild dyspnea on exertion is a non-specific symptom at some stage in almost all patients with far advanced cancer. Severe dyspnea at rest is surprisingly rare even with lung cancer patients. Similarly, towards the end of life almost all patients will complain of weakness.

Most patients have several different physical symptoms at the same time.

Symptom	%
Weight Loss	77
Pain	71
Anorexia	67
Dyspnea	51
Cough	50
Constipation	47
Weakness	47
Nausea/Vomiting	40
Edema/Ascites/Pleural Effusion	31
Insomnia	29
Incontinence/Catheterized	23
Dysphagia	23
Bedsore	19
Hemorrhage	14
Drowsiness	10
Paralysis	8
Jaundice	6
Diarrhea	4
Fistula	1

Some very important problems are not included on this list. About 70% of patients complain of soreness or dryness of the mouth. Some less common physical symptoms are also missing: hiccups, pruritis, sweating, thirst. Psychological and spiritual problems (confusion, anxiety, depression) are also not included. Nevertheless, this list provides a useful over-view of common problems.

Since patients tend to have several symptoms, polypharmacy is unavoidable. **Skillful prescribing** is essential and often makes the difference between poor and excellent symptom control. (see *Prescribing*)

ABDOMINAL DISTENTION

Abdominal distention is a common complaint in cancer patients.

It may be due to:

- Hepatomegaly
- Tumor masses
- Ascites
- Intestinal obstruction
- Constipation
- Gas
- Steroid side effects
- Perforated bowel

Examine the abdomen for the **liver edge** (which may be near the right iliac crest in massive hepatomegaly), **tumor masses**, and for shifting dullness which may indicate **ascites**. An ultrasound scan may occasionally be useful to diagnose the cause of distention.

Intestinal obstruction causes distention (unless the obstruction is high) and increased bowel sounds. Retroperitoneal tumors can cause neurogenic dilation of the colon and abdominal distention. (*see Intestinal Obstruction*)

Constipation is usually obvious from a careful history. Feces may be palpable in the descending colon (unlike other masses, they indent). Plain x-ray may demonstrate fecal material throughout the colon, indicating constipation. (*see Constipation*)

Distention due to **gas** can occur after prolonged treatment with lactulose (consider changing the laxative), and is also a feature of malabsorption in pancreatic cancer which responds to pancreatic enzyme supplements. Distention due to gas can also be caused by anxiety and repeated swallowing (of air). (*see Diarrhea, Pancreatic Cancer*)

Prolonged use of **steroids** produces abdominal distention (due to increased fat and weaker muscles) which can be distressing. Reduce steroid dose where possible.

Rarely a patient with advanced cancer can develop a bowel **perforation**, which is usually a terminal event. There is sudden abdominal pain with generalized abdominal tenderness and rebound tenderness. The abdomen may become distended. Treat with adequate doses of morphine by injection (since patients will usually have nausea and vomiting). **Avoid** the mistake of passing nasogastric or flatus tubes which add to the patient's discomfort.

ACUPUNCTURE

Acupuncture is mainly used to relieve pain in a variety of chronic conditions such as arthritis or migraine. Most studies show some benefit in around 60% of patients, suggesting it is more than simply a placebo (which usually improves about 30%). The shorter the duration of the pain the better the response.

Acupuncture has been used to relieve pain in terminal malignant disease. It is a time-consuming procedure, but can sometimes reduce opioid analgesic requirements.

The **mechanism of action** may be release of endogenous opioids, which inhibit the central transmission of pain. (Acupuncture analgesia can be reversed by naloxone.) An early study showed cerebrospinal fluid (CSF) from rabbits receiving acupuncture could raise the pain threshold of normal rabbits after intra-ventricular injection. Recent studies using specific antisera to encephalins (in order to abolish their specific effects) suggest high frequency electro-acupuncture (100Hz to 200Hz) may be mediated by dynorphin, and low frequency electro-acupuncture (2Hz to 6Hz) by metenkephalin. 5HT levels (in brain and CSF of experimental animals) also rise after acupuncture, and 5HT is known to inhibit transmission of pain in the spinal cord.

Traditional Chinese acupuncture (acu = needle) practiced for over 4,000 years is based on the theory that needle insertion alters the flow of energy (Chi) along certain lines (meridians) on the surface of the body. This is said to restore the balance of positive and negative forces (Yin and Yang) in the internal organs, resulting in cure of pain or disease. Modern acupuncture also uses electrical stimulation or laser stimulation in addition to needles. Many Western practitioners believe in focal points rather than the meridian theory.

ADJUSTMENT REACTION

Anyone facing loss or change has to **adjust**. The concept of an "adjustment reaction" is a helpful way of understanding the transient episodes of anxiety and depression in terminal illness, bereavement, or any major crisis. (see *Crisis Theory*)

The term **"psychosocial transition"** describes a sudden major change in lifestyle that permanently alters a person's

assumptive world (the set of assumptions we make about the world, based upon past experiences, and expectations of the future). The assumptive world not only contains a model of the world as it is, but also as it might be. Giving up hopes or dreams for the future can be more difficult than giving up objects which actually exist. (Psychotherapy can be described as a painful reviewing of prior assumptions.)

Changes can occur in:

- Familiar environment
- Physical or mental capacity
- Role or status
- Expectations of the future
- Personal relationships

Several changes often occur simultaneously, making adjustment all the harder.

Elderly persons can become very disturbed and even confused by changes in their physical environment. Loved possessions can become an extension of self — the tools by which we function in the world. Losing them can produce a profound sense of insecurity and loss of confidence.

Increasing **dependence** can be seen as "giving in" and can cause increasing frustration. Giving permission to "regress" to a more dependent state can bring satisfaction to both the patient and carers. Sometimes this need to regress in illness has to be explained (for example, when a mother-child relationship is re-established and pushes out a new husband or wife).

Changes in role are painful but they can be coped with. A man who is ill may feel threatened by further loss of role if his wife needs to learn to drive, but can be helped to see that he can assist in teaching her and take pride in her new achievement.

Unrealistic hopes about the future bring frustration. **Unrealistic fears** can bring crippling anxiety. Meeting a patient more seriously ill than oneself who is coping well and cheerfully can enable a person to look to the future in a more optimistic and realistic way. (see *Day Hospice*)

Illness often involves **restructuring of a family unit**. The amount of time spent with different family members may suddenly change. New bonds strengthen, others weaken. Helping family members communicate with each other about all the changes facilitates adjustment. (see *Communication Problems, Talking with Families*)

Good hospice and palliative care can largely be seen in terms of facilitating this process of psychosocial transition. Encouraging communication allows people to close the gaps between their internal assumptions and their real situation. (see *Crisis Theory, Grief, Support*)

ADVICE

★ **Advice is like medicine: easy to give, hard to take.** (Al Silverman)

Giving advice is an essential part of medical and nursing care, but in advanced disease the patient has often been through many investigations and treatments, and may therefore have strong views about his past experiences and future management. It becomes increasingly important to **discuss options** with the patient.

★ **Patients listen to you, if you listen to them.**

Compliance with advice is improved if:

1. The advice is consistent with the patient's beliefs. ("Do you have any thoughts about what might be causing it?")
2. The patient feels involved in making decisions. ("What have you tried already?")
3. The patient is satisfied with the consultation. ("The doctor seems to understand how I feel.")
4. The advice is clearly and simply explained. (see *Explanation*)
5. The advice is given with authority and conviction.

★ **Avoid the expression "If I were you..." which can sound patronizing. It is sometimes helpful to share your honest feelings about "If it were me..."**

★ **Good advice seldom hurts anyone because so few people take it seriously.** (C.G. Jung)

AGONIST/ANTAGONIST ANALGESICS

This group of drugs includes:
- Buprenorphine
- Pentazocine
- Nalbuphine

These are effective analgesics for moderate pain. Buprenorphine has a small place in the management of cancer pain, but the other drugs have no advantages over buprenorphine in this situation, and **should be avoided**.

Buprenorphine is a strong narcotic, but has a low ceiling effect. It is rapidly metabolized by the liver, and (where available) the sublingual route allows systemic absorption which is almost as potent as by IM injection. About 20% of patients complain of unacceptable nausea or dizziness.

All three drugs have **two disadvantages**. First, above a certain dose the incidence of side effects increases with no increase in analgesia (the ceiling effect). Second, their high affinity for morphine mu receptors (agonist action) blocks the effect of morphine (antagonist action).

★ **Buprenorphine and morphine should never be given together. If buprenorphine is given to a patient on morphine it can displace morphine from the receptor and cause pain (and sometimes withdrawal symptoms of yawning, sweating, rhinorrhea, nausea and restlessness).**

AIDS

Background information — Acquired Immune Deficiency Syndrome (AIDS) was first described in 1981, and the virus was discovered in 1983. The virus is transmitted in blood products, by sexual intercourse (either anal or vaginal), or from mother to child. The virus infects T4 lymphocytes, monocytes and brain cells. Antibodies to human immunodeficiency virus (HIV) are usually, but not always, detectable within 1 to 2 months of infection. A high proportion of seropositive individuals (current evidence suggests around 75%) progress to develop AIDS over a number of years (the median time currently is 8 years).

50% of patients present with dyspnea due to **pneumocystis carinii pneumonia** (PCP). Any system may be affected.

Other common features at presentation are the raised, painless bruise-like spots of **Kaposi's sarcoma** (KS), persistent oral thrush, lymphadenopathy, weight loss, fevers, diarrhea and mental changes.

Treatment — The median survival from diagnosis of AIDS is around 24 months (but this is likely to extend as treatment improves). Treatment with zidovudine (formerly AZT) 250mg every 6 hours prolongs survival, but it causes bone marrow suppression and 50% of patients eventually need blood transfusions. Numerous drugs and regimens are currently being evaluated for possible prophylaxis and treatment of AIDS.

In the early stages of AIDS there can be a good response to vigorous treatment with antiviral, antifungal and antibiotic drugs and almost full recovery of weight and energy levels. As the disease progresses opportunistic infections recur, with a shortening interval between each episode of infection. Vigorous treatment can produce some improvement with intervening periods of relatively good health. As the disease progresses weight loss and fatigue become marked and the HIV virus can cause dementia and visual loss. Infections tend to become more frequent despite vigorous treatment.

The decision to stop treating infections needs to be made only after discussion with the patient, even when the focus has shifted to symptom control and supportive care. Interventions such as blood transfusions and antiviral infusions for cytomegalovirus (CMV) retinitis to prevent blindness may still be appropriate.

A large number of opportunistic infections can occur (most of them rare in people with intact immune systems). Some are treatable, some are not. The drugs used to treat these infections have many complicated side-effects and expert consultation is essential.

Common problems in AIDS include:
- Weight loss, fever, lymphadenopathy
- Dry cough (PCP, tuberculosis, conventional organisms)
- Persistent oral and esophageal thrush
- KS purple skin lesions
- Diarrhea (salmonella, cryptosporidium, CMV, anerobes)
- Peri-anal ulceration (herpes simplex)
- Headaches (toxoplasmosis, cerebral lymphoma, abscess)
- Meningitis (cryptococcus, tuberculosis)

- Dementia (HIV)
- Blindness (CMV retinitis)
- Peripheral neuropathy
- Arthralgias
- Eczema, psoriasis, drug eruptions
- Multiple warts or molluscum contagiosum

Intellectual deterioration occurs terminally in more than 50% of AIDS patients. Primary HIV infection of the brain can cause cerebral atrophy and dementia before other physical signs of AIDS appear. The early features may be subtle, with poor concentration, mental slowing, personality changes and loss of memory. It is characterized by slowing of movements and speech, and Parkinsonian features. Patients may progress to severe dementia with mutism, incontinence and paraplegia. In about 20% of patients the onset is more acute, and the course is rapidly progressive.

Opportunistic infections can also cause intellectual deterioration and it is important to exclude treatable conditions such as cryptococcal meningitis, viral encephalitis or toxoplasmosis (which like cerebral metastases can present with personality change).

About 20% of AIDS patients develop **Kaposi's sarcoma** (KS) in mucosae, skin or internal organs. KS is an endothelial neoplasm (hence bruising and edema can occur around lesions). Purple lesions occur on any part of the skin, and they are usually multiple and rapidly progressive. They are also common on the hard palate. Secondary edema occurs and is most noticeable on the face. The tumor is multi-focal and develops simultaneously in different sites (skin, gut and lung). Depending upon their site, KS lesions may be life-threatening. Large lesions can be painful, especially in the mouth, and cosmetically unsightly. Lesions can bleed, presenting as hemoptysis, rectal bleeding or hematuria, and hollow viscera may obstruct. Radiotherapy, usually as a single treatment, can cause shrinkage of lesions and also stops bleeding. Pleural KS can cause pleuritic pains or pleural effusions. Gut lesions can cause colicky pain that may respond to high dose steroids. KS involving a pressure area can be very painful.

Treatment options for KS include:
- Camouflage make-up
- Surgical excision or cryotherapy
- Intra-lesional vinblastine
- Radiotherapy
- Systemic chemotherapy (if widespread)
- Interferon

Radiotherapy should be considered early for large or troublesome lesions. It is best given before surrounding edema occurs. It is avoided for oral lesions (mucositis is severe in AIDS patients). Expert consultation is essential in planning management.

Nursing the AIDS patient — The Centers for Disease Control has issued "Recommendations for Prevention of HIV Transmission in Health-Care Settings" (MMWR 1987;36 #2S) whose guidelines should be observed.

There is no need for routine isolation of AIDS patients unless there is profuse diarrhea.

Gowns and masks are not routinely necessary. Gloves should be worn when dealing with blood or body fluids. The routine measures for dealing with material infected with hepatitis B (which is much more infectious than HIV) are more than adequate. HIV is fragile, and is destroyed by household bleach or the hot water of a washing machine at 70°C for at least 3 minutes.

Basic hygiene precautions:
- Cover abrasions or eczema with waterproof dressing
- Wash off any contaminating fluid immediately
- Use gloves if dealing with blood or body fluids
- Gown and mask are needed only if splashing is anticipated

Only 0.3% of documented needlestick injuries from AIDS patients have caused seroconversion.

Common problems in terminal AIDS:

1. Most patients will need **prophylactic drugs**. Ketoconazole to prevent recurrence of thrush, prophylactic acyclovir for herpes infections and Bactrim or pentamidine for PCP. Whether to continue zidovudine is debatable, and the chance of prolonged survival versus bone marrow suppression and the need for blood transfusions should be discussed with the patient.

2. **Altered body image** is often a major issue:

- Cachexia, pressure sores
- Weakness and dependence
- Rapid aging process (wrinkling, gray hair)
- Disfiguring KS lesions

3. **Intellectual deterioration** eventually occurs in 50% of patients, sometimes with confusion, memory loss and incontinence.

Common symptoms in terminal AIDS:

- Thrush
- Weakness, weight loss
- Anemia (secondary to drugs)
- Headaches
- Arthralgia
- Painful peripheral neuropathy
- Dyspnea
- Pleuritic chest pains (KS)
- Anorexia
- Nausea
- Diarrhea
- Colic (KS)
- Dental problems
- Blindness
- Anxiety
- Depression

Pain in advanced AIDS:

- Headaches
- Arthralgia
- KS (oral, pleuritic, colic)
- Peripheral neuropathy
- Post-herpetic neuralgias
- Pressure sores

People with AIDS tend to be young (average age 35) and are often very knowledgeable about their condition.

Their special needs can be summarized as:

A — Acceptance
I — Information
D — Disease control
S — Social and spiritual support

Acceptance — The biggest problem for many AIDS patients remains the ignorance and fear prevalent among the general public. Discrimination occurs. Social ostracism is a terrible plight for anyone. Unconditional acceptance of people need not imply acceptance of their lifestyle, but our own deep-seated fears of contagion and our attitudes about sexuality (our own and others') need to be examined. Drug abusers with AIDS present special management problems, but **all** persons with AIDS are entitled to competent, compassionate and respectful care.

Information — The need for explanation and reassurance is as important in AIDS as in any chronic condition, but even more so because it is such a complicated disease. The implications of AIDS are so broad (physical, psychological, social, legal) that the patient needs access to a team of professionals and volunteers with many different skills. Local and national support groups for persons with AIDS are developing special skills and resources, and are available for advice and practical assistance.

Disease control — Any hope of cure is at present extremely remote once AIDS is diagnosed. (An equivalent situation for the cancer patient is not diagnosis, but when recurrence of the cancer occurs.) For this reason skilled psychological, social and spiritual support is needed from the beginning.

The progression of AIDS differs from cancer. It is not a relatively steady decline, but a series of acute, life-threatening illnesses requiring intensive treatment, between which the patient may be quite well.

Persons with AIDS therefore need **easy access to good acute medical care** and **multi-disciplinary team support** throughout the illness.

Social and spiritual support — Housing and health insurance problems abound. Persons with AIDS have been summarily (and illegally) evicted by ignorant and fearful landlords, and even by their own families. There is a shortage of AIDS residences, home health care, hospices and specialist in-patient units. Where does the person with AIDS wish to live, and with whom?

Family dynamics are particularly complex when homosexual or bisexual relationships have occurred, and family counseling is often necessary to resolve some of the conflicts. If the person with AIDS is in a sexual partnership, the partner may be HIV antibody positive, or have intense fears about the future.

Above all, the person with AIDS is facing up to the prospect of death, often in the prime of life, with plans and hopes shattered.

ALZHEIMER'S DISEASE

About 15% of people over 65 have some form of dementia. Alzheimer's Disease is by far the most common cause of pre-senile dementia.

The main causes of dementia are:

- Alzheimer's Disease (50%)
- Multi-infarct dementia (20%)
- Combination Alzheimer's and Multi-infarct (15%)
- Rarer causes (15%)

Alzheimer's Disease is rare before the age of 45. The duration of the disease is between 3 to 20 years, with an average of 7.5 years from diagnosis to death. It causes progressive and irreversible damage to brain cells (with brain shrinkage visible on CT scans). Confirmation of the diagnosis requires examination of brain tissue (usually at autopsy). The cause is unknown and there is no treatment.

The onset is usually gradual and can mimic depression with:

- Decline in initiative
- Memory failure (especially recent memory)
- Poor concentration

The patient is usually distressingly aware of these early failings. It is at this stage that a formal evaluation of mental state is helpful as a baseline to detect later changes.

The condition gradually progresses to affect:

- Personality (suspicion, delusions)
- Behavior (violence, wanderings)
- Intellect (loss of memory)
- Language (aphasia)

The level of consciousness remains normal (there is no drowsiness). Psychiatric problems are common (depression, psychotic features).

Finally, the person loses personality ("the loss of self") and becomes:

- Incapable of self-care
- Disorientated
- Incontinent
- Mute
- Bedbound (bedsores, contractures)

Death is usually from bronchopneumonia or other infection. Life-prolonging measures are not appropriate at this stage.

The burden on carers is long-term and can become all-consuming and exhausting. Most carers are elderly spouses (often with their own health problems) or adult daughters (with other responsibilities).

Carers need:

- Good medical support and interest
- Emotional support
- Nursing assistance
- Time off (respite care)
- Financial support (laundry, equipment, loss of earnings, home help)
- Social contact with other carers
- Regular help (volunteers, neighbors)
- Family communication (agreement about levels of care)
- Advice in the terminal phase (symptom control, place of care)
- Bereavement support (grief can be intense)

Hospice philosophy and practice can be adapted for Alzheimer's Disease patients and their families. However, extra support given only during the terminal phase (when the patient is often bedbound, mute) is not enough. **Carers need long-term assistance (particularly emotional support).** Hospices can extend their skills to include Alzheimer's Disease (and other conditions) by learning from, working with and teaching other caring organizations, rather than by necessarily increasing their own patient load.

AMYOTROPHIC LATERAL SCLEROSIS

Background information — Amyotrophic Lateral Sclerosis (ALS) is a rare neurological disease characterized by progressive muscular weakness, dysphagia and dysarthria. It is also called **Lou Gehrig's Disease**, and (in Britain) **Motor Neurone Disease**. There is no known cause and no specific treatment. It is invariably fatal. Patients benefit considerably from skillful, supportive management.

It is rare under the age of 30. The peak age of onset is 50 to 70 years.

The early symptoms are usually clumsiness in one hand, falls or slurred speech. As the disease progresses weakness tends to spread and become bilateral.

The pattern of involvement varies. Some patients have weak limbs only, some have bulbar symptoms only, but most patients progress to both.

Bulbar symptoms affect speech and swallowing. Emotional lability can occur, with uncontrolled crying (or laughing) due to loss of control of reflexes (**not** intellectual impairment). This can be partially controlled by breathing exercises.

The patient becomes progressively more dependent on the help of others for transport, transfer, feeding, washing and eating. (Regular respite care is essential to avoid exhaustion of family carers.)

Eventually the respiratory muscles are involved, with poor basal expansion of the chest (a clinical clue to a shortened prognosis), and either a chest infection supervenes or the patient develops terminal dyspnea for 24 to 48 hours (controllable with morphine), or sometimes dies suddenly while being moved.

Choking is very rarely the cause of death, occurring in only 1% of patients.

Many patients remain mentally alert right up to the moment of death, and explanation and encouragement continue to be important.

Diagnosis relies on clinical examination (there are no diagnostic tests).

The classical features are:
- Fasciculations
- Flaccid weakness in the arms
- Spastic weakness in the legs
- Bulbar signs

Generalized fasciculation is diagnostic and occurs in no other disease. It is most easily seen in the tongue and deltoid muscles. A fasciculation is a visible muscle twitch. (Compensatory branching of normal nerve fibers occurs so each nerve now stimulates a whole group of muscle fibers.)

The combination of lower motor neuron weakness and wasting (**Amyotrophic**) with upper motor neuron weakness and spasticity (due to **Lateral Sclerosis** of the spinal cord) is highly suggestive of ALS — especially if wasting and spasticity occur in the same muscle group. A myelogram is occasionally necessary to exclude cervical spondylosis which can mimic ALS by causing wasted arm muscles (due to nerve root damage) with spastic leg weakness (due to cord pressure).

Prognosis varies. The majority of patients die within 4 to 5 years after diagnosis. 25% of patients present with bulbar symptoms, and their prognosis is worse (2 to 3 years). In some patients the disease is confined to the limbs and respiratory muscles, and they have a better prognosis (10% survive 10 years).

Explanation of the cause of weakness is valuable (for patient and family). Explanation is supportive. Patients who are getting weaker, falling, and fearing what is wrong, are always relieved to know that it is a recognized condition with a name. Isolating a person from the truth increases his despair. It is essential to be open, and then to provide support. The diagnosis is not grasped in a moment. It usually takes the patient several weeks or months to adjust to the new situation.

It is especially helpful to explain which functions are not affected:

- Sensation (pressure sores unlikely)
- Intellect (unlike multiple sclerosis)
- Eyesight
- Hearing
- Bladder control
- Bowel control
- Sexual potency

(Many persons mistakenly confuse ALS with multiple sclerosis.)

There are many types of **specialized equipment** available to help someone with ALS. These can improve a patient's quality of life.

The key is skillful assessment and timely prescribing of appropriate equipment. Introduction of equipment before it is necessary can be demoralizing, but there is no point in equipment arriving too late for the patient to use because the disease has progressed. This increases the patient's sense of frustration. ("If only I'd had this two months ago.")

Some helpful equipment can include:

- Communication aids (printer, computer equipment)
- Mobility aids
- Transfer aids (boards, hoists, slings, turning disc)
- Armchairs, Spenco cushions
- Wheelchairs (push, powered, reclining)
- Mobile arm supports
- Bathing aids (shower chair, bath lift)
- Special toilet equipment
- Eating aids (heated plate, 2-handled mug, straws)
- Special beds and mattresses
- Backrests, bed elevators
- Special car equipment (car hoists, rotating seats)
- Collar, head and neck supports
- Page turner
- Various environmental control systems

As the disease progresses, a patient usually needs differing types of particular aids and appliances (for example, one person may need 4 or 5 different types of communication aids at different times).

Expert advice from a skilled occupational therapist is essential.

Teamwork among professionals and family carers, especially including good communication, is essential.

The best way of co-ordinating care and involving appropriate professionals at the right time is by means of a **key worker** supporting the family.

Symptom control — A retrospective review of 100 patients with ALS at St. Christopher's Hospice emphasized the differences that a determined program of symptomatic treatment coupled with a positive attitude can make to a patient's quality of life and to the support of the family.

★ **Attention to details is essential: What helps one patient may be unbearable for another.**

80% of patients benefited from oral opioids, often initially only at night, with excellent results. (Being unable to turn over in bed causes very uncomfortable "bedache".)

Morphine does not have to be reserved for the terminal stages. Low doses can transform a patient's condition by abolishing the generalized aching that occurs if a person cannot change position frequently. Some patients take 5mg to 10mg of morphine at night for months with no danger of tolerance. Laxatives are essential with morphine. (see *Analgesics, Morphine*)

Common symptoms in ALS are:

- Weakness (100%)
- Communication problems (90% eventually)
- Dysphagia (75% eventually)
- Dyspnea (60% eventually)
- Falls
- Muscular aching
- Night cramps
- Muscle spasms
- Stiff joints
- Constipation
- Swollen legs
- Poor sleep
- Dribbling from mouth
- Choking episodes
- Sore eyes (reduced blinking)
- Sore bottom
- Anxiety
- Panic attacks
- Boredom

Dysphagia is often partially relieved by sucking ice before meals and applying an ice pack to the front of the neck for a few minutes, which reduces muscle spasm and improves the swallowing reflex. The patient should eat slowly and focus on lip closure (the first part of the reflex). Food must form a firm bolus to initiate the pharyngeal reflex (semi-solid foods are usually best). Food may need to be placed at the back of the mouth (tongue movement is usually poor). Neck position is important (it is difficult to swallow with the neck either too flexed or too extended).

Dehydration or taking an unacceptably long time to eat are indications for a nasogastric tube. Fine bore tubes are well tolerated. Some patients like to try to eat normally again once they are rehydrated and rested, and some succeed. Severe persistent dysphagia is an indication for a gastrostomy.

Choking is a defensive cough reflex to prevent aspiration of food into the lungs. Explanation of this fact can help to overcome some of the fears. Choking can usually be considerably relieved by skillful nursing care. Meals need to be slow and relaxed to avoid muscle fatigue. Cough can be made more forceful by abdominal compression. Cricopharyngeal myotomy is likely to be helpful only if there is pharyngeal spasm (which tends to cause choking after eating as pooled food spills into the larynx). Repeated severe choking is an indication for a gastrostomy, although most patients can be successfully managed without one.

Dribbling (due to an inability to contain or swallow saliva) is a common problem. Normally 1 to 2 liters of saliva are produced and swallowed automatically each day. Some patients with ALS fear that the disease is making them produce excessive saliva, and that they may drown. Others fear that dribbling is a sign they are losing their minds.

Explaining the causes of dribbling can reassure the patient.

Atropine can be very useful. The patient may prefer the tablets or the liquid preparation. The dose must be carefully titrated (up to 1.2mg every 4 hours on occasion). Excess dosage will cause the equally unpleasant problem of a dry mouth. (It is important to warn the patient that blurred vision may occur as a side effect of atropine, and not as a progression of the disease.)

Sucking ice can sometimes reduce spasm and bunching of the tongue, and allow saliva to be channeled to the back of the throat.

A palatal lift (a plastic disc attached to an existing denture or removable plate) can help to close the soft palate during the first phase of swallowing, and can improve swallowing and reduce dribbling.

A portable suction machine used a few hours a day can improve comfort if saliva is pooling at the back of the throat. Carers need to be carefully instructed on the proper use of the machine.

Polo-neck bibs ("dickies") with velcro fasteners can be changed regularly to prevent soiled clothing. These are more comfortable and less demeaning than regular bibs.

Bilateral neurectomy of the chorda tympani nerves (which innervate the salivary glands) is possible via the middle ear, and may be considered in cases of severe dribbling. Other techniques (including irradiation of the salivary glands) are rarely necessary.

Terminal phase — The patient must be comfortable, repositioned regularly, free of pain and dyspnea, and sleeping well. Regular mouth care is essential after every meal.

As the patient gets weaker and more dependent, communication and companionship become even more important. It is essential to support the family to enable them to support the patient. These patients become overwhelmingly dependent and vulnerable. They are often unable to communicate, yet remain mentally alert. Extra effort by carers is needed to maintain the patient's self-esteem and sense of control.

A continuous subcutaneous infusion of drugs can be very useful in the terminal phase. (see *Subcutaneous Infusions, Terminal Phase*)

Artificial ventilation for terminal dyspnea is contra-indicated. The patient can be kept free of distress with titrated doses of morphine. Ventilation simply prolongs the process of dying.

★ **"It is madness to demand from medicine a cure which it cannot give, or for the body to resist a disease which is irresistible."** (Hippocrates)

These comments, made by patients with ALS, may help to draw attention to their special needs (and to the needs of many other patients, too):

"When a person is paralyzed quite ordinary discomforts assume the character of minor tortures."

"For the average homebound invalid, conversation with visitors is the highlight of the day."

"Loneliness is not so much a matter of being alone as of not belonging."

"It is not realized that fear amounting to panic occurs by day or night, and it is therefore essential that help should be readily available. Contact can be made by means of a bell or buzzer which responds to the slightest touch."

"Being told the disease was a progressive one enabled me to do things while I could."

"I feel that patients and families should be told as much as possible in the home, in preference to the doctor's office or the rather tense atmosphere of a hospital clinic."

"I find it difficult to talk to people who tower above me, because of difficulty with neck control."

"Breathing exercises combined with simple speech exercises have not only kept my speech understandable but have also helped me with my swallowing."

"An understanding of my unusual tiredness is very important. This illness needs rest during the day and lots of sleep at night. Over a period of time I have come to recognize within myself waves of energy, which are followed by long periods of exhaustion. Things can be tackled while my energy lasts which should not be attempted once the exhaustion has set in."

"With the practical help and prayers of others I have found it possible to set aside the physical and let the mental and spiritual take over. This is a very enriching experience."

"Doctors of today should not feel that because they cannot cure patients with ALS they cannot help them. They can indeed help them by their compassionate understanding and friendship."

ANALGESICS

(see Agonist/Antagonist Analgesics, Brompton's Cocktail, Heroin, Meperidine, Methadone, Morphine, Subcutaneous Infusions)

★ **Continuous pain needs continuous pain relief. The cardinal rule is to give regular analgesia to keep pain away. Never prescribe PRN. (In hospice medicine, PRN means "Pain Relief Negligible".)**

Regular analgesia should ideally be oral, easy to take, and with few side effects, so that the patient can live as normal a life as possible once pain is controlled.

There are three basic analgesics:

- Acetaminophen (non-opioid)
- Codeine (weak opioid)
- Morphine (strong opioid)

Other analgesics are alternatives to these.

Mild pains need mild analgesics. Acetaminophen (1g every 4 hours) is an effective analgesic for mild pains.

Moderate pains respond to weak opioid drugs such as codeine. If oral codeine 60mg every 4 hours does not abolish pain, the patient should be started on oral morphine. If weak opioids reduced the pain, it usually means that the pain is opioid-responsive, and will be well controlled on the correct dose of oral morphine.

It is illogical and ineffective to try several drugs from the same group (morphine with another opioid drug).

When weaker opioids prove ineffective, **start oral morphine**. The principle is to start with a low dose, and to titrate, increasing promptly in steps until the pain is controlled. The usual starting dose for 4-hourly oral morphine is 5mg. The dose may be increased every 4 hours in steps: 5mg, 10mg, 20mg, 30mg, 45mg, 60mg (or more as needed). Once the patient's pain is well controlled on 4-hourly oral morphine, it is possible to stop the 4-hourly morphine and change to an equivalent dose of MS-Contin (morphine sulfate controlled-release) every 12 hours. (Do not use 4-hourly oral morphine and MS-Contin together. It is unnecessary and tends to confuse both patient and carers.) If the patient is pain-free and drowsy, reduce the dose of morphine. The aim is to have a **pain-free and alert patient**. (see *Morphine, Prescribing*)

Never prescribe opioid agonist/antagonists (buprenorphine, nalbuphine, pentazocine) with opioid agonists (codeine, morphine). (see *Agonist/Antagonist Analgesics*)

Always start a laxative and anti-emetic at the same time as morphine or any of the opioids, weak or strong. (see *Constipation, Laxatives, Nausea & Vomiting*)

Polypharmacy in hospice and palliative care is unavoidable and necessary. However, fixed mixtures of drugs which have not been individually titrated should be **avoided**. (see *Brompton's Cocktail, Prescribing*)

★   **There is no place in terminal care for patient-controlled analgesia. The aim is to achieve total pain control with as simple a regime as possible, releasing the patient to think about more important things than pain.**

If the patient is unable to swallow (for example, due to dysphagia or vomiting), change to one of the following:

- Morphine suppositories
- Morphine by IM injection (for the short term only)
- Morphine by continuous **subcutaneous** infusion

Many analgesics are not suitable for management of chronic pain, and include:

- Dihydrocodeine (constipating)
- Pentazocine (dysphoriant effect)
- Meperidine (too short-acting)
- Methadone (too long-acting)

★ **There is no known opioid superior to morphine. Pain that does not respond to carefully titrated doses of morphine will not respond to other opioid analgesics. Other opioid analgesics should generally be avoided.** (see *Morphine*)

The table below is a guide to equi-analgesic oral doses. It is useful when changing a patient from **regular** oral analgesia with one of the other opioids to **regular** oral analgesia with morphine, in order to avoid prescribing too much morphine (drowsiness) or too little (pain breakthrough) at time of changeover. The table does not apply to single doses.

CONVERSION TABLE FOR STRONG ORAL OPIOIDS **Applies to Oral Use Only**		**4-hourly morphine**
Meperidine	50mg	5mg
Pentazocine	50mg	5mg
Methadone	5mg	20mg
Hydromorphone	5mg	25mg

Opioid is a term meaning any compound (natural or synthetic) which has morphine-like activity and which is antagonized by naloxone. No known opioid analgesic is superior to morphine, but since the elucidation of the structure of morphine in 1925, much effort has gone into producing new chemical entities with equal analgesic effect but without the side-effects.

Opioids act at receptors in the brain (especially the midbrain) and at the spinal cord to inhibit the transmission of pain. There are several different types of receptor.

Most opioid drugs in clinical use (like morphine, codeine, methadone, and meperidine) act at the mu-receptors. They are selective mu-receptor agonists (causing strong analgesia but also other side effects). The structure of all these drugs (and the naloxone molecule) is similar, with a phenyl-N-methyl piperidine backbone which "fits" the mu-receptor. Some analgesics (pentazocine, for example) also stimulate sigma-receptors, causing dysphoria.

If an opioid selective to kappa-receptor agonists could be developed there is some evidence that the result would be strong analgesia with fewer side-effects.

Clinical differences between opioids concern:

- Analgesic ceiling
- Oral efficacy
- Speed of onset
- Duration of action
- Side-effects
- Potential for abuse

The potency of the drug (the amount in milligrams needed to achieve a given analgesic effect) is not as relevant as the **analgesic ceiling** (the highest strength of the drug which can be given in order to achieve the needed analgesic effect). Morphine has a high ceiling, so increasing the dose can increase the analgesic effect even at high doses. Agonist/antagonist drugs have a low ceiling. (see *Agonist/Antagonist Analgesics*)

Oral efficacy depends on lipid solubility (rate of absorption) and susceptibility to first-pass metabolism in the liver. Methadone is well absorbed and slowly metabolized and therefore has a long half-life. More lipid-soluble drugs have a more rapid **onset of action** (crossing the blood-brain barrier more easily), but also leave the CNS more readily (and thus have a shorter duration of action).

Duration of action also depends on receptor affinity. The duration of pain relief varies from about 1 to 2 hours (meperidine) to 4 hours (morphine) to 8 hours (buprenorphine, methadone).

Side-effects depend not only on the receptor profile of the drug, but also on the receptor profile of the patient, which explains, for example, why some patients develop severe nausea with buprenorphine or constipation with dihydrocodeine, and others do not. (If a patient cannot tolerate one opioid analgesic it is still worth trying another.)

Physical dependence can occur with most opioids after 3 to 4 weeks in a person without pain, but **does not occur in a patient with pain**.

ANEMIA

Any chronic illness can cause anemia, which is typically normocytic (normal MCV in the range 76-96). A hemoglobin (Hb) level below 8g/dL [5.0mmol/L] suggests another cause (usually bleeding or bone marrow involvement) in addition to that of chronic disease. In one study of 110 patients with advanced cancer who were admitted to St. Christopher's Hospice, only 6 had a hemoglobin level below 8g/dL [5.0mmol/L].

The chronic anemia of advanced disease is usually asymptomatic because the patient is not active (and because there is a compensatory shift in the oxygen dissociation curve, so that the Hb molecule gives up its oxygen more easily in peripheral tissues). Symptoms of anemia only tend to occur with severe anemia (Hb less than 7g/dL [4.3mmol/L]) or if blood loss is sudden.

A common question is this: are the symptoms due to advanced disease and debility, or due to anemia?

Anemia can cause the following symptoms:
- Dizziness
- Fainting
- Palpitations
- Angina
- Dyspnea
- Heart failure
- Fatigue

If anemia is causing distressing symptoms, in a patient with a reasonable prognosis (e.g., expected to live at least two weeks), blood transfusion may be indicated.

With some symptoms (dizziness, exertional dyspnea) it can be very difficult to know whether these are due to the anemia or to the advanced malignancy. If the patient has a prognosis of weeks (rather than days) it is justifiable to transfuse and to monitor symptoms. If symptoms improve significantly it has been worthwhile: if symptoms are unchanged the situation is clarified and further transfusions are not indicated.

Blood transfusions do not significantly improve the weakness and fatigue of advanced malignancy.

A transfusion can be used to give a patient a boost for a special occasion (to attend a wedding, for example) but any beneficial effects may be very short-lived (1 or 2 days).

One unit of blood raises the Hb level by about 1g/dL [0.6mmol/L]. Normally 4 units of packed cells are given over 16 hours, with a dose of oral furosemide 40mg in the early stage of transfusion to prevent the increase in circulating volume precipitating heart failure.

A retrospective study at St. Christopher's Hospice over four years (1980-1983) showed that only 23 patients had blood transfusions (out of about 2,500 cancer patients admitted), only 13 showed improvement, 7 had mild reactions (fever, heart failure, raised urea levels with transient confusion) and 1 had a severe transfusion reaction. Blood transfusion carries risks, and an iatrogenic disaster is the last thing needed when coping with a terminal illness.

If the patient has been receiving multiple transfusions with little benefit, he may welcome a frank discussion and the opportunity to stop. Stopping regular transfusions does not inevitably hasten death — the patient can sometimes adjust to a low Hb level and live for weeks or even months.

Active bleeding that cannot be controlled is not usually an indication for transfusion, which simply causes heavier bleeding.

If the patient is iron deficient, as shown by a hypochromic hypocytic anemia (low MCH and MCV), it can be worthwhile giving iron if the patient has a reasonably good prognosis. Ferrous sulfate tablets should be taken with food to avoid gastritis. In far advanced disease the disadvantage of constipation due to the iron can outweigh any benefits.

ANOREXIA

Anorexia occurs in about 65% of hospice patients.

Management options include:
1. Consider causes
2. Consider steroids
3. Consider metoclopramide
4. Increase attractiveness of meals
5. Explain to patient and family
6. Seek advice from dietitian

1. **Causes** — Exclude oral thrush, nausea, constipation, hypercalcemia. Stop all unnecessary drugs. Anorexia occurs after chemotherapy or radical radiotherapy, but it is rare after low-dose palliative radiotherapy. Often no cause

can be found. In some cases anorexia may be due to tumor peptides that affect metabolism (since plasmapheresis has been shown to improve appetite for 24 hours). Psychological factors are important, and anorexia may reflect the morale of the patient; it is common to see patients who have had severe anorexia eat well as soon as they enter the secure environment of a hospice or a day-care program.

2. **Steroids** — Patients often find anorexia upsetting — a daily reminder that they are "fading away". Eating well often boosts morale. Steroids (dexamethasone 4mg per day or prednisolone 30mg per day) help about 80% of patients. Cyproheptadine is sometimes used as an appetite stimulant, but it is rarely effective. There is some evidence that megestrol acetate (480mg to 1,600mg per day) improves appetite and produces weight gain in patients with advanced breast cancer. There is some evidence that high dose Vitamin C (500mg 4 times a day) for 6 weeks or more may improve appetite and well-being.

3. **Metoclopramide** — If anorexia is due to a feeling of fullness or heartburn, it may be due to a small stomach, and metoclopramide 10mg before meals can help. (see *Small Stomach Syndrome*)

4. **Meals** — Attractive preparation and serving of favorite foods with strong tastes (salty or spicy) often helps. An alcoholic drink with the meal is appropriate if that is the patient's usual practice. Small portions are important. Large helpings are a demoralizing reminder of healthier days, and can bring on nausea in some patients. Eating whenever hungry is better than observing strict traditional mealtimes. (A microwave oven can be helpful for a quick response). Eating in a room other than the sickroom can also help.

Avoid strong smells of cooking food at mealtimes. As the patient becomes less well, ice-cold food is sometimes preferred. Patients sometimes need permission to eat less. Liquid supplements may suffice. (see *Diet*)

5. **Explanation** — It is very important to explain anorexia to the family. Rejection of lovingly prepared food can feel like rejection of love. Explain that taste abnormalities are common in the very ill, and therefore the patient may develop new preferences. The body needs less food when inactive. There is no danger of wrong foods — the patient senses what he needs. Family members can encourage fluids right up to the end, but eating can become a difficult event, so do not allow family members to force food on a dying patient.

6. **Dietitian** — Advice from a dietitian is usually welcomed. The dietitian can give advice about a balanced diet, provide suggestions on overcoming problems from taste changes or a sore mouth, and advise on the use of the growing number of available oral nutritional supplements.

★ **Hyperalimentation and/or intravenous parenteral feeding do not improve appetite or weight experimentally, and have little or no place clinically in far advanced illness.** (see *Nutrition*)

ANTIBIOTICS

Antibiotics have an important place in controlling symptoms in advanced disease. **If an infection is causing symptoms it should be treated promptly** (after a swab or specimen has been taken for bacteriology) with an appropriate antibiotic (always ask about drug allergies).

A broad-spectrum antibiotic is indicated for cellulitis, pulmonary or urinary tract infections, sometimes as a trial in a patient with sweating that may be secondary to bacteremia, or while awaiting laboratory sensitivities.

Chloramphenicol 500mg 4 times a day is very useful as a broad-spectrum antibiotic which is active against anaerobes. It is refreshingly free of side effects. (Bone marrow damage is rare, occurring in about 1 in 30,000 patients, which is an acceptable risk for an individual patient with advanced disease.)

It is occasionally correct practice to withhold antibiotics for a potentially fatal pneumonia (and treat any symptoms of dyspnea, cough or pleuritic pains with morphine and scopolamine). Sometimes during a discussion about quality of life the patient requests no further active treatment of pulmonary infections. At other times the decision has to be made by the doctor (preferably one who knows the patient well) that further active treatment would be prolonging dying and "officiously striving to keep alive" rather than promoting quality of remaining life.

ANTI-CHOLINERGICS

Scopolamine is an important drug in terminal care. It dries up secretions and usually prevents terminal respiratory bubbling. It is also powerfully sedative. The usual dose is 0.4mg to 0.6mg IM every 4 hours.

Scopolamine is available as a **trans-dermal patch**. The patch is applied to the hairless area of skin behind the ear. It contains 1.5mg of scopolamine, delivers 0.5mg per day over 3 days, and is principally intended for the control of motion sickness, when it should be applied 4 hours before the effect is required. (Carers should wash their hands after applying a patch, to avoid inadvertent contact with eyes and possible temporary blurred vision.)

Since the usual dose of scopolamine in terminal care is 0.4mg to 0.6mg IM every 4 hours (or 2mg to 4mg per 24 hours by continuous subcutaneous infusion), and one trans-dermal patch delivers only 0.5mg per 24 hours, it may be necessary to use 3 to 5 trans-dermal patches simultaneously to achieve an adequate dosage.

Atropine is indicated if an anti-cholinergic effect is required without sedation — for example, to decrease salivation in patients with amyotrophic lateral sclerosis (ALS).

ANTI-COAGULANTS

Anti-coagulants reduce blood clotting. Heparin has a short action. It is given by continuous IV infusion or by subcutaneous injection. Warfarin acts by antagonizing Vitamin K (necessary to synthesize clotting factors) and takes 36 to 48 hours to take effect.

Indications:
- Deep vein thrombosis
- Pulmonary embolus
- To prevent embolic stroke
    - In atrial fibrillation
    - In valvular heart disease
    - With arterial grafts or valve prostheses
    - Following myocardial infarction

Patients with advanced cancer may require anti-coagulant therapy for a venous thrombosis or pulmonary embolus to **control symptoms of pain or swelling**. Treatment needs to be carefully monitored if there is co-existing liver damage. Treatment does not need to be continued for more than 3 to 4 weeks.

Warfarin is **potentiated** by certain drugs (including cimetidine, chlorpromazine, naproxen, chloramphenicol, allopurinol and aspirin), which may cause bleeding.

Occasionally patients are already taking long-term warfarin therapy when they enter hospice or palliative care. There may come a time when this therapy becomes inappropriate. It can be a difficult decision to stop treatment because the patient has usually been told by the hematologist that treatment must not be stopped. If the tumor itself is causing troublesome bleeding this is usually a clear indication to stop warfarin. If a terminally ill patient, after discussion with the doctor and nurse, is reluctant to stop warfarin altogether it can be reasonable to compromise by halving the dose and monitoring less frequently.

If a patient who is dying is still on warfarin there can be problems. IM injections of warfarin can cause large hematomas. There is a risk of gastrointestinal bleeding with altered blood coming from the mouth during and after death. This is very distressing for the relatives. If a patient is dying, warfarin can be reversed with Vitamin K. Oral phytonadione 10mg is effective within 4 hours. By IV injection (given slowly to avoid nausea) phytonadione takes almost immediate effect. (see *Bleeding, Terminal Phase*)

ANTI-DEPRESSANTS

The question is often: appropriate sadness or depression? Endogenous depression is surprisingly rare in terminal illness.

A truly depressed terminally ill patient can respond very dramatically within 7 to 10 days after starting a tricyclic anti-depressant in proper doses. Start with a low dose, then increase the dose as quickly as the patient will tolerate the side effects, particularly the dry mouth. (For example, start imipramine 10mg to 25mg, usually at bedtime, increasing the dose by steps to 75mg to 150mg per day.) (see *Depression*)

A useful guide to the speed of increase in daily doses of imipramine is:

Day 1	10mg to 25mg
Day 3	25mg to 50mg
Day 7	50mg to 100mg
Day 10	100mg to 150mg

Note: Elderly or frail patients need lower doses. Side-effects often limit the tolerated dose.

Tricyclics can be categorized according to their sedative properties:

Sedating:	Trimipramine
Moderately sedating:	Amitriptyline
Less sedating:	Imipramine
	Desipramine
	Nortriptyline
Stimulant action:	Protriptyline

Agitated patients respond best to sedative tricyclics. Withdrawn patients benefit from less sedating or stimulant tricyclics. The newer tricyclics have fewer anti-cholinergic side effects, but some can cause bone marrow depression and monthly full blood counts are required.

Patients with chronic pain tend to get depressed. There is some evidence that long-term morphine causes depression. There is some evidence that imipramine has a morphine-potentiating effect. Therefore, in any patient who has suffered severe pains for more than a few months, consider a trial of imipramine.

Being anti-cholinergic, almost all anti-depressants can cause dry mouth, blurred vision and urinary retention, and can sometimes contribute to the patient's confusion. (*see Depression*)

ANTI-EMETICS

The theory — Anti-emetics can be divided into 3 groups:

1. Anti-emetics acting mainly on the **vomiting center in the mid-brain**. These are anti-cholinergic drugs (which can cause dry mouth, drowsiness, blurred vision). Anti-histamines are also anti-cholinergic.

This group includes:
- Scopolamine
- Cyclizine
- Promethazine (sedating)

2. Some anti-emetics act mainly on the **chemoreceptor trigger zone** (CTZ). (The CTZ is in the medulla, close to the vomiting center.) The CTZ has dopamine receptors, therefore these are anti-dopaminergic drugs (which can have Parkinsonian side effects of stiffness and dystonic movements).

This group includes:

- Prochlorperazine
- Thiethylperazine
- Haloperidol
- Chlorpromazine
- Methotrimeprazine

3. **Gastro-kinetic anti-emetics** which act on the CTZ and also **increase gastric emptying and gut peristalsis**.

This group includes:

- Metoclopramide

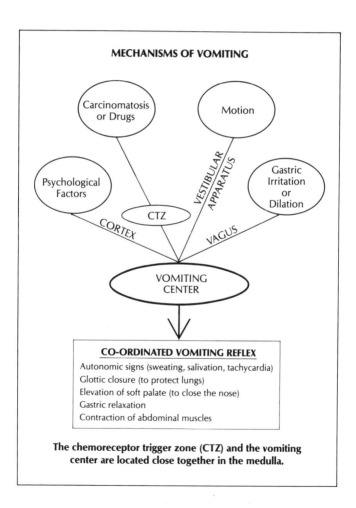

MECHANISMS OF VOMITING

The chemoreceptor trigger zone (CTZ) and the vomiting center are located close together in the medulla.

The neurophysiology of vomiting is complex, and has been investigated mainly in the cat. A human is not a cat and the pathways may be different. For example, in the cat motion sickness is known to be mediated via the CTZ whereas in humans anti-cholinergics are more effective than phenothiazines in preventing motion sickness, suggesting motion in humans acts directly on the vomiting center.

Useful drugs:

1. **Prochlorperazine** 5mg 3 times a day is useful to prevent nausea when starting morphine. It has few side effects and causes little or no drowsiness.

2. **Thiethylperazine** is a phenothiazine that is similar in clinical usage to prochlorperazine, and is less sedating than chlorpromazine. It is a useful drug in preventing and controlling nausea. The usual oral dose is 10mg 2 to 3 times a day. It is available in suppository form (usual dose, 10mg every 12 hours).

3. **Haloperidol** is a strong anti-emetic. It is a narrow-spectrum anti-emetic, with a powerful antagonist action at the dopamine receptors of the CTZ, but with no action at cholinergic or histamine receptors. It is the strong anti-emetic of first choice, causing little drowsiness. The usual starting dose is 1.5mg at bedtime. The dose can be increased to 5mg 2 times a day, or for short periods to 5mg 4 times a day, but extrapyramidal effects (stiffness initially) are common. It can be used in a continuous subcutaneous infusion.

4. **Chlorpromazine** is a strong anti-emetic but can cause drowsiness and dry mouth. It is indicated for the nausea of uremia, if the patient also has hiccups, and is used if anxiety is contributing to the nausea, or if the patient also needs some sedation. The oral dose is usually 10mg to 25mg 3 times a day.

5. **Cyclizine** 50mg every 8 hours either orally or by intramuscular injection is a very useful and logical addition to drugs that act at the CTZ, since it has a different site action, acting on the cholinergic or histamine receptors of the vomiting center. It is therefore indicated for nausea due to intestinal causes or due to brain metastases causing raised intracranial pressure. It is also particularly indicated if there is an element of motion sickness, e.g., nausea that is worse on turning over in bed. It causes some drowsiness and dry mouth. Cyclizine can be used alone in a continuous subcutaneous infusion up to a concentration of 15mg/ml. Mixed with morphine, however, there is a risk

of precipitation if the concentration of each drug exceeds 10mg/ml.

6. **Metoclopramide** is particularly useful if there is poor gastric emptying, e.g., hepatomegaly compressing the stomach and causing heartburn, wind and fullness as well as nausea. Metoclopramide is particularly effective in high doses for the nausea of cytotoxic therapy. It acts at the CTZ but also causes gastric emptying, by relaxing the pylorus, tightening the lower esophageal sphincter, and causing peristalsis of the stomach and of all the small bowel. It is useful if there is reflux esophagitis or hiccups due to gastric distention. It should be avoided if there is colicky pain. It can be used in continuous subcutaneous infusions, and has been used in high dosage (up to 240mg per day) to overcome gastric stasis.

7. **Methotrimeprazine** is a powerful anti-emetic and sedative. It is used in a continuous subcutaneous infusion (50mg to 200mg over 24 hours) for severe nausea, but can cause marked drowsiness and dry mouth. In ambulant patients it can also cause postural hypotension. It is also particularly useful for terminal agitation and restlessness. (see *Subcutaneous Infusions, Terminal Phase*)

ANXIETY

Important points in the history include:
- Drugs
- Any new symptoms
- Specific fears or phobias
- Patient's knowledge of disease
- Previous experience of cancer or illness
- Previous personality
- Previous crises ("How did you cope?")
- Relationships ("Who do you rely on?")
- Pattern of anxiety ("When?", "Where?" — not Why?)
- Sleep (dreams, nightmares, insomnia)
- Behavior (attention-seeking, panic)
- Views of family members

Drugs such as albuterol and aminophylline can cause shakiness. Anti-cholinergics can cause palpitations. Metoclopramide and haloperidol can make some people feel restless. High dose steroids occasionally cause excitation. It may be necessary to exclude thyrotoxicosis, which can mimic anxiety, by measuring serum thyroxine levels.

Long-term users of benzodiazepines may take high doses (diazepam 40mg to 60mg per day, for example) with no drowsiness, but they may suffer severe anxiety if the dose is reduced.

It can be helpful to try to classify the anxiety:

1. Chronic
2. Specific fears
3. Adjustment reactions
4. Separation
5. Excessive denial

1. **Chronic anxiety** — In severe anxiety states important questions are: What was the patient's previous personality? Is there a history of chronic anxiety? Does the patient have a particular phobia about illness?

2. **Specific fears** — Anxieties due to specific worries can almost always be relieved. They may relate to the family ("How will they cope without me?"), to financial concerns or to spiritual matters. It is useful to ask a general question ("Are you a worrier?" or "Are you a sensitive person?") to broach the subject. Asking "What is the thing you are most worried about?" often enables a patient to analyze and reality-test fears, and so reduces anxiety.

3. **Adjustment reactions** are transient episodes of anxiety or depression that are normal features of adapting to life changes, and to a different role and future. Patients (like bereaved family members) should be supported emotionally and practically as they grieve for what is lost. Most patients cope with losses and fears one step at a time. Anxiety is minimized by maintaining the patient's morale and self-respect in a secure and loving atmosphere where communication is encouraged. (see *Adjustment Reaction*)

4. **Separation anxiety** — Many patients feel worse in unfamiliar surroundings, and when separated from their family and friends. Separation anxiety is the first emotion we experience in life, and it is easily re-awakened. Frightened people need physical contact to reassure them. Feelings of insecurity and anxiety may only resolve with contact from a family member, lover or trusted friend.

5. **Excessive denial** — Denial, used intermittently, is a normal way of coping with overwhelming difficulties as a person learns to adjust. Used excessively, however, denial usually increases anxiety. The terminally ill patient who denies excessively has usually coped with previous crises by denial (presenting very late with the symptoms of cancer,

for example), and is in effect saying "I am frightened, and I feel I cannot cope." That patient never benefits from the self-confidence which comes from facing problems and working through grief. (see *Denial*)

Complete denial often results in increasing anxiety, which is also denied, and thus may manifest itself as symptoms (nausea, tremor), nightmares, insomnia, or very demanding behavior. Attention-seeking is usually due to anxieties that resolve if the patient is given sympathetic attention and time. Asking about nightmares in detail (without attempting interpretation) is a very useful way of allowing a patient to express fear, and can help the patient to discuss how he normally copes with fears.

Denial of severe anxiety can occasionally mimic confusion as the patient withdraws from an intolerable reality.

Patients who have previously coped with anxieties by being busy and competent can find terminal illness intolerable and may (very rarely) develop hysterical conversion symptoms like becoming mute or feigning coma.

The anxiety of denial is reduced by improving the patient's acceptance of his illness and situation. Any deterioration in physical condition tends to increase anxiety, and is the time to give the patient plenty of opportunity to ask questions and express fears. Avoid forcing information on patients about matters they clearly do not wish to discuss. They usually deny the conversation and just feel more anxious.

Management options:
- Counseling
- Relaxation therapy
- Visualization
- Cognitive methods
- Drug therapy

Allowing the patient **time** to ask questions and express fears, and supporting the patient with **skilled and sympathetic personal attention** remains the management option of choice. Carers must learn the extent and limits of their abilities in counseling and, when necessary, seek consultation with specially trained psycho-social professionals.

Relaxation therapy is very useful for almost all patients. Features of anxiety such as dyspnea and palpitations can make the patients fear that the disease has advanced. This can escalate into hyperventilation and panic. Relaxation practiced regularly can abort panic attacks. (see *Relaxation*)

Visualization (usually practiced 2 times a day) can help patients set boundaries to the amount of time spent worrying about their disease, and can reduce anxiety by giving them a feeling of control. (see *Visualization*)

Cognitive methods focus on the thoughts that are associated with feelings of anxiety. In pathological anxiety the patient tends to overestimate a feared event (in terms of both probability and severity), and to underestimate coping resources (in self and others). By changing habitual modes of thought or behavior an individual can reduce his own distress. Automatic thoughts can be interrupted by distraction or positive thinking, or by positive self-statements.

It can be helpful to ask the patient to keep a log of mood, thoughts and activity as they occur during the day and night. These patterns can then be reviewed by the patient and carers (in cooperation with a psychologist or other psycho-social professional), restoring a feeling of control and providing a basis for behavioral and social modification.

A **beta blocker** (such as propanolol 20mg to 40mg 4 times a day) can be useful if there are physical manifestations of anxiety such as sweating, palpitations or tremor.

If **anxiolytics** are required diazepam 10mg at bedtime is effective. Lorazepam 0.5mg to 2mg every 3 to 6 hours is less cumulative.

Haloperidol 1.5mg to 5mg 1 to 3 times a day can be helpful if benzodiazepines are ineffective or cause drowsiness, or if there is an element of paranoia or severe agitation. On doses above 3mg 2 times a day, tremor and rigidity can occur. This is drug-induced Parkinsonism, and can be partially controlled by oral procyclidine 2.5mg to 5mg 3 times a day (slightly sedating) or orphenadrine 50mg to 100mg 3 times a day (slightly stimulating). Chlorpromazine 10mg to 25mg 3 times a day is a useful alternative if sedation is also required.

A **tricyclic anti-depressant** may be necessary for patients with agitated depression.

AROMATHERAPY

Massage with fragrant oils has biblical precedents. It is now practiced to relieve stress as part of a holistic approach to health and self-healing. Some of the essential oils (camomile, basil) may be absorbed in minute quantities. Touch and smell are primitive senses and focusing on them can induce **relaxation**. (see *Relaxation, Touch*)

The sense of smell can evoke powerful **memories** and can be used to trigger emotional memories, or to help induce a state of relaxation (for example, evoking memories of a seaside holiday with cassette tapes of seagulls and waves, combined with seaside smells).

Aromatherapists usually make recommendations about diet, massage, breathing and relaxation exercises, as well as the use of inhalations, bath oils and lotions.

ASCITES

Ascites means free fluid in the peritoneal cavity. It causes abdominal distention. It is detected clinically by the sign of "shifting dullness" (the line of dullness to percussion shifts laterally as the patient turns on his side), but there must be at least 500cc of free fluid. Ultrasound scans will detect as little as 100cc.

Pathophysiology — The subphrenic lymphatic plexuses become blocked with tumor. Fluid is exuded by both tumor-involved and normal peritoneum, mediated locally by vasoactive products. Sodium retention also occurs in malignant ascites which explains why diuretics can be effective. Ascites due to peritoneal deposits can occur with almost any carcinoma, but is seen most often in carcinomas of breast, ovary, colon, stomach, pancreas and bronchus.

Symptoms are due to pressure:
- Abdominal discomfort
- Inability to bend or sit upright
- Leg edema
- Dyspnea
- Heartburn

Summary of management options:
- Analgesia for discomfort or dyspnea
- High dose diuretics
- Paracentesis
- Peritoneovenous shunt

There is no place for intra-peritoneal instillations of cytotoxics, which are usually ineffective. A wide variety of agents have been used (including bleomycin, fluorouracil, thiotepa and quinacrine). Several studies have shown a partial response in about 30% of patients, but in practice the results are usually disappointing. Ascites can sometimes resolve in response to systemic chemotherapy (for example, fluorouracil for gastrointestinal malignancies).

1. **Analgesics** — Ascites can sometimes cause a feeling of tightness and discomfort which responds well to low doses of opioid analgesics. (see *Analgesics, Dyspnea*)

2. **Diuretics** — The recommended starting dose is spironolactone 200mg per day with furosemide 40mg per day. It usually begins to work within 5 days, and the ascites resolves over 2 to 4 weeks in about 70% of patients. Girth measurements are taken twice weekly and should decrease. If there is no decrease after one week, increase the doses to spironolactone 200mg 2 times a day with furosemide 120mg per day. Follow-up is needed with these high doses to avoid dehydration. Spironolactone may cause nausea.

High dose diuretics can effectively reduce malignant ascites. In one study 13 of 15 patients with malignant ascites had an excellent response to spironolactone started at 150mg per day, and increased by 50mg per day if average daily weight loss was less than 0.5kg. All patients showed increased sodium excretion.

There is a case report of intravenous infusions of furosemide (100mg in 100ml saline at 5ml per hour) effectively reducing ascites when oral diuretics had failed.

If the patient has a short prognosis (gross hepatomegaly and jaundice, for example) then paracentesis to relieve symptoms quickly is indicated, rather than starting diuretics.

★   **Do not give potassium supplements with spironolactone (which is potassium-sparing) because hyperkalemia can occur.**

3. **Paracentesis** is a useful emergency measure when a patient has a tense ascites causing severe discomfort, dyspnea or inability to sit up. It occasionally needs to be repeated. It is safe to drain off the first 4 liters quickly, and then a further 6 liters more slowly at 2 liters per hour.

Procedure:
- Use 0.5% bupivacaine as a local anesthetic, which prevents pain at the drainage site from 6 to 8 hours.
- The bladder should be empty. Marked bowel distention is a **contraindication** to paracentesis.

- The ideal site is the left ileac fossa (10cm from the mid-line to avoid the inferior epigastric artery). Puncture sites should be away from scars.

- A good method is to use a pediatric trocar and cannula which connects straight into a urinary drainage bag.

- Ascitic fluid occasionally continues to dribble from the paracentesis site. Explain to the patient that this may occur, and apply a colostomy bag to collect the leaking fluid. If leakage has not stopped within 48 hours, consider suturing.

- Paracentesis can easily be performed in the home.

4. **Peritoneovenous shunts** — A shunt can effectively control malignant ascites. The use of a shunt for ascites due to cirrhosis was first introduced in 1962. In 1974 Leveen developed a shunt with a one-way pressure-sensitive valve, and in 1979 Denver developed a shunt which has the advantage of a pumping chamber to reduce the incidence of occlusion (which occurs eventually in about 30% of patients).

The shunt can be inserted under local or general anesthesia. The fenestrated peritoneal tube is inserted in the right or left hypochondrium, the valve chamber is placed over a lower rib, and the venous end of the shunt is led subcutaneously to a neck incision above the clavicle and introduced through the internal jugular vein into the superior vena cava. The operation is covered by antibiotics for three days.

The insertion of a shunt is **contraindicated** if the ascitic fluid is particularly viscous due to infection or blood, or if it is loculated.

There is no evidence that the shunt increases distant metastases.

Occlusion due to fibrin deposition or omental plugging can usually be detected by ultrasound. If it does not respond to pumping, the shunt has to be replaced. Rarely occlusion may be due to thrombosis around the venous end of the shunt, which may respond to anti-coagulation.

Insertion of a shunt does not affect prognosis. It can produce excellent palliation of symptoms even though the abdomen is not totally emptied of fluid. The shunt can remain patent and effective for months and years.

Mrs. R.T., age 27, was diagnosed as suffering from carcinoma of the ovary in November, 1982 and treated with chemotherapy. She developed ascites, and a peritoneovenous shunt was inserted in July,

1985. She was referred for hospice care in November, 1986. She developed rigors and the shunt was removed in March, 1987 (after being in place for 1 year and 10 months). The rigors settled and the abdominal distention did not recur, possibly because the skin of the abdominal wall had become indurated and less able to distend. She continued her part-time job until the week she died, two months later.

ASSESSMENT

The aims of a full and detailed assessment are:
- To identify and tackle problems (physical, mental, social, spiritual)
- To increase trust
- To plan for the future

Patients usually have many different problems. A full assessment demonstrates a serious intent to be in control of all the facts. The way it is done is a powerful message.

It is possible to ask questions at a first assessment that can be difficult to ask ever again.

Assessment includes:
- History of illness
- List of physicians involved
- Inquiry about present symptoms
- Discussion of drugs prescribed
- Physical examination
- Occupational history
- Questions about financial worries, will
- Family tree
- List of forthcoming events (anniversaries, graduations)
- Principal carers
- Daily routine (?self-care)
- Home conditions
- Religious beliefs, church membership
- Insight
- Assess priorities (What are your aims now?)
- Make a plan
- Follow up

A full assessment may take an hour or more, but it lays the foundation for a relationship of trust. Encourage joint assessments, but avoid repeated assessments by different team members. ("I've said all this twice already!")

Make a note of any **explanations** you give. This improves team communication. Different explanations by team members can destroy the patient's trust.

Avoid assumptions. When assessing a patient's needs and priorities, remember that no two people are the same. The patient will often have very different priorities from your own (sometimes surprisingly so).

BENZODIAZEPINES

Benzodiazepines are useful drugs in terminal care, provided they do not become substitutes for the counseling, discussion and continuing reassurance needed by an anxious and distressed terminally ill patient.

★   **Writing a prescription for benzodiazepines is not an appropriate reply to the difficult questions a terminally ill patient often asks the doctor.**

General uses:
- Night sedation (temazepam, triazolam)
- Anxiolytic (diazepam, lorazepam)
- Muscle relaxant (diazepam)
- Anti-convulsant (clonazepam, diazepam)

Special uses:

Clonazepam is reserved for use as an anti-convulsant.

Diazepam (usual dose 5mg to 10mg at bedtime) is useful to reduce anxiety and control muscle spasms.

Rectal diazepam enema 10mg is useful for control of seizures and works as quickly as an IV injection. (Diazepam enemas are not available commercially in the United States, but enterprising pharmacists can prepare them for use in hospice and palliative care.)

Lorazepam is less cumulative than diazepam, and is usually the anxiolytic of choice. The oral dose is 0.5mg to 2mg, usually every 4 to 6 hours (but may be needed every 2 to 3 hours). Lorazepam 1mg to 2mg IV is useful for urgent sedation.

Midazolam is water soluble, and can be used in a continuous subcutaneous infusion (usual starting dose is 20mg to 30mg per 24 hours).

Temazepam (15mg to 60mg) is the most useful drug for night sedation for the majority of patients. A few patients find even temazepam 15mg causes a "hangover" effect the next morning, in which case use triazolam 0.125mg to 0.5mg at bedtime.

Some long-acting benzodiazepines (those with half-lives above 25 hours) are converted into active metabolites with very long half-lives. Diazepam is converted into desmethyldiazepam with a half-life of about 150 hours!

Half-lives of some commonly used benzodiazepines:

Diazepam	40 hours
Lorazepam	20 hours
Temazepam	13 hours
Triazolam	3 hours
Midazolam	3 hours

BLADDER SPASMS

Bladder spasms (hyperactivity of detrusor muscle) cause intermittent suprapubic pain together with urinary urgency. Bladder spasms occur due to radiation cystitis or tumors (bladder, prostate). An indwelling urinary catheter usually worsens the discomfort. It is important to exclude urinary tract infection or fecal impaction.

The most useful drug is **oxybutynin**, a powerful antispasmodic with local anesthetic properties. Oxybutynin 5mg to 10mg 3 times a day can be very effective in reducing bladder spasms. Anti-cholinergic side effects (particularly a dry mouth) can be severe.

The tricyclic drugs also reduce bladder spasms (for example, imipramine 25mg to 50mg at bedtime). NSAIDs can sometimes reduce detrusor hyperactivity (naproxen 500mg 2 times a day). Bromocriptine, starting at 1.25mg per day and increasing up to 2.5mg 2 times a day can reduce urinary urgency and frequency (presumably via its dopamine agonist effect) but may cause nausea, headache and postural hypotension.

BLEEDING

Management of bleeding depends on its site and severity.

Management options may include:

1. Topical adrenaline and/or alginate dressings
2. Palliative radiotherapy
3. Tranexamic acid
4. Reversal of warfarin
5. Transfusion
6. Laser
7. Alum solution
8. Radiation menopause
9. Sedation in severe bleeding

1. Liberal use of **topical adrenaline** (1 in 1,000) on a dressing, applied with firm local pressure, is a good first aid measure for surface bleeding. If infection is contributing to bleeding give a broad spectrum antibiotic. **Alginate dressings** are hemostatic and can be useful for surface bleeding. (*see Pressure Sores*)

2. **Palliative radiotherapy** can dry up surface bleeding from fungating breast cancer or malignant nodes and is often effective for hemoptysis. It cannot be given if the area has already received radical doses of radiation.

3. Oral **tranexamic acid** 1g per day can stop capillary bleeding. It is an anti-fibrinolytic and acts by stabilizing the fibrin plug. It can cause nausea. Anti-fibrinolytics are said to increase the risk of clots forming in the bladder in patients with hematuria. Clots in the bladder can be lysed by citrate bladder washouts.

4. If the patient is taking warfarin the effect can be reversed by giving Vitamin K, phytonadione 10mg orally (which reverses warfarin in 4 hours), or 10mg IV by slow injection to avoid nausea (which has immediate effect). **Warfarin should be reversed in the terminal phase of illness** to prevent the distressing bleeding that can occur as the patient dies, causing altered blood to trickle from the mouth. If warfarin overdosage has caused hypothrombinemia and bleeding, fresh frozen plasma replaces clotting factors immediately.

5. **Blood transfusion** is not usually considered for active bleeding in terminal illness, unless the bleeding is controlled and the patient is left with symptomatic anemia. (In fact, transfusion can make bleeding heavier for a time.)

6. **Laser therapy** can coagulate bleeding tumors in the bronchus and rectum. It can be performed through an endoscope and has the advantages of immediate relief of symptoms without systemic side effects. It usually has to be repeated.

Standard (no-touch) laser techniques may not control heavy bleeding from large, friable tumors. Such bleeding has been controlled in gastric cancers using low-power interstitial laser coagulation. (*see Lasers*)

7. A **1% alum solution** (100mg alum dissolved in 1,000ml sterile water, then diluted x 10 with normal saline) is the best styptic solution for bladder washouts to control bladder hemorrhage, and on ribbon gauze to control hemorrhage from carcinoma of the rectum. (*see Bladder Cancer, Rectal Cancer*)

8. Heavy menstrual bleeding can be troublesome for a disabled patient (with ALS, for example) and can be stopped by inducing a **radiation menopause**.

9. If severe bleeding and shock occurs, the patient should be **sedated** (with an injection of morphine, scopolamine and chlorpromazine). If a sudden massive hemorrhage is a strong possibility, these drugs should be kept ready in a syringe. A red blanket should also be readily available to reduce the visual effects of massive hemorrhage. (*see Terminal Phase*)

BODY IMAGE

Old photographs of a patient can be valuable in patient care. These help carers relate to the patient as a person, seeing him as he was before he became ill. (*see Weight Loss*)

Photography can help a patient become more **accepting of disfigurement or disability**. A family photograph emphasizes that the ill person is still part of the family, possibly the most important part. A photograph can also enable the adjustment process, by making the event an undeniable reality.

If a couple are having **difficulties in communication**, particularly where one partner is reluctant to discuss dying, it can be very helpful for them to look through old family photographs together. This integrates the past and present, and can help them to grieve together for their lost future. (*see Spiritual Pain*)

Videos, home movies and photographs can be very helpful ways of including a patient who is too ill to attend an important family occasion (such as a baptism, a bar mitzvah, or a wedding).

BONE MARROW TRANSPLANT

Bone marrow transplant is a technique used in treating relapsed leukemias (and more recently in lymphomas and neuroblastomas). Residual tumor along with the patient's bone marrow is destroyed by a combination of alkylating agents and total body radiation. Bone marrow previously obtained from the patient (**autograft**), or from a related or non-related donor (**allograft**), is then infused intravenously. The cells migrate from the blood stream into the bone marrow.

This technique is useful in diseases which are chemo- or radio-sensitive, where intensive treatment would increase the chances of cure, but where bone marrow toxicity limits the dose. Bone marrow can often be obtained from family members (siblings have a 1 in 4 chance of tissue compatibility). Graft rejection is rare but the marrow cells can attack the recipient's normal cells (graft vs. host disease) causing skin and liver disease. This is reduced by removing the T-lymphocytes from the bone marrow with monoclonal antibodies.

In autografting, the marrow is taken from the patient during a remission, when it is free of demonstrable malignant cells, and frozen. There is a risk that undetected malignant cells may still be present in the marrow, which is therefore pre-treated in various ways in an attempt to eliminate malignant cells.

BONE METASTASES

The clinical consequences of bone metastases are:
- Pain
- Fractures
- Cord compression
- Hypercalcemia (in around 10% of patients)

Bone is the third most common site for metastases. 80% of bone metastases are from breast, bronchus and prostate, and 20% from other cancers (including kidney, thyroid, pancreas, stomach, colon and ovary). Kidney and thyroid are less common cancers but commonly metastasize to bone. 75% of myeloma patients have bone metastases at diagnosis.

In a series of 1,000 autopsies bone metastases were found from the following primary cancers:

Site	%
Prostate	84
Breast	73
Thyroid	50
Kidney	37
Lung	32
GI tract	13
Pancreas	9
Ovary	9

Metastases occur most commonly in the axial skeleton (spine, pelvis, skull). Spread occurs through the blood stream. Typically the spine, pelvis and ribs are the earliest sites of metastases. Skull, femur, humerus, scapula and sternum are later sites. In the spine, the vertebral bodies are involved more often than the pedicles. Lumbar and thoracic involvement is more common than cervical. Metastases to the bones of the hands are rare. Renal tumors tend to involve the humerus.

The mechanism of bone destruction by tumor cells involves a disturbance of the normal remodeling process in bone, rather than direct destruction of bone cells. The tumor cells release chemicals, including prostaglandins and parathyroid hormone-like factors, which stimulate bone resorption by osteoclasts (probably by means of carbonic anhydrase). It may become possible to use drugs which inhibit osteoclasts (biphosphonates), to decrease bone resorption or to protect bone from further metastases, since bone resorption may release chemotactic factors that attract tumor cells (the "metastatic cascade"). Most metastases also cause increased osteoblastic (bone forming) activity as well, which shows as "hot spots" on a bone scan.

Diagnosis of bone metastases relies on imaging techniques:

- X-rays
- Bone scans
- Computerized tomography (CT)
- Magnetic resonance imaging (MRI)

X-rays can detect defects if at least 50% of cancellous bone is replaced by a soft tissue mass (contrast difference). Most metastases are multiple. Metastases not visible to x-ray may show up on a radionuclide bone scan.

Radionuclide bone scans can detect 2mm lesions. Hot spots indicate increased osteoblastic activity from any cause, including degenerative disease. Ideally, both x-ray and scan need to be positive to confirm bone metastases. Bone scan be negative in purely lytic lesions, sometimes found in myeloma and renal carcinoma.

CT scan is useful to detect early bone destruction, and can visualize lesions undetectable by other means.

MRI scan is particularly useful to detect lytic metastases or involvement of the bone marrow. It can accurately visualize the entire skeleton.

Bone biopsy (needle, trephine or open) may be necessary if a patient presents with bone pain and bone lesions and the diagnosis is in doubt. Biopsy may indicate the primary site (kidney, thyroid).

Bone marrow involvement can occur without cortical bone involvement, but is rare in solid tumors. In one study, 2 out of 213 breast cancer patients had bone marrow involvement with no other evidence of metastases in cortical bone or elsewhere. The bone marrow is an organ site susceptible to metastatic involvement. The patient may require transfusions and may be more susceptible to infections.

The mean survival after diagnosis of bone metastases is around one year, but longer with bone metastases from breast or prostate cancer. Occasionally patients with renal or thyroid carcinoma, who undergo excision of a bone metastasis together with the primary tumor, can survive for years.

BONE PAIN

Bone metastases commonly occur in carcinomas of the prostate, breast and bronchus. Bone pains (and related nerve compression pains) account for 40% of cancer pains.

Assessment — The pain is typically worse on movement, often well-localized, and tender to pressure or percussion. There may be a dull ache, even at rest. However, bone pain is occasionally vague and poorly localized with no obvious bony tenderness. There can be radiating pains due to nerve compression in the arm, leg or around the chest (often bilaterally).

Metastases on x-ray can be both lytic and sclerotic. Sclerotic metastases are particularly common in carcinoma of the prostate. Pure lytic lesions occur in myeloma, leukemia and lymphoma. Where x-rays are negative or equivocal, an isotope bone scan is the investigation of choice.

Management options:
  1. NSAIDs
  2. Opioid analgesics
  3. Palliative radiotherapy (localized or hemi-body)
  4. Radio-isotopes
  5. Chemotherapy
  6. Hormone manipulation
  7. Calcitonin

★ **Palliative radiotherapy is the treatment of choice whenever possible.**

1. **NSAIDs** should be first choice as analgesics for bone pain. Anti-inflammatory drugs (prostaglandin inhibitors) can reduce pain from bone metastases. There is some evidence that osteolytic activity in bone metastases is mediated at least in part by prostaglandins. There are no comparative controlled trials demonstrating their efficiency. Clinical experience suggests that about 80% of patients show a response to NSAIDs (about 20% complete, and 60% partial). The drug of first choice is naproxen 500mg 2 times a day. About 10% of patients complain of dyspepsia, which can sometimes be controlled by adding ranitidine. (see *NSAIDs*)

2. **Opioid analgesics** — Mild bone pain may respond to acetaminophen 1g every 4 hours. More severe bone pain can be reduced by morphine, in titrated doses as always. **Morphine will reduce any constant aching pain, but is ineffective for the sharp pains on movement typical of bone pain, which respond better to an NSAID.** (see *Morphine*)

3. **Radiotherapy** — Local external radiotherapy is the treatment of choice for local painful bone metastases. 80% of patients get a response (50% complete, 30% partial) within 1 to 2 weeks (occasionally it takes 3 to 4 weeks).

A single radiotherapy treatment of 800cGy can be just as effective as multiple fractions. In one prospective study of 288 patients with bone pain randomized to either 800cGy in a single treatment, or 3,000cGy in ten daily fractions, there was no difference in speed of onset or duration of pain relief, and pain relief was independent of the histology of the primary tumor.

For patients with a short prognosis, the difference between a single visit and 10 visits for radiotherapy is considerable. Some radiotherapists have used a single treatment of 800cGy for painful bone metastases for years. It is safe and effective and all patients should be offered this simpler treatment.

Many patients have multiple bone metastases and several areas of pain, particularly in carcinoma of the prostate and myeloma. **Wide field irradiation can be used.** 800cGy in a single treatment is given to either the upper or lower hemibody followed, if necessary, with treatment to the other half six weeks later. (Only half of the body can be treated at one time.) This provides useful pain relief in 75% of patients, usually within 24 to 48 hours, with a duration of several months.

Wide field irradiation produces side effects:

- Nausea and vomiting (especially upper half)
- Radiation pneumonitis (especially upper half)
- Neutropenia (especially lower half)
- Malaise

Patients must be carefully selected for wide field irradiation, and in-patient admission is necessary. Pre-medication is given (anti-emetics and steroids), and the blood count must be monitored for 2 weeks, with hematological support if necessary. Isolated painful areas that persist or arise can still be treated with local radiotherapy.

4. **Radio-isotopes** — Treatment with radioactive phosphorus has been replaced by treatment with radioactive strontium (87Sr) which is given intravenously. It is preferentially concentrated in areas of increased osteoblastic activity, but delivers a lower dose to the bone marrow than radioactive phosphorus. About 70% of patients get a response, and pain relief can occur rapidly within 1 to 2 days. Treatment can be repeated after several weeks. Local sites can still be treated with local radiotherapy. Further research is needed into this treatment.

5. **Chemotherapy** — No effective chemotherapy is available for carcinomas of the lung, prostate or kidney (except for small (oat) cell lung cancer). In myeloma or breast cancer with bone pain, chemotherapy may be considered, particularly if there is active disease elsewhere.

★ **The relief of bone pain by chemotherapy can take weeks or months, so the correct use of analgesics and NSAIDs to control bone pain is necessary as well.**

6. **Hormone manipulation** — Bone pain in metastatic breast cancer will respond to:

- Aminoglutethimide in 35% of patients
- Tamoxifen in 20% of patients
- Progestogens in 20% of patients

Bone pain in metastatic prostate cancer responds to the first hormone manipulation in 85% of patients. For this reason, use of hormone preparations should be delayed until symptoms occur.

★ **The response to hormone manipulations can take up to 6 weeks to occur, so the correct use of analgesics and NSAIDs to control bone pain is necessary as well.**

7. **Calcitonin** can produce useful pain relief in about 40% of patients, but it has to be given as an injection 2 times a day, and causes very severe nausea and vomiting in a significant number of patients. It is expensive. It has no place in routine management. (New oral biphosphonates may prove useful for bone pain, but are presently experimental.)

Mr. L.I., age 59, had carcinoma of the stomach with chest pain. Increasing doses of MS-Contin had failed to relieve the pain, and a specialist in symptom control was asked by the family doctor to visit the patient at home. Clinical examination revealed that the inappropriately high doses of morphine were causing drowsiness, confusion, falls and severe constipation, and the main finding in the chest was severe bilateral rib tenderness due to bone involvement. An anti-inflammatory drug was prescribed (naproxen 500mg 2 times a day). The dose of MS-Contin was reduced from 120mg 2 times a day to 30mg 2 times a day, because his wife remembered that previously this dose had reduced the pain without causing drowsiness. Within 24 hours Mr. L.I. was much less confused, which meant that his wife now felt able to continue looking after him at home, which was his particular wish. He was pain-free at rest, with minimal pain on movement. A visiting nurse gave enemas to clear the lower bowel, and the dose of oral laxatives was increased. He died peacefully at home two weeks later.

BOREDOM

Boredom is a real problem for many patients who remain limited by disability or lack of energy.

The most important aspect of caring for patients with advanced illness, once symptoms are controlled, is helping them to enjoy the time they have left. **Patients usually want to go on feeling as useful and independent as possible.**

Social activities require the ability to communicate. This depends upon eyesight and hearing.

A new prescription for eyeglasses, or even readjusting a loose frame, can make a difference. A new hearing aid, or repair of an existing one, can help to expand a patient's world. (In severe deafness, specialized communication equipment should be rented, especially if the patient cannot lip-read.) Even spending some time writing messages down on paper reduces loneliness a bit.

Despite increasing weakness some patients want to continue working. Part-time employment, or employment at home, can often be arranged. Patients may want to remain useful in the home, take up old hobbies, or create something to leave behind. (For example, knitting for an expected baby, or writing a diary for a young child to read later, can be very important activities.) Whenever possible, patients should continue to enjoy social, civic and fraternal affiliations.

Special aids can help the patient to enjoy leisure time. Some hospices use art, music and creative writing as tools. At home, a radio, VCR, stereo or remote-control TV can be helpful, as can a simple reading stand and carefully arranged lighting.

We all need something to look forward to. Day trips, or visits to a day hospice, can break up the monotony of advanced illness. Sometimes a short holiday can be arranged. Narrow horizons are not necessarily boring. Some patients are content with very simple pleasures, like a visit to a nearby shopping mall.

Opportunities for entertainment or creative activities should be encouraged — with the emphasis on "doing" rather than "being done to".

★   **A skillful occupational therapist can sometimes transform the life that is left.** (see Occupational Therapy, Quality of Life)

BRAIN METASTASES

Only 10% of all cancers metastasize to the brain.

Tumors that most commonly metastasize to the brain are:

Site	Approximate % with brain metastases.
Melanoma	60
Lung	40
Breast	20
Kidney	20
Digestive tract	6

Lung cancers that most commonly develop brain metastases are small (oat) cell and adenocarcinomas.

Many other tumors can occasionally spread to the brain. Brain metastases are multiple in over 80% of cases.

Sites of metastases:

Site	%
Cerebral hemispheres	80
Cerebellum	15
Pituitary	6
Brain stem	1

Clinical features:
- Raised intra-cranial pressure (ICP)
- Epilepsy
- Stroke
- Focal signs

The early features of **raised ICP** are early-morning headaches (worse on coughing or straining) and vomiting (often with little preceding nausea). Papilledema may be absent.

About 25% of patients present with **seizures**, either focal (often starting in the thumb or hand, or corner of the mouth) or generalized, however, for most patients routine prophylaxis with **anti-convulsants** is unnecessary, and usually need only be started after the first seizure.

About 15% of patients present with an **acute stroke-like illness**, due to sudden hemorrhage around a metastasis. Unlike a cerebro-vascular accident (CVA) a continued stepwise deterioration then tends to occur. (Remember, cancer patients can also suffer an ordinary stroke.)

Focal signs include:

- Personality change or confusion (frontal)
- Disorientation (parietal)
- Dysphasia (parietal dominant)
- Hemianopsia (parietal, occipital)

Diagnosis is confirmed by CT or MRI scan.

★ **Multiple cranial nerve lesions suggest carcinomatous meningitis.** (*see Meningeal Metastases*)

Management options:

In one study median survival varied with treatment:

No treatment	1 month
Steroids	2 months
Radiotherapy	5 months
Surgery plus radiotherapy	6.6 months (30% had 1-year survival)

High dose steroids (dexamethasone 16mg per day) can dramatically reduce cerebral edema and ICP and can often alleviate focal neurological signs. In lymphomas steroids can shrink the cerebral deposits themselves. 75% of patients experience short-lived symptom relief with steroids. (*see Steroids*)

The usual indications for radiotherapy are:

- Relatively fit patient
- No other symptomatic metastases
- Disease-free interval of 1 year

Cranial irradiation can be helpful for brain metastases from carcinoma of the breast, or small (oat) cell lung cancer, or lymphoma. It is usually indicated for troublesome focal symptoms such as hemiparesis or cerebellar ataxia. It is not indicated if the patient's condition is deteriorating rapidly unless it is considered that the treatment would facilitate nursing care.

Patients who show a good response to steroids are likely to benefit from radiotherapy. Most studies show that about 75% of patients selected for radiotherapy derive worthwhile benefit, with neurological improvement from 3 to 6 months. Median survival is around 16 weeks (double the life expectancy without treatment) and 10% will live at least a year. Breast cancer patients tend to survive the longest.

The whole brain should be irradiated because of the high probability of multiple lesions. Hair loss occurs, but few other immediate problems occur if steroids are given simultaneously. A high dose can be used (for example, 3,000 cGy over 10 days) because brain cells do not divide. However, if the patient should survive 2 years or more a dementia-like syndrome can occur.

The usual indications for neurosurgical excision are:

- Relatively fit patient
- No systemic metastases
- Solitary deposit on CT or MRI scan
- Disease-free interval of 1 year

Other indications for surgery may be uncertain diagnosis, or relatively radio-resistant solitary metastasis (especially in melanoma, renal cell cancer or sarcoma).

Surgery should be followed by radiotherapy.

BREAKING BAD NEWS

★ **Bad news is any information that drastically alters a patient's view of his future. It may include information about symptoms ("Your breathing will not get completely better.") or prognosis ("This disease will shorten your life.").**

★ **The way the diagnosis of life-threatening illness is first imparted can affect the family's ability to cope.**

★ **Adjustment to bad news, to a different future, takes time and is similar to a process of grief. The person is shocked and needs support.**

Comments from a patient on how not to do it:

(Mrs. S.C., is 35. Advanced cancer of the ovary was diagnosed at laparotomy 2 days after delivery of her first child.) "The way I was told the diagnosis is still a very painful memory. It still hurts very much. It was not my own gynecologist, it was a doctor I had never seen before. He didn't wait for my husband or even ask if I wanted him there. He started right away telling me about the chemotherapy and said 'Yes, you may lose your hair, but don't be vain.' You can't remember the details of the information. It needs to be repeated again and again. People are shocked when they are told something is wrong with them. It takes time to adjust."

Comment from a relative on how not to do it:

> *"I found out one evening after visiting Fred. My son and I were walking down the corridor and a medical resident stopped us and said 'I'm afraid I think this effusion is serious' I asked him what he meant and he said 'Can't you guess?' I asked if he meant cancer. Just then his beeper went off and we had to wait in the corridor for him to come back. My son looked gray. When he came back my son suddenly fainted and we spent the rest of the evening in the emergency ward. The resident came down there later and said he was sorry, and told the emergency doctor that he had just given us some bad news. It was a nightmare. Then we had to decide how to tell Fred."*

These doctors broke most of the rules of common sense and common courtesy. Breaking bad news is never easy (and never should be easy). It does not necessarily need to be time-consuming to be done satisfactorily.

Basic principles:

- Set aside time (give your beeper to someone else!)
- Arrange for privacy and quiet
- Convey empathy ("You must be worried.")
- Ask questions first and listen
- Explain using kind words
- Give information in a graded way
- Avoid jargon (it confuses)
- Arrange emotional support ("Who will be at home?")
- Offer to meet with family members (a disaster happens to a whole family)
- Offer availability ("Let's meet again next week.")

The person must be **ready to hear** the information. The person may react with anger or may deny having heard the information and yet become very anxious. Telling people something unpleasant that they do not want to hear can be a risky business (the ancient Greeks used to kill the bearers of bad news).

It is often possible to **gauge the information** a person needs and wants. On walking into an out-patient clinic for the first time, one lady with cancer said "Now don't go telling me anything I don't want to hear." This is a clear message which should be honored. Most patients are less forthright but the signs are there to be read nevertheless. Changing the subject, looking out of the window, a slight widening of the eyes — all say "this conversation is becoming increasingly frightening" — and are messages to be noted.

Avoid making assumptions. Even if a patient asks a direct question, ("What do you think is wrong with me?") it is important not to start giving information based on assumptions about what data is wanted and needed. Reflect the question back ("What have you been thinking is wrong with you?") and ask questions until the person has expressed his knowledge and some of his feelings. In this way you can develop a intuitive feel for the right approach and for what to say or not to say.

A common dilemma is sensing that more knowledge would reduce a patient's uncertainty yet sensing also his fear of hearing bad news. It is possible to test feelings with questions like "Are you a worrier?" or "Have you been worrying about yourself?" The initial answer is usually "No", but if a friendly silence is allowed to linger, the patient may say something relevant, making it clear whether more information would be helpful. Information must be clear and simple and free of jargon. A person receiving bad news is shocked and often remembers virtually nothing of facts and figures.

Use kind words. It is tempting for professionals to hide behind technical explanations and jargon to spare themselves emotional distress. But detailed explanations (or discussion of treatment options) should usually take place later. Patients often comment "Once he told me I didn't hear anything else."

The words **do** make a difference. One couple whose child had cancer asked for a second opinion. Afterwards, they said "He only said what the other doctor said, but somehow it didn't seem so bad." A "**hierarchy of euphemisms**" can be helpful to test how much the person can take at that time ("problems, illness, lump, tumor, cancer").

Be as optimistic as possible. **"No one knows enough to make a pronouncement of doom upon another human being."** (Norman Cousins)

The purpose of breaking bad news is to **reduce uncertainty** about the future and enable appropriate adjustments to occur. Uncertainty is the hardest of all emotions to bear. A common reaction to bad news is "It's a relief now that I know." Reducing uncertainty enables a person to make sensible decisions about the future.

A common myth about bad news is "Don't tell him, it will destroy all his hope." **Inappropriate hope** can be an exhausting and depressing business. Watching someone spending his last weeks hoping for an operation to cure him, or hoping to wake up feeling well again, as he gets weaker day by day is a sad sight. It usually causes the patient anxiety ("What is happening to me?") and guilt ("Am I doing something wrong?"). It cheats him of the opportunity to use his remaining time for things that are important.

Bad news obviously **affects the whole family**. It often helps to have family members present. On-going support from family and friends is very important in the patient's process of adjusting to bad news. It is essential that all family members be given similar information to enable and encourage mutual support. (see *Communication Problems, Talking with Families, Telling the Truth*)

★ **The breaker of bad news may also need support (time to share his own feelings with colleagues or friends).**

★ **If bad news is explained completely and compassionately, anxiolytics are rarely needed.**

BROMPTON'S COCKTAIL

Brompton's Cocktail is now **obsolete and should not be used**. It was introduced in the 1920s at the Brompton Hospital in London for post-thoracotomy pain, and was in widespread use by the 1930s. The active ingredient was morphine. The "cocktail" latterly consisted of morphine, cocaine, chlorpromazine, 90% alcohol and flavored syrup.

Cocaine was added as a stimulant to reduce drowsiness. It is not an analgesic and can cause agitation and confusion. Chlorpromazine causes too much sedation for routine use. 90% alcohol causes an unpleasant stinging in patients with a sore mouth, and causes confusion in the elderly.

Fixed "cocktails" of drugs should generally be avoided because the correct dose of one component will usually result in inappropriate doses of the others. Other fixed solutions ("Schlessinger's Solution", "Oncology Mixture") should not be used. (see *Analgesics, Morphine*)

BURN OUT

Burn out (a term chosen by Freudenberger in 1974) is the current jargon for **work-related emotional exhaustion**. A much better term is Mary Vachon's "**battle fatigue**" because it suggests a reversible symptom, not a terminal event. It occurs not only to health care professionals, but wherever people try to relieve the emotional distress of others for a sustained period.

Emotional support is given most effectively when carers recognize their own needs. An emotionally exhausted person cannot provide emotional support for others. **Perpetual giving is not possible.** Each person needs to recognize personal limitations. The number of people each carer can support and become attached to will vary, but everyone has a maximum tolerated dose! Taking on too much causes not only battle fatigue, but also ineffective care.

The effects of work-related stress, where emotional demands exceed resources, include:

- Irritability
- Criticism or cynicism
- Feelings of failure
- Social isolation or depression
- Insomnia, exhaustion
- Poor concentration
- Seeing patients as objects
- Poor staff relationships

Paradoxically, in battle fatigue the job can become the sole source of satisfaction, and detaching from it becomes increasingly difficult.

The cause of emotional exhaustion is an imbalance between output and input.

Output of emotional energy goes with:

- Counseling
- Grieving (anger, guilt, sadness)
- Communicating
- Problems outside work

(Communication problems with other team members ranks high on the list of work-related stress, made worse if a person has unrealistic expectations, gets little encouragement or cooperation, and feels unrecognized or not making a useful contribution.)

Input of emotional energy comes from:

- Patients (who often encourage us)
- Personal philosophy or religion
- Developing our skills
- Being appreciated ("Thank you")

- Exercise
- Recreation ("re-creation")
- Outside interests
- Expressing emotions

★ **A "personal support system" usually means having friends who will listen to us for a change!**

It can be helpful to use the principles of **transactional analysis** to consider the balance in our own lives. (*see Talking with Patients*)

Ego State	Negative Aspect	Positive Aspect
Controlling "parent"	Persecuting	Setting boundaries
Nurturing "parent"	Rescuing	Affirming
Vulnerable "child"	Being a victim	Playing

We need to keep these three aspects of our personality positive. Under stress they tend to become more negative. Even the three positive elements need to be kept in balance. Carers are often good at two areas and neglect the third.

CANCER SUPPORT GROUPS

"I finally met a fellow young patient with ovarian cancer. We shared our experiences ... I realized that other patients could give me something unique which I could not obtain from my doctors or nurses, however caring." (Vicky Clement-Jones, a doctor and cancer patient)

Support groups are informal meetings of cancer patients, which may include families, friends and carers. They can provide valuable emotional and practical support. (There are also support groups for bereaved family members and friends.)

A support group can provide opportunities to:

- Obtain information
- Express and share feelings (anxiety, fear, isolation)
- Discuss frustrations
- Improve communication with professional staff
- Discuss problems of communicating with others
- Exchange practical advice
- Learn complementary approaches or visualization techniques

Anxiety and depression are common in cancer patients, fueled by treatment, or fear of recurrence, or progression of disease. Information given in a supportive environment can reduce stress. Groups can enable people to feel supported without the intensity of one-to-one counseling. People often feel supported even if they do not actively participate, although giving support (as well as receiving it) increases the benefit. Most people feel happier and relaxed after attending a group, and clearer about ways of coping with cancer.

The death of a group member causes sadness and (sometimes) other emotions, but provided these feelings are discussed the morale of the group members is not usually affected. (see *Coping with Dying*)

CANDIDIASIS

Candidiasis (thrush) occurs in about 70% of patients with advanced cancer.

It can cause:
- Sore mouth
- Dysphagia
- Hoarseness
- Misery!

It is particularly likely to occur if the patient has been on steroids or antibiotics, and is common after radiotherapy involving the buccal cavity.

Oral thrush — The mouth typically has white patches (pseudomembraneous variety) but may just look reddened (atrophic variety). Angular stomatitis is also common. The white patches are easy to diagnose, but can easily be missed if the mouth is not completely inspected, including the roof of the mouth, the inside of the cheeks and lips, and the back of the throat.

Treatment of oral thrush can be with nystatin suspension 1ml to 2ml every 6 hours, but this is a contact agent and needs to be swilled round the mouth, with no drinks for 30 minutes after. Dentures should be soaked in diluted Clorox (1 in 80). Alternatively, ketoconazole tablets 200mg per day can be given, which can clear even very severe thrush in 24 hours. (Ketoconazole is estimated to cause hepatitis in 1 in 15,000 individuals — an acceptable risk in a patient with advanced cancer.)

Esophageal thrush — Severe esophageal candidiasis can occur without any evidence of oral thrush. This usually causes painful dysphagia, and patients usually complain particularly of discomfort with hot drinks. Treat with keto-conazole 200mg per day which usually relieves the dysphagia within 24 to 48 hours.

CAUDA EQUINA DAMAGE

The cauda equina is a leash of nerve roots extending from the end of the spinal cord (at the lower level of L1) to the intervertebral foramina (where they leave the spinal canal).

Compression of the cauda equina causes **lower motor neuron lesions** in the lumbar and sacral nerves supplying the lower limbs, bladder and rectum. Interruption of the bladder-emptying reflex (S2, 3, 4) causes retention of urine.

The clinical features include:

- Sciatic pain (often bilateral)
- Peri-anal numbness ("saddle anesthesia")
- Urinary hesitancy or retention
- Weak, flaccid legs

("Saddle anesthesia" means loss of cutaneous sensation in perineum, buttocks, back of thigh, leg and sole of the foot.)

Often the clinical situation is not clear-cut and the cauda equina damage remains suspected rather than proved (a myelogram often appears normal).

Radiotherapy and/or high dose steroids can help, but the results are often disappointing in relieving pressure and reducing nerve damage.

CELIAC PLEXUS BLOCK

The celiac plexus block (CPB) is the most useful of all the nerve blocks. (see Nerve Blocks)

Indications:

1. Visceral abdominal pain uncontrolled by correct doses of morphine (mainly in carcinomas of the stomach, pancreas or liver)
2. Severe colic due to malignant intestinal obstruction (rarely indicated)
3. Intractable nausea (rarely indicated)

CPB is a very successful technique, and at least 90% of patients get good pain relief, following which morphine can be reduced or stopped altogether. Its effect is usually permanent.

Technique — CPB is performed under sedation and local anesthetic, and x-ray control is necessary to position the needles. The 15cm needles are inserted 7cm from the midline, below the 12th rib. The plexus lies behind the peritoneum, at the level of L1, just anterior to the aorta (which is just anterior to the body of the L1 vertebra). 10ml of neurolytic (phenol or absolute alcohol) preceded by 10ml of 0.5% bupivacaine, is injected. **Absence of post-block postural hypotension indicates failure of the technique.** CPB can also be performed at open laparotomy provided the plexus is not obscured by tumor, or via an anterior approach under CT scan control.

Side effects of CPB:

- Postural hypotension for 1 to 2 days
- Increased gut motility
- Backache for 24 hours
- Loss of ejaculation (sometimes)

Potential complications (as follows) are rare:

- Hematoma (from aorta or IVC)
- L1 neuritis (numbness of anterior thigh)
- Pneumothorax
- Paraplegia (injection into spinal artery)
- Sudden death

CENTRAL PAIN

Central pain is due to permanent neuronal changes in the spinal cord or brain.

Longstanding pain can cause permanent changes in **cortical neurons**. In patients with chronic pain, electrical stimulation of large areas of the cortex that normally have nothing to do with pain, can reproduce the same pain.

Longstanding pain may set up a memorized pattern for pain, possibly in the **thalamus**. (One patient continued to experience the pain of an ingrowing toenail after a traumatic cord transection.)

Damage to the **spinal cord** may remove spinal inhibition of a pain pattern. (A cordotomy for cancer pain resulted in one patient re-experiencing the severe pain of a patella fractured six years earlier.)

Treatment of central pain can be with psychotropic or membrane-stabilizing drugs, but a combination of a tricyclic and a phenothiazine is probably the most helpful. (see Nerve Pain)

Mr. B. C., a 37 year old with a thoracic glioma, became paraplegic. He then started to complain of severe sacral pain. After several months of pain he underwent a therapeutic spinal cord transection which failed to control the pain. The pain fluctuated in severity but was constant, worse on sitting up, and disturbed his sleep. It was overwhelming at times, so that he was unable to think of anything other than his pain. 5mg, 10mg and 20mg of morphine every 4 hours caused increasing drowsiness, but did not affect the pain. NSAIDs had no effect. X-rays of the sacral area were normal. The pain was eventually well controlled for the last two months of his life by a combination of chlorpromazine 75mg 4 times a day, and imipramine 100mg at bedtime, which caused virtually no drowsiness. This severe pain can only be explained on the basis of a central mechanism. (see Pain Pathways)

CHEMOTHERAPY

60% to 70% of all cancer patients develop distant metastases. In the majority of patients metastatic disease is incurable, and the realistic aim of any chemotherapy treatment is palliation (control of symptoms and improved survival).

Tumor response may be:
- Partial (regression of measurable lesions)
- Complete (disappearance of all evidence of tumor)

High dose chemotherapy regimes are used to treat sensitive tumors in the hope of cure. Tumors that are **usually curable** by chemotherapy include Hodgkin's Disease, testicular cancer, choriocarcinoma, Burkitt's lymphoma, childhood leukemias and nephroblastoma. Tumors that are **sometimes curable** include non-Hodgkin's lymphomas, sarcomas, ovarian cancer, neuroblastomas and acute leukemias.

Most **solid tumors** (bronchus, breast, esophagus, stomach, pancreas, colon, bladder, etc.) respond poorly to chemotherapy. High dose regimes therefore have little place in palliation of solid tumors. The tumor cells will not be eradicated and survival is rarely prolonged, and is sometimes shortened by toxic effects. Chemotherapy that produces toxic side-effects is not justified when the main aim is symptom control. **Metastatic small (oat) cell cancer of the bronchus is an exception.** Combined chemotherapy can reduce symptoms and prolong survival from a few weeks up to 12 months (and occasionally 2 to 3 years). Three courses of combined chemotherapy will produce improvement in 75% of patients.

In breast cancer 50% of patients with soft tissue and lung metastases respond after three courses of combined chemotherapy, but only occasional patients achieve prolonged survival.

In **adenocarcinomas** of the stomach, pancreas and colon 20% of patients respond to single-agent treatment with fluorouracil, and combined chemotherapy does not increase the response rate.

Metastases from non-small cell lung cancer, melanoma, or from an unknown primary site respond very poorly to chemotherapy.

In patients who do respond and achieve a stable remission of disease, the next question is whether the patient should receive **maintenance therapy**. All chemotherapy has side-effects, and maintenance therapy has no proven benefit in terms of survival.

★ **It is important to control symptoms simultaneously, and not to wait to see if chemotherapy will produce a response which may take weeks.**

Chemotherapy-related side effects can develop after the course of treatment, the usual time-scale being:

Nausea	during, and 1 to 2 days later
Bone marrow suppression	7 to 10 days later
Malaise	7 to 14 days later
Neuropathies	Several weeks later
Lung fibrosis	Several weeks later

Stopping chemotherapy — When chemotherapy fails to control disease, treatment becomes a burden. A decision clearly and kindly explained to change the focus of care to symptom control, and to stop inappropriate chemotherapy, usually brings welcome relief to patient and family.

Patients are often more realistic than their physicians, who sometimes tend to prolong chemotherapy unrealistically because they wrongly assume that stopping treatment will make the patient feel helpless, or because they have invested personal emotional energy in the treatment.

Stopping treatment can be explained to patients in terms of the principle that "chemotherapy that is not doing you good is doing you harm". When this is not explained the patient may continue with debilitating treatment ("so I don't let my family down") and endure unnecessary suffering.

Timely consultation with colleagues who understand the principles of hospice and palliative care can help change treatment goals to restore control to the patient and to maximize his remaining potential. This reduces the feeling of helplessness, and helps to restore morale.

★ **Teaching doctors about symptom control, communication skills and spiritual support empowers them to help patients without resorting to inappropriate therapy.**

CHILDREN

(see Talking with Children)

There are many special issues involved in caring for children with advanced diseases. (This book deals primarily with the care of adults.)

Some of these special issues are:

1. Diseases
2. Drug doses
3. Family needs
4. Educational needs
5. Play
6. Concepts of death
7. Hospice care
8. Support services
9. Terminal phase

1. Carers need to be familiar with the **range of diseases** in children that threaten life. These include congenital anomalies, CNS degenerative disorders, mucopolysaccharidoses, degenerative neuromuscular disorders, cystic fibrosis, liver and heart failures and AIDS, as well as certain malignancies (leukemias, CNS tumors, nephroblastoma, retinoblastoma).

2. **Drug doses** are calculated according to the weight of the child and carers need to be familiar with correct dose ranges and pediatric prescribing. The percentage of adult dose is **approximately** 15% at 2 months, 25% at 1 year, 33% at 3 years, 50% at 7 years and 75% at 12 years. Cytotoxic drug doses are based on surface area.

3. **The family's needs** are generally similar to those in adult care (practical help, information, explanation and opportunities to express feelings) but there are two special issues:

- The parents
- The siblings

The divorce rate is very high after a child dies. Tension arises because of the needs of each parent to grieve (both before and after the death). Unless a couple can "alternate their grief" while supporting their partners, communication problems arise.

Siblings have their own needs which can too often be neglected. Siblings need explanation at every stage, and need to be included. Their grief can be complicated and family counseling can be helpful. (see *Family Therapy, Grief, Talking with Families*)

4. Sick and dying children continue to have **educational needs**. Carers must be aware of the importance of continued stimulation and learning. Children's hospitals often have on-premises schools. Children who are terminally ill often feel quite well and need to go on being as normal as possible. Children who are dying should go on learning new things right up to the time they die.

5. Carers must understand how **children play**. Children develop and communicate through play. Play used to be considered just "release of excess energy" but is now understood as essential to normal emotional development. Children learn new skills, solve problems, adjust to change and develop social relationships through play. Professional carers involved with children have to be familiar with how children play at different ages. A sick child is at a disadvantage in terms of normal play. Children's hospitals often have a play specialist to catalyze play for ill children. Explanation about illness or procedures has to be through play (involving objects or symbolic language) and preparation through play (with real medical equipment) reduces anxiety. Children's fears and misconceptions are best understood by observing them at play, and can only be addressed through play. Siblings of terminally ill children also have powerful emotions and adjustment problems.

Dolls and puppets may be used to symbolize negative feelings in a safe and indirect way. ("She doesn't love me any more, she's gone away.") They can be used to re-enact experiences. Even the way dolls and puppets are handled can convey the child's feelings.

Drawing and painting can be useful ways of seeing a child's view of experiences, and allowing the child to express feelings (both through drawing and painting, and through play or conversation that stems from the activity).

Many adults have forgotten how to play. Play is enjoyable, spontaneous, voluntary, involves active participation, has no goal and has a systematic relationship to non-play. **(Play is also therapeutic for adults — children teach it free of charge!)** (see *Talking with Children*)

6. Carers need to understand **childhood concepts of death**. Young children (under 5 years) see death as separation or desertion, and imagine it is somehow reversible (an idea reinforced by cartoon stories). The dead can see, hear and feel. A 4-year old boy driving past a cemetery asked his father what it was. His father explained that people who had died were buried there. After a pause the boy replied "They must be starving!"

Older children (about 5 to 8 years old) search for a cause for death. They may imagine an angel or a dreaded figure taking the person away, or they may believe that something they said or did caused it ("magic thinking"). They begin to understand that death is permanent and begin to realize it will happen to them one day. They usually have some concept of heaven. ("Will there be bicycles in heaven?") Children's concepts of death depend on their experience, intelligence and emotional development, and whether their natural curiosity is encouraged and their questions answered. Some 5-year old children have quite a mature concept of death.

7. **Hospice care** can be helpful. **For most children, home is the right place to die.** The parents will want to do most of the caring themselves, but at times will need intensive support from the home care team. A few families need the facilities of an in-patient hospice, either to provide respite care for exhausted parents, for the terminal phase, or occasionally for symptom control or the needs of the siblings. One mother said "When at home there was a lot of fear with each crisis, at the hospice that almost dissolved. We were safe, cosseted, loved. There was peace. Beth died in bed between us, in my arms, with our other children safely asleep in the adjoining room."

"The (in-patient) hospice should feel like going on holiday or staying with friends." (Mother Frances Dominica)

8. **Support services** for dying children and their families tend to be poorly coordinated. There can be confusion among the many helping organizations about who is responsible for what. There can be poor communication among hospital staff, pediatric specialists, family doctor and visiting nurses. Medical, nursing and psychosocial professionals sometimes fail to share information together, or with the parents. This erodes the trust of the family. It can help greatly to have one professional act as **liaison worker**, making appropriate contacts and keeping all team members involved and informed. Parents may wish to keep a "shared care card" listing names and telephone numbers of all professionals and volunteers, and the responsibilities of each.

9. **Most dying children prefer to stay at home.** Since relatively few family physicians will have cared for a child dying at home, good liaison and communication with pediatricians, palliative care specialists and the hospice team is important.

Parental distress can create strong emotional pressure to contrive and continue inappropriate treatments. The decision to abandon aggressive and unpleasant modes of treatment, and focus instead on symptom control and quality of life, can come too late if a clear decision is avoided. (see *Chemotherapy, Leukemia*)

Procedures such as repeated venipunctures or injections can be traumatic for children. A central venous line can be established under general anesthesia and can be useful for administering drugs, although tolerance can sometimes develop to IV morphine. A continuous subcutaneous infusion is a very useful alternative. The principles of care are the same as for adults. (see *Morphine, Terminal Phase*)

COLOSTOMY CARE

A colostomy is an artificial opening of the colon onto the anterior abdominal wall. There are two types of colostomy: **end** (defunctioning), and **loop** (decompressing).

An **end colostomy** is a defunctioning colostomy. It is commonly sited in the sigmoid colon (in the left iliac fossa). It is usually permanent (for example, following abdomino-perineal resection for cancer of the rectum).

A **loop colostomy** can be created from any segment of the colon (but usually the transverse or sigmoid colon). It is a decompressing colostomy to relieve obstruction. It is usually temporary (although in advanced cancer an emergency loop colostomy to relieve obstruction may remain as a definitive procedure). A loop of colon is brought to the surface and supported for 5 to 7 days on a bridge. The stoma tends to be large and irregular. Leakage can be a problem. A loop colostomy does not always totally prevent the passage of feces into the distal colon.

The site for the stoma must be carefully chosen and the method of care discussed and explained. A stoma therapist should always be involved. The type of ostomy pouch must be carefully selected to suit the patient. Provided they have the manual dexterity, patients are encouraged to manage their own colostomy as soon as possible. In the postoperative period the stoma tends to be swollen and the effluent thin. During this phase a drainable bag can be useful so it does not have to be changed frequently resulting in soreness.

Skin care — Inflammation of the peri-stomal skin affects 50% of patients at some time.

There are two causes:

- Contact dermatitis (allergy)
- Effluent dermatitis (ill-fitting appliance)

An allergic reaction to the appliance causes itching and redness with a distinct margin. Change the type or brand of appliance.

Effluent dermatitis is due to prolonged contact with intestinal contents. Desquamation and secondary infection can occur, which may require steroid and antifungal creams. Inflamed skin is protected with a layer of stomahesive paste. Irregularities in the skin contour can be filled with Karaya gum, if necessary.

Fecal consistency — Stomal diarrhea is managed by:

- Bulking agents
- Opioid anti-diarrheals (if severe)
- Diet modification

Foods that constipate include potatoes, white bread, rice, noodles, cheese, bananas and peanut butter.

Stomal constipation is diagnosed by digital examination and can be managed by an oil or phosphate enema followed by regular oral laxatives and increased intake of fluid and dietary fiber.

★ **A colostomy will not retain suppositories.**

To control **flatus and smell**, modify diet. Reduce or banish onions, cabbage, cucumbers, beans, lentils, fizzy drinks and (sometimes) milk products. Fish, eggs and cheese also tend to produce smell. Oral chlorophyll tablets can reduce smell. Activated charcoal or unscented deodorizers can be added to the bag. Odor-proof disposable bags are available, or flatus can be allowed to escape through a charcoal filter fitted to the appliance.

Prolapse is seen most often with a temporary loop colostomy. The stoma suddenly increases in size and protrudes. It can be reduced manually as a temporary measure. It seldom recovers spontaneously and requires surgery (to close or re-fashion). If the protruding mucosa becomes purple or black the patient will die of intestinal ischemia and necrosis without prompt surgery.

Parastomal hernia causes a bulge near the stoma on straining. It can be left alone unless it causes difficulty fitting the appliance or intermittent intestinal obstruction. The stoma is best re-sited unless the patient's prognosis is short.

Obstruction can be due to impacted feces, adhesions or malignant involvement.

Bleeding is quite common and usually trivial, due to mucosal irritation. It stops with local pressure from a gauze pad. It can (rarely) be due to a stomal secondary deposit, and local cryosurgery can be helpful.

Rehabilitation — The psychological implications of a stoma are immense. Anxiety, depression, awareness of altered body image and sexual problems are all common. Counseling by a stoma therapist is important before and after surgery to overcome the psychological problems.

COMMUNICATION AIDS

Communication aids provide alternative ways of communicating for patients who have lost the function of speech, usually due to dysarthria in progressive neuromuscular diseases, and occasionally after head injuries or with brain tumors.

If a patient is still able to move his arms, writing messages usually remains the best option, and a wipe-off screen is often very useful.

If arm weakness begins to become a problem, alternatives to writing have to be considered, including:

- Miniature typewriter
- Typewriter with large keyboard
- Patient-operated selector mechanism
- Transparent chart
- Word board

★ **Referral to an experienced speech therapist or occupational therapist with up-to-date knowledge of communications equipment is essential, so that a suitable device can be obtained and future needs assessed.**

A patient who cannot even point may still be able to operate "Possums" (**patient operated selector mechanisms**) activated by very slight movement or suck-blow, used to stop and start a light scanning over a number of words or phrases.

If the patient has only eye movement, he may still be able to spell out words using a transparent letter board. The patient is viewed through the board and uses eye movements to spell out words. Alternatively, a word or symbol chart that a companion can point to can be very helpful.

Computer ingenuity and microchip technology is improving all the time. In addition to assistance with communications, it will someday offer disabled patients more opportunities for continued employment.

Important points:

- Make sure all equipment is accessible, as the patient can't ask for it.
- Converse with the patient, don't simply admire the equipment! It takes courage to change from normal speech to dependence on a machine. Have a positive attitude and be encouraging.
- Allow time. The patient may have spent a long time preparing questions or comments in advance. Try to avoid speaking for the patient and thus closing conversation down.
- Encourage graded use well before all function is lost. Skillful timing in introducing communication aids is essential.
- Mobile arm supports can prolong the usefulness of communication aids.
- Remember that using communication aids is tiring for both the user and listener.

COMMUNICATION PROBLEMS

★   **"Poor communication causes more suffering than any other problem except unrelieved pain. It is also the easiest problem (in terms of the therapist's time and skill) to treat."** (Averil Stedeford)

Communication problems are common. The emotional crisis of an ill or dying person within a family tends to reduce its members' ability to communicate.

This can cause:
- Misunderstandings
- Disagreements
- Emotional upsets
- Emotional coldness
- Altered behavior
- Poor adjustment to change (see *Adjustment Reaction*)

The most important factor in a family's coping and adjustment is the degree of openness in the family. **Openness** is the ability to communicate thoughts and feelings to each other. Families vary considerably in their level of openness. In any family the longer and more intense the stress, the more difficult it is for relationships to remain open.

There are 3 main reasons why communication problems are so common in families facing death:
1. Avoidance
2. Lack of emotional energy
3. Fear

1. Family processes operate to reduce emotional tension and maintain equilibrium. The usual "emotional reflex" concerning death is to **avoid the issue** and hope that the disruption will not occur. "We didn't want to upset each other..." is a commonly heard comment when families are finally helped to communicate together.

2. Families become **emotionally exhausted** by the stress of permanent **uncertainty**. In a changing situation emotions may alternate between hopes of life, and fears of death. Uncertainty reduces the energy available for communication, at a time when a great increase in the normal level of communication is needed to adjust to changing roles and powerful emotions.

3. Family members often **fear expressing emotions.** ("He mustn't see me crying.") Some families feel very unsafe with the idea of expressing their deepest feelings, in case it results in embarrassment or anger, violence or even madness. There is sometimes a feeling that to "break down" in tears may somehow cause a mental "break-down". These attitudes may be reinforced by family myths. ("Men in our family don't cry.")

Collusion ("Please don't tell . . . ") is a common problem. Family members often fear telling the sick person the truth, usually to protect the person they love and to spare him anguish. ("What's the point of upsetting him?" "He'll give up hope.") Sometimes family members fear the patient's anger about earlier deceits. ("We've known for months but we couldn't tell her.") Sometimes family members know that the patient has always coped with life crises by denial. Denial is therefore the family's best attempt at coping — the situation in which they feel most comfortable. Never-theless, "comfort" is costly. **Collusion distorts all com-munication.** Family members have to adjust all their con-versations. ("She mustn't see I'm upset.") Important emotional business is left unresolved, which makes it more difficult for the family members to resolve their grief. The patient becomes increasingly isolated, which can cause anxiety and/or depression, and lowers the threshold for symptoms (especially pain and nausea).

One way of managing the situation is to talk separately, first with the family members, then with the patient:

- Encourage family members to ventilate their feelings and worries.

- Elicit their good reasons for not telling. ("I'd like you to tell me your reasons for deciding not to tell him.")

- Establish the emotional cost. ("What effect is all this having on you?")

- Ask permission to talk to the patient alone to discover his feelings. Usually the family reluctantly agree be-cause their own "solution" to the problem is uncom-fortable. They may say "You won't tell him, will you?" Emphasize that you want to ask questions only to find out how the patient feels.

The patient is often greatly relieved to be able to share worries and feelings in answer to your questions, and to ask you his own questions. Occasionally the reaction is anger. ("Talking about it won't change it.") Occasionally the patient wants to deny the illness (and it is his denial which has led to the collusion).

It is essential to see the whole family together again, usually briefly, to facilitate communication and to interpret what each member understands. A comment such as "You've all been finding it difficult to talk about this illness — I guess you've not wanted to upset each other ", often brings visible relief. It allows family members to start sharing the one issue that has been worrying all of them. (see *Denial, Talking with Families, Talking with Patients*)

Denial by the patient can disrupt family communications and can often be the main cause of collusion. ("Don't talk about it.") Some couples, particularly couples who have been very close, may know the truth but find discussing their impending separation too sad and painful. It can be easier for each to talk to professionals about separation and death than for the couple to speak to each other. In this situation it can be helpful to set the couple a practical task. Looking at old family photographs can allow some couples to share feelings of sadness without actually having to discuss them.

"Don't be morbid." Some families fear what might happen if sad or upsetting subjects are mentioned. They may dread mentioning certain words, like "making a will" or "priest" in case the patient assumes death is near. A counselor may need to be careful, returning gently to sensitive words to encourage further discussion, and not being put off by the obvious avoidance of the family. Another method is to grasp the feared word and simply ask "Have you ever thought of making a will?" If the response is "Don't be morbid ", a comment like "Most people find it takes away a lot of worries ", can encourage the family to realize it is safe to discuss such things.

"Should we tell the children?" The worry about telling children in the family also commonly applies to telling elderly parents. The sooner a person finds out, the sooner he can start the process of adjustment. The more time there is to adjust, the less of a shock the outcome will be.

Parents also need to know that:

- Children can cope very well provided they are included and feel it is safe to ask questions.
- Children can mask their distress from their parents.
- Children who are included in the situation can be very supportive.
- Children who are denied the opportunity to be supportive often regret it or resent it later. ("If only I had known . . . ")

- 50% of children have major problems in bereavement. Anticipation and preparation reduce later psychological problems.

It is important for the counselor to acknowledge that parents understand their children better than anyone else. A family meeting can be offered to help parents to talk to their children and to realize how much their children already understand or want to know. It is usually best to leave the timing of the meeting to the parents. (see *Grief*)

The use of metaphor (talking about a situation which resembles this one) can make it possible to discuss distressing events.

Mrs. E.S., a teacher for many years, was dying in a private hospital room with her husband and teen-age son and daughter present. It was probably the last time they would all be together (the son was leaving the next day for college). It was difficult for them to talk meaningfully because the woman denied her short prognosis, and would not allow words like "cancer" or "dying" to be used. This meant that her husband and children did not really know what to say (in case they said the "wrong thing") and there was an atmosphere of tension and awkwardness. The doctor asked them all to imagine a political situation where each of them might be taken away by the secret police at any moment and asked "What would you each say to the other members of your family?" (a good question to consider whether a person is well or ill). They began to express their love for each other, to say good-bye and to cry together. Having been sitting widely separated, they ended up cuddling together on the bed. The woman died two days later.

It is often safe to ask "**if questions**". ("If your life were short what would you say to . . . ?") This is useful for patients who want to deny and yet need to make adjustments or arrangements. ("If you needed a lot more nursing help and became weaker, would you want to stay at home?")

★   **"Considerable suffering is caused by poor communication and much of this is avoidable."** (Averil Stedeford)

COMPLEMENTARY THERAPIES

Patients and families turn to complementary therapies looking for care as much as cure. "Complementary therapy" is a description preferred to "alternative therapy", as there is every reason to use such methods **alongside orthodox medical care** if the patient finds them helpful.

All patients need ways of coping with cancer. If they find non-harmful complementary therapies supportive they should be encouraged to participate, providing they can afford the costs, and provided the practitioners are not leading them to hope inappropriately for a cure. There is no evidence that any such therapies are effective, and they occasionally cause side effects (for example, laetrile can cause a neuromyopathy due to cyanide intoxication).

Before a doctor or nurse decides to advise against a complementary therapy it is important to ask "How is this therapy helping the patient and family to cope, and what will we provide in its place?"

"I would like to see doctors and practitioners of complementary therapies come together — anything that improves the quality of life must be strived for." (Maggie H., a cancer patient)

CONFUSION

Confusion affects about 30% of cancer patients at some stage in their illness. It is especially common in elderly patients when their environment is changed (for example, by admission to a hospital or in-patient hospice).

The features of confusion are **reduced level of consciousness, disorientation** and **misperceptions**. Usually the patient appears drowsy, easily startled and frightened, or is rambling and behaving inappropriately. Concentration is poor. Disorientation is easily assessed by simple questions, but remember that not knowing the day or time is common in hospitalized patients. Misperceptions can be elicited by asking "Has anything frightened or puzzled you recently?"

Causes of confusion — The following check-list should be considered in assessing the patient:

- Drugs
- Pain or discomfort
- Full bladder

- Impacted feces
- Brain metastases or cerebrovascular accident
- Infection (pulmonary, urinary, septicemia)
- Heart failure
- Biochemical imbalance (urea, calcium, sodium, glucose)
- Alcohol or benzodiazepine withdrawal ("delirium tremens")
- Extreme anxiety (facing approaching death)

★ **Confusion appears worse if the patient is deaf.**

Psychotropic drugs (phenothiazines, benzodiazepines, tricyclics) can cause confusion (due to deteriorating liver or renal function, even if the patient has been on them a long time and the dose has not been changed).

Other drugs that can cause confusion include:

- Pentazocine
- Indomethacin
- Digoxin
- Beta-blockers
- Diuretics
- Atropine
- Anti-Parkinsonian drugs
- Sulfonamides
- Phenytoin
- Cimetidine

Assessment — In severe agitated confusion (delirium) there is exaggeration of underlying emotions and memories. The patient may be aggressive and paranoid or alternatively timid and terrified. Urgent sedation may be needed (for example, haloperidol 10mg IM or chlorpromazine 100mg IM repeated every hour if necessary).

When talking with a confused patient, it may not be possible to understand the content of speech, but it may be possible to sense the person's mood. ("You seem to be feeling sad.")

Information needed includes:

- Patient's previous personality
- Alcohol history
- Fluid balance (examine for a full bladder)
- Bowel history (and rectal examination)

- Capillary blood glucose (if diabetic)
- Signs of infection (fever, sweats, flushing, tachycardia)
- Neurological signs (weakness, poor coordination, dysphasia)
- Mid-stream clean catch urine specimen
- Blood tests (urea, electrolytes, glucose)

Hyponatremia is a rare cause of confusion. Plasma sodium concentration below 120mEq/L [*120mmol/L*] can be a cause of nausea, drowsiness, confusion or seizures. It can be due to excessive doses of diuretics.

Very rarely, hyponatremia results from the syndrome of inappropriate secretion of anti-diuretic hormone (ADH) in small (oat) cell carcinoma of the bronchus, and is diagnosed by a low plasma osmolality (less than 275mosmol/Kg), a urinary osmolality higher than the plasma level (usually around 500mosmol/Kg), and a urinary sodium above 20mmol/L. Treatment is by restricting fluids or giving demeclocycline 600mg 4 times a day, which inhibits the tubular effect of ADH.

★   **Signs of infection can be masked by steroids, and are often absent in the elderly.**

Management options:

- Exclude physical causes (pain, retention, infection)
- Explain to patient
- Quiet, well-lit familiar room
- Familiar people (staff or family)
- Stop unnecessary drugs
- Provide alcohol if habitual
- Avoid sedation if possible
- Start drug treatment if confusion is uncontrolled

★   **Confusion is the most difficult problem of all to cope with at home.**

Confusion is **distressing to family members**. They usually need detailed explanation and a lot of support. ("It is part of the illness, she is not losing her mind.") Confusion often fluctuates, so there may be **lucid intervals**.

Drug treatment — Psychotropic drugs cannot reverse confusion, but may be needed to quiet distressing agitation, paranoia or hallucinations. Haloperidol 5mg 2 to 4 times a day is usually effective and not too sedating. (In the elderly or frail, haloperidol 1.5mg 2 times a day may be sufficient.) Chlorpromazine 10mg to 50mg 3 times a day is more sedating. If tremor or rigidity becomes troublesome add trihexyphenidyl 1mg to 2mg 4 times a day (build up dose slowly), which is anti-cholinergic.

Anxiety or agitation not associated with hallucinations or psychosis is best treated with diazepam. Agitated depression requires a tricyclic.

Very occasionally an agitated aggressive patient needs urgent sedation with chlorpromazine 100mg IM repeated if necessary every 1 to 6 hours.

Distressing terminal confusion **in the last hours of life** is best treated with morphine, chlorpromazine and scopolamine. For severe terminal agitation methotrimeprazine 50mg to 75mg every 4 hours is very useful. (It is a phenothiazine with about twice the potency of chlorpromazine.) (see Terminal Phase)

CONSTIPATION

Constipation means **hard** or **infrequent** feces. Constipation is undoubtedly one of the biggest problems for terminally ill patients. In a study of 200 patients admitted to a hospice 75% needed rectal measures (suppository, enema or manual evacuation) within the first week.

A hospice patient wrote a journal about her experiences in facing up to terminal illness. She wrote:

"If I mention constipation to most people, even friends, who are concerned about the tumor, they grin... I understand their amusement but I feel anger, too. For most terminally ill people, constipation is one of the most dreadful aspects of their lives. Analgesics freeze your pain, but they freeze up your bowels, too. I want people and doctors to understand the plight of the terminally ill who have so much to cope with, never mind this most basic of functions. Feeling very, very bunged up is so terrible."

Causes of constipation:
- Low fiber diet
- Dehydration
- Drugs (opioids, anti-cholinergics, diuretics)
- Reduced defecation (weakness, confusion, pain)
- Depression
- Hypercalcemia

★ **The commonest cause of constipation in cancer patients is opioids used without adequate doses of laxatives.**

History needs to be detailed:

- Bowels last moved?
- Time before that?
- Motions hard, soft or liquid?
- Normal amount each time?
- Laxatives: how much, how often?
- Suppositories?
- Do you ever have to chip it out with your finger?

An important question is whether laxatives were started at the same time as opioids (or only later once constipation had occurred). Alternating constipation and diarrhea is usually due to the incorrect use of laxatives (intermittently instead of regularly) in a patient on opioid drugs.

On **examination** the abdomen may appear distended. Fecal masses (which indent on steady pressure) may be palpable in the descending colon (left iliac fossa). The constipated colon is usually moderately tender. In severe constipation the cecum can become distended with pain and tenderness in the right iliac fossa. It is sometimes difficult to decide whether abdominal masses are fecal (which move after treatment to clear the bowel) or neoplastic (which do not). Rectal examination may reveal hard impacted feces, a malignant stenosis, or an empty ballooned rectum (suggesting impaction higher up). Note any painful hemorrhoids or fissures.

X-ray is not usually necessary, but will show the colon loaded with fecal matter with no gaseous distention or fluid levels.

Important points:

1. Opioids constipate from the moment they are started, and high doses of laxatives need to be started simultaneously with any opioid analgesic.

2. Patients can still get severely constipated on inadequate doses of laxatives.

3. Patients who are not eating continue to produce waste in the bowel (gut secretions, desquamation, bacterial matter), continue to need to pass motions, and can still get impacted with feces.

4. It is an important working rule that the bowel should move at least every three days. If a patient goes longer than three days without a bowel movement, he or she should have a rectal examination, and a suppository or micro-enema should be considered.

5. An empty ballooned rectum on rectal examination can be a sign of impaction with feces higher up in the colon. If the history is suggestive of constipation, the patient should have high enemas.

6. Constipation can cause anorexia, nausea, vomiting, abdominal pain, rectal pain, confusion, abdominal distention and sometimes even obstruction. Pain tends to be colicky. ("It comes in waves.") It can radiate to chest, back and upper legs. (see Tenesmus)

7. Severe constipation can present as spurious diarrhea with small amounts of liquid feces leaking past the fecal mass.

8. Prescribe **both** a fecal softener and a stimulant laxative (Peri-Colace or Senokot-S, for example) whenever starting an opioid analgesic.

9. If maximum doses of laxatives are still ineffective, add oral magnesium sulfate 5mls to 10mls in the morning (taken with plenty of water), which flushes through the small bowel and is a very effective fecal softener.

10. If the patient has fecal masses palpable throughout the colon, he will need either oil retention enemas, or soap and water enemas to soften the feces, followed by phosphate enemas to stimulate the bowel.

11. Constipation often causes painful anal fissures. Bulk-forming agents can be useful and analgesic suppositories can be used before defecation.

12. If rectal examination reveals a large clay-like lump in the rectum that is too big to pass through the anal sphincter, this needs to be removed manually. This is painful, and the patient should be given morphine and diazepam prior to the procedure.

Impacted feces can be suspected from:
- The history (although the patient may be too embarrassed to give the full story)
- Prolonged constipation (5 to 20 days)
- Patient's chipping out feces with a finger
- Small liquid feces (spurious diarrhea)
- Fecal leak or incontinence
- Pain (colic or tenesmus, or both)

Note on bowel physiology:
The **small bowel** daily pours out several liters of digestive secretions which are mostly reabsorbed. The ileum probably acts as a reservoir releasing small bowel contents into the colon through the ileo-cecal valve.

The **colon** absorbs water (about 1.5 liters per day). Semi-liquid motions in the cecum gradually become harder as they move round the colon. The hardness of the motions depends upon water content. Feces contain about 50ml to 150ml of water per day. Transit time through the colon normally varies from a few hours to several days.

Both longtitudinal and ring contractions (haustrations) occur, and contents can be propelled in either direction. Opioid drugs increase ring contractions, thus lengthening fecal transit time.

The **rectum** acts as a reservoir for the storage of feces until evacuation is socially convenient. In fact, sigmoidoscopy shows that the rectum is often empty. The acute angle at the rectosigmoid junction acts as a valve, and the rectum is usually empty until there is active propulsion of feces from the sigmoid colon. The awareness of rectal filling is due to stretch receptors which initiate the emptying reflex.

A bowel movement normally consists of the contents of the rectum only, but, with strong laxatives, can be from the whole descending colon. The evacuation of a large movement requires less effort than a small one. Sitting on a commode requires less effort for an evacuation than sitting on a bedpan.

The **internal anal sphincter** is responsible for fine control of flatus or liquid feces. Rectal distention causes reflex transient relaxation of the internal anal sphincter. This allows the fecal bolus to contact the sensory area of the anus which distinguishes flatus from feces. (Damage to this region of the anus prevents the distinction between flatus and feces.) Further relaxation of the internal anal sphincter will then allow passage of flatus.

Following internal sphincterotomy continence of solid feces is still possible. The anorectal angle (maintained by the pubo-rectalis muscle) acts as a flap-valve preventing the passage of solid feces. The pubo-rectalis muscle relaxes during defecation.

The **external anal sphincter** can only contract continuously for about 60 seconds. It serves as an emergency measure to control incontinence. (see *Laxatives*)

COPING WITH DYING

How does a person respond to the process of dying?

Relatively little is known about psychological responses to dying. Kübler-Ross, in *On Death and Dying* (1969), described the reactions in terms of **denial** and isolation, **anger**, **bargaining**, **depression** and **acceptance**. This framework provided helpful new insights into the emotions of those facing death, and emphasized that emotional distress is normal.

Dying (like other life crises) causes varied emotions. Each can produce a **range of responses** (psychological defenses) and these can change with time. The extremes of these responses can be classified as "open" or "closed". A **dynamic (changing) model of coping responses** is therefore more helpful.

Emotion or Need	Closed Response	Open Response
1. Fear	Denial	Facing fears
2. Anger	Guilt, blame	Fighting the illness
3. Sadness	Misery	Grieving, adjusting
4. Dependency	Helplessness	Participation
5. Search for meaning	Hopelessness	Seeking sense of purpose

This dynamic (non-sequential) model emphasizes that a person often has **several simultaneous emotions** to cope with, and that the methods of coping are not necessarily fixed, but can vary (sometimes from day to day) in degree of openness.

The dynamic model is **task-orientated** and can help to pin-point a particular area of difficulty. It can then facilitate coping by encouraging a shift towards openness. (While closed responses are effective for some people at some times, they are more likely to become maladaptive, and to result in **anxiety** or **depression**.) (see *Anxiety, Depression*)

Mrs. M.F., a woman of 42 with four teen-age children, had advanced cancer of the colon. She was referred to the hospice out-patient clinic for pain control. She looked frightened and anxious. Her distress about her pain seemed to exceed the abdominal pain she described, which was already quite well controlled with moderate analgesics. The doctor asked if she was afraid. Mrs. M.F. talked of being frightened for her children's futures. She talked about the children, who were in their late teens and almost independent. The doctor suggested that her emotions about leaving the children were really sadness (and that she and her family were grieving for their lost future), and did not account for her apparent fear. With great difficulty, Mrs. M.F. then began to talk of her childhood, when an elder brother died in severe pain from bone cancer. They discussed this, and her own current fears of a painful death. Following the discussion she became visibly more relaxed and in control.

A person's **coping strategy** (the overall pattern of coping responses) will depend on attitudes, family experiences, previous crises, level of support, degree of illness, and current emotions and problems.

Each coping response is like a door — open, closed, or partly open. Very rarely can a person keep all doors open all the time, nor is this necessarily healthy. Closed coping responses are not necessarily harmful. (Any coping response that allows a person to function without harming others, and to adjust to illness, should be encouraged.) Most people keep some doors open, and others partly closed, to maintain equilibrium. An open response in one area can facilitate openness in others.

"Good copers" tend towards open responses. They tend to be optimistic, resourceful, willing to express feelings, knowledgeable about their illness, socially well supported, and to have both a sense of purpose and realistic short-term goals.

★　　　**Strong emotions are normal, and varied coping strategies are normal.**

★　　　**Coping strategy may need to change as the situation changes.**

A patient may cope very well at first by adopting the sick role and becoming excessively dependent, but the closed response of helplessness may become maladaptive in time (if, for example, family members become exhausted and resentful). The caring team might then encourage a change in strategy by suggesting a family meeting, by discussing with the patient things he can do to help himself, and by supporting the patient as he accepts more responsibility for his own health.

coming fears). But the closed response of denial can become maladaptive, if it causes increasing anxiety or when fears are masked by distracting activities (such as heavy drinking or irresponsible spending) that damage the family. The patient then needs help in facing his fears (by means of encouragement, support and communication). Denial of fears may resolve as the illness progresses and as imagined fears (concerning the future) dimish. (see *Denial*)

★   **Major modification of coping responses is usually only possible if a crisis (a temporary inability to cope) has occurred.** (see *Crisis Theory*)

★   **It is possible to improve a patient's ability to cope.**

"Most patients cope better when they experience friendly professional interest that is sincere and sustained." (Thurstan Brewin)

The following can facilitate coping:
- Control symptoms and rehabilitate
- Explain and discuss
- Listen (and gently encourage openness)
- Encourage family communication
- Allow patient and family participation in care
- Offer occupational therapy
- Offer support in crises (see *Support*)
- Teach relaxation, visualization
- Encourage realistic short-term goals
- Encourage positive thinking
- Address spiritual issues (see *Spiritual Pain*)

It is always possible for carers to be both realistic and optimistic. Encouragement ("to fill with courage") can be extremely helpful. Focus on the strengths of the patient.

Your words can be powerfully therapeutic:
- "You are doing very well at the moment."
- "I admire the way you are handling this."
- "Look at what you have already coped with."

★   **Emotions occur in no particular sequence, may coexist simultaneously, and may recur at any time.**

Commonly encountered emotions in terminally ill persons are:

- Fear
- Anger
- Sadness
- Dependency
- Search for meaning

1. **Fear** (with episodes of anxiety) is almost universal in patients with advanced illness. The "door" to fear can be opened and closed. A patient may realistically discuss one aspect of his illness one day, but deny it the next. Facing and overcoming fears, usually step by step over a period of time, brings relief and an increase in confidence and self-esteem. A certain amount of denial usually facilitates gradual acceptance without the patient being overwhelmed by fear, but the closed response of complete denial demands constant psychic energy (leaving less energy for other things). Complete denial can occasionally result in extreme personality changes. For example, one patient became manic and talked continuously of how happy she felt, in order to block other thoughts. Another patient refused to speak for the last three weeks of her life. (see *Denial*)

2. **Anger** is common, but not universal. (For example, a patient tormented by chronic hypochondria can initially feel relief at a firm diagnosis of serious illness.) Anger is a normal response. Its expression can be positive and helpful, or negative and destructive. Anger often abates when it is expressed. Anger can also be internalized ("I feel so useless!" — causing guilt or depression) or transferred (blaming the carers). The energy created by anger can sometimes be usefully channeled (into fighting the illness, investigating treatment options, or focusing on complementary approaches to maintaining health). These all restore a feeling of control ("using your energy to fight the illness"). Taken too far these responses can become maladaptive (for example, visiting many medical centers at great expense to confirm the diagnosis, or searching unrealistically for a new cure). (see *Spiritual Pain*)

3. **Sadness** is appropriate. If it is not acknowledged it causes misery and sometimes clinical depression (including low self-esteem). Adjusting to losses takes time and involves a process of grief. Normal adjustment may involve withdrawal for a time and this reaction can resemble depression (but self-esteem remains normal). The dying person needs to be able to share his feelings of sadness and begin to adjust to his losses. (see *Adjustment Reactions, Grief*)

4. **Dependency** is the hardest aspect of illness for many people. Some patients cope by adopting a passive sick role, but for many the helplessness of dependency brings frustration and depression. Focusing on rehabilitation (after symptoms are controlled) can boost morale. As strength and function fade, a patient can remain active and in control by deciding how to relinquish responsibility, by handing over his roles and duties, and by seeing dependency as a role in itself. Even a totally dependent person can still have an important role in a family or community and can still help others. We are all interdependent. (see *Occupational Therapy, Rehabilitation*)

5. The **search for meaning**, to find some sense of purpose in living and dying, is an important quest. (Failure to find some meaning often leads to hopelessness and depression.) The purpose may be to help or contribute in some way, to leave something behind, or to prepare family members for their changed futures. It is often helpful for a patient to have realistic short-term goals. As death approaches goals will change. The dying patient tends to focus on the present, to recall and then relinquish the past, and to begin to let go of the strong instinct to survive. He often prepares himself for death, through gradual withdrawal from life. Some people derive their sense of purpose from their religious beliefs, and religious support may be especially important as death approaches. (see *Spiritual Pain*)

CORDOTOMY

A cordotomy involves destruction of pain fibers in the anterolateral quadrant of the spinal cord (where the sensory fibers run in the spino-thalamic tract) resulting in contralateral analgesia (pain fibers cross to the opposite side of the cord). Surgical cordotomy was described in 1912. Percutaneous cervical cordotomy (PCC) was introduced in 1963.

Cordotomy is rarely required. The only indication is severe unilateral cancer pain below C5 unresponsive to analgesia or other techniques. The effect can wear off after several months. It is usually only indicated when the prognosis is short. (Its successful use requires considerable expertise, and it is an infrequent procedure even at major medical centers.)

About 80% of patients get good long-term pain relief, in expert hands. In some people not all the sensory fibers cross over in the cord, which explains why pain relief can be partial.

PCC is performed under local anesthetic and fluoroscopic x-ray control. A needle is inserted (just below the mastoid process) via the C1-C2 space into the spinal cord. Its position is checked by electric stimulation of the needle which should cause sensory changes in the contralateral half of the body. A radio-frequency electric current then produces a heat lesion. The power is increased until the area of analgesia covers the whole painful area.

★ **The patient has to be able to talk and cooperate during the procedure.**

The procedure has a 6% mortality rate and several complications:

- Numbness and tingling - 100%
- Horner's syndrome - 100%
- Ipsilateral weak leg - 40%
- C2 neuritis - occasional
- Urination affected - rare
- Respiration affected - rare
- Ataxia - very rare
- Impotence - very rare

Motor weakness can occur due to damage to the corticospinal tracts.

Urination can be affected (especially if a pelvic tumor has already damaged bladder nerves). Cordotomy is performed contralateral to the tumor and the pain.

There is often a short-lived weakness in the muscles of one side of the body which can adversely affect respiration, especially if the patient has chronic obstructive pulmonary disease (COPD). Bilateral cordotomy is **avoided** because of the danger of Ondine's syndrome (loss of the involuntary breathing reflex and, therefore, resultant inability to sleep).

Morphine should be stopped following a cordotomy, then re-titrated (starting with low doses) if some pain persists. This prevents possible occurrence of respiratory depression. (*see Morphine*)

COUGH

About 30% of patients with advanced cancer admit to some cough, but as a troublesome symptom it is surprisingly uncommon.

Persistent coughing can cause anorexia, nausea or vomiting, insomnia, musculo-skeletal pain, cough fracture of a rib, exhaustion or cough syncope.

A **recurrent laryngeal nerve palsy** (usually due to a bronchial carcinoma) causes vocal cord paralysis and a "bovine" cough. The normal expulsive force of the cough is lost and the patient may need help to cough up tenacious sputum. (see *Hoarseness*)

Cough productive of sputum is easier to manage than a dry cough. The usual causes are **bronchitis**, **pulmonary infection** or **lung abscess**.

Rarely an **alveolar cell carcinoma** can produce large volumes (500cc to 1,000cc) of clear watery sputum (bronchorrhea).

Left ventricular failure can develop (due to an infarct or arrythmia), causing frothy sputum, orthopnea, nocturnal cough, tachycardia, gallop rhythm and fine basal crepitations. It responds to diuretics.

If sputum is green and infected, sputum culture and antibiotics may be indicated. A broad spectrum antibiotic can be started while awaiting results of sputum culture.

Physiotherapy 2 or 3 times a day, shaking or gently percussing the chest with forced expiration can help loosen sputum, and is a useful form of active therapy. There is no place for postural drainage in very ill patients. (see *Physical Therapy*)

Other treatments that are sometimes useful include steam inhalations, expectorants and mucolytics.

Dry cough — A persistent irritating cough without sputum production can be difficult to manage. The usual causes are **bronchospasm**, **pleural effusion** or **bronchogenic carcinoma**.

Management options:
1. Bronchodilators
2. Pleural aspiration
3. Radiotherapy
4. Steroids
5. Humidified air
6. Soothing syrup
7. Opioids
8. Nebulized lidocaine

1. **Bronchospasm** can cause a troublesome cough. There may be no history of asthma and no audible wheeze. Peak flow rate may be reduced although it may be intermittent (nocturnal coughing, for example). Treatment includes albuterol (by nebulizer or inhaler), slow-release aminophylline or steroids. (*see Dyspnea*)

2. A **pleural effusion** can occasionally present as a cough due to diaphragmatic irritation. It is confirmed by chest x-ray and treated by aspiration. (*see Pleural Effusion*)

3. **Radiotherapy** may be indicated if there is a large untreated carcinoma.

4. **Oral steroids** (dexamethasone 4mg to 8mg per day) can reduce wheeze and may reduce cough due to a large bronchial abscess.

5. A **humidifier** can help. Dry air and irritants like cigarette smoke worsen coughing.

6. **Simple linctus** (5mg to 10mg 4 times a day) can reduce pharyngeal irritation.

7. **Opioids** are the most powerful central cough suppressants. Codeine linctus 5ml to 10ml 4 times a day may be sufficient. Oral morphine starting with 2.5mg every 4 hours, and increasing to 5mg, 10mg or 20mg every 4 hours will suppress cough in patients not already taking morphine. For patients already taking morphine, methadone linctus (2mg in 5ml) 3 times a day can sometimes help to reduce cough (for unknown reasons).

8. **Nebulized lidocaine** 2% can bring dramatic relief, used for 10 minutes every 2 to 6 hours (maximum of 10ml per 24 hours). Numbness of the mouth may persist for about 30 minutes after each treatment, therefore the patient must be told not to eat or drink for this time.

Terminal phase coughing — If the patient is too weak to cough up secretions, atropine 0.6mg up to 4 times a day can reduce distressing bubbling without causing sedation. For terminal bubbling use scopolamine 0.4mg IM every 4 hours. Suction is occasionally helpful if the patient is distressed by tenacious sputum at the back of the throat, but repeated suction is distressing and should be avoided. (*see Terminal Phase*)

COUNSELING

Counseling is a **therapeutic dialogue** intended to increase a person's self-understanding and emotional independence. Sigmund Freud spoke of the "talking cure".

It involves:

- Support and encouragement
- Non-possessive warmth
- Listening skills
- Ventilation of feelings
- Non-judgmental attitudes

At its simplest, counseling is help that anyone with warmth and common sense can give to help restore a person's self-confidence. Counseling skills are now seen as important to many different professionals.

A trained and experienced counselor will have a repertoire of approaches and styles to draw upon. Unskilled counselors tend to overuse directive counseling and may dabble dangerously in confrontation and catharsis.

The counselor's approach must fit the situation. For example, if a person has a short time to live then lengthy insight-orientated psychotherapy is inappropriate.

At a deeper level counseling can help a person make sense of conflicting thoughts and feelings which may be causing irrational (neurotic) behavior. This takes more time and skill and tends to be called psychotherapy. Counseling alone cannot help if there is total disruption of the personality as in a psychosis, or if a person does not want to be helped or changed.

The aims and expectations of the counselor need to be realistic and in agreement with the client or patient.

The effectiveness of counseling depends largely on the personality and skill of the counselor, who should ideally have:

- Genuine concern
- Little interest in status
- An understanding of his own emotional needs
- Support and supervision

Counseling involves a number of essential skills which can be listed as:

- Information-giving (*see Explanation*)
- Information-receiving
- Clarifying
- Probing
- Empathy
- Confronting (with reality)
- Sharing
- Reassurance (*see Reassurance*)
- Listening without speaking (*see Listening*)
- Giving alternative frames of reference
- Interpretation
- Reflection
- Acceptance, affirmation
- Noticing body language (*see Non-verbal Communication*)
- Giving feedback
- Supporting (*see Support*)

Problems arise if the counselor is trying to resolve his or her own un-met emotional needs. (Ventilating your own feelings and attitudes is **not** counseling.)

Skills are best acquired by the practice of counseling, while being supervised by an experienced counselor. Counseling is emotionally demanding and needs to be structured and supported to avoid exhaustion. (*see Burn Out*)

Short workshops to teach basic counseling techniques, using group work, video filming and feedback on performance, can effectively improve basic skills.

It is estimated that up to 50% of hospice patients and their families want counseling help in dealing with their emotional problems. The few studies that exist support the assumption that emotional support and improved communications reduce anxiety and depression, improve satisfaction and self-esteem, and have a positive effect on the family. More work is needed to measure the effectiveness of these interventions, to assess the different types of interventions, and to develop ways of targeting those patients and family members at high risk. (*see Communication Problems, Listening, Talking with Families, Talking with Patients*)

CRISIS THEORY

A crisis can be defined as a temporary inability to cope with change.

"During a crisis, even though the person does not have at the start the way of dealing with the problem, he may work out a way of dealing with it before it is over . . . remember those little experiments . . . in the biology laboratory with a paramecium, where you put a glass plate in front of it, and the paramecium bumps its nose against the glass plate, and then does a lot of trial and error running about to try and find a way around this." (Gerald Caplan)

Adjusting to illness or having an ill family member involves many changes. Some of these can provoke a crisis. In a crisis we must use problem-solving skills to find new solutions. We can usually develop solutions, provided those around us provide support. Struggling to solve a problem involves trying several different approaches. This demands energy, which means there is less energy for other aspects of life, both practical and emotional. (see Support)

Most life crises involve loss and change. If two crises occur simultaneously it can be much more difficult to find effective solutions. A crisis may be developmental (child leaving home, retirement), emotional (bereavement) or situational (promotion, illness, burglary). Some events require both social (external) and psychological (internal) adjustments (the birth of a first child, for example).

A crisis is an opportunity for growth and the development of new skills to solve problems. Therapists sometimes aim to provoke a degree of crisis in a person or family in order to bring about change. There is a danger of a maladaptive response to try to avoid the crisis (a suicide attempt, for example) which makes matters worse.

A crisis causes increasing anxiety and failure to cope until the person acknowledges the severity of the difficulty and looks for solutions, both within the self and from helpful others. At this point there is maximum **potential for change** when the person recognizes the need for solutions. A small amount of professional help can now catalyze a change for the better, often a change in attitude.

★   **"A crisis is not an abstract imposition from without, but a high point in the life of the person concerned . . . a dynamic interaction between a person and an extreme event."** (Lily Pincus)

DAY HOSPICE

A "day hospice" provides a very useful half-way stage of support for the terminally ill patient. It often enables an ill patient, who might otherwise need admission to an in-patient facility, to stay at home. It provides rest and relief for family carers. It is particularly helpful for the isolated, the anxious and the house-bound. Medical and nursing involvement is important, because patients have advanced disease and problems can occur suddenly, but **the principal goal of the day hospice is social support and recreation**.

Good liaison with the family physician, home care nurses and other members of the caring team is important. They should be encouraged to visit the day hospice.

Most day hospices are open for part of the day, once or several times each week. If a free-standing in-patient hospice exists, it should be the site of the day hospice, as familiarity with the building and staff helps to overcome fears of admission for terminal care. (In-patients may participate in day hospice activities, and home care patients attending the day hospice can visit friends now admitted to the in-patient unit.)

If no in-patient facility exists, the day hospice can use any easily accessible community facility, such as a senior citizens' center, a church, a hospital lounge, etc. (Medical and nursing input remains important.)

Day hospice is a useful way of introducing a patient to the entire hospice team.

Ideally, a patient is driven back and forth between home and the day hospice by the same volunteer each time, so that a useful "one-to-one" friendship can develop.

Sometimes family members wish to attend the day hospice with the patient, and they should be allowed to do so. However, a common function of a day hospice is to give a couple space from each other (sometimes important even in the most loving relationship). Illness and dependency can bring unaccustomed and excessive closeness, and a few hours apart can often restore normality.

Day hospices can offer:
- Social contact and mental stimulation
- Relief for caring family members
- Psychological support

- Basic nursing care (change dressings, catheters)
- Access to a doctor for symptom control
- Bathing facilities
- Hairdressing and barber facilities
- Physical therapy (mobilization, breathing, relaxation)
- Occupational therapy
- Group recreational activities
- Hobbies and handicrafts
- Family support
- Spiritual support (chaplain, church services)
- Access to a social worker

Discussion — The aim of the day hospice is to help the patient remain as independent as possible. Personal development is encouraged as part of holistic rehabilitation. The emphasis is social and recreational, rather than medical or narrowly therapeutic. Patients (and the occasional family member who wishes to attend) **enjoy** day hospice activities. (see *Occupational Therapy*)

Day hospice care can give physical and psychological relief to caring family members, plus "time off". It can function as an effective support group for patients to discuss their feelings and frustrations.

A day hospice program facilitates discharge of in-patients who after symptom control and rehabilitation are well enough to return home, but can benefit from added support. (see *Rehabilitation*)

Mr. N. J., an extremely anxious man of 56 with lung cancer, was admitted to an in-patient hospice for pain control, but was too frightened to go home. ("What will I think about all day?") He started attending the day hospice while still an in-patient, and learned woodworking which he found totally absorbing. This gave him the confidence to get home and continue his hobby there. Returning to the day hospice twice a week, he remained at home for the last 6 weeks of his life. It was a fulfilling time for Mr. N. J. and his wife.

DEHYDRATION

Terminal dehydration is not distressing, and the only symptom of dehydration is a dry mouth. Patients do not feel thirsty, just as starving people do not feel hungry. (Intravenous fluids are rarely administered to patients dying in a British hospice, and then only if the **patient** is complaining of thirst — which is rare.)

Intravenous fluids tend to exacerbate discomfort in the patient close to death, and may actually add to the emotional distress of the family.

Terminal dehydration is not inevitable. During a study on hypercalcemia, 22 patients had blood taken within 48 hours of death, and 12 had essentially normal urea and electrolyte results.

Dehydration actually has a number of advantages in the patient near death. It reduces pulmonary secretions and the likelihood of vomiting, reduces urine output and the possibility of incontinence.

Careful mouth care every 2 hours is important.

DENIAL

Denial is normal. It is an exaggeration of the normal process of selective attention. We have to be able to select information in order to function normally. (For example, to focus on the potential dangers around us all the time could bring disabling anxiety.)

Denial is a normal coping mechanism for a person with advanced cancer, who will fluctuate in the degree of acceptance of illness and impending death. (see *Coping with Dying*)

★ **"Neither the sun nor death can be looked at with a steady eye."** (La Rochefoucauld)

Life-changing news ("You have cancer.") is overwhelming if all the consequences are immediately considered. The only way to adjust is to deny certain elements and focus on others. Normal adjustment to bad news takes time.

It is not possible or healthy to think continuously of bad news. This is seen most clearly in grieving children who can seem sad one minute and happy the next. Children facing death can be greatly helped by relaxation techniques or hypnosis (for example, taking them on an imaginary journey in a space ship where they are back in control and having fun, thus giving them a rest from their emotions). Some adults facing death do this for themselves, continuing to plan for the future, (scheduling holidays, designing renovations to their homes, etc.) while also knowing they only have a short time to live.

It can sometimes be helpful to ask a patient "If someone could wave a magic wand and make you better, what would you do today?" This helps to discover some of what has been important to that person, and also encourages him to take a brief rest from his emotions.

Denial is helpful when used appropriately, and when it does not hinder other adjustments (practical, financial, emotional, spiritual).

Excessive denial — Persistent refusal to discuss an illness is due to fear. Some people adopt an attitude of total denial (for example, calling a fungating breast cancer a "rash"). Asked a question like "What did the surgeon say about the operation?" they quickly change the subject. Such people are usually lacking confidence in their own abilities and never benefit from the boost in confidence that comes from facing and adjusting to problems.

Confronting someone with information he does not want is not helpful and can be unkind. Often the patient forgets he has heard the information and yet may demonstrate increased anxiety, or sometimes anger. It is usually unhelpful to confront repeated denial, but it is important not to collude.

> Mrs. L.E., 66, who had never wanted to discuss her illness, was getting very weak due to advanced colon cancer with liver metastases. As the doctor stood up to leave her bedside one day, she said "So you think I'm getting better." The doctor sat down with her again. He agreed that her nausea and vomiting were better, but said the illness was about the same and could not be completely cured. This enabled future conversations to remain honest. To collude would have made it uncomfortable for the doctor to go back again as she became progressively weaker. She soon began to talk about her dying and said she felt relieved to do so.

Denial must be respected as a coping mechanism. Some people refuse to discuss or think about their illness right up to the time they die. However, most people reach a stage when it becomes a relief to discuss some of their fears. Extreme denial prevents the sharing and discussing of unrealistic fears, and anxiety tends to escalate. It also blocks meaningful communication with the family. (see Communication Problems)

The aim of discussing a person's illness is to reduce anxiety. The skill is in choosing the right moment and the right words. Remember that a person who prefers denial to discussion tends to be frightened and under-confident. Careful explanation can reduce anxiety (which, however, may be replaced with appropriate sadness). A patient will convey verbally or non-verbally whether the information or explanation is excessive or unhelpful at that particular time.

Testing denial — Ask "Can you help me by explaining what you understand about your illness?" The most common immediate reply to this question is "Nothing." Avoid the temptation to give premature explanations. Continue to **ask questions and listen**. (see Talking with Patients)

★　　　**Ask how the person felt at each stage. ("How did you feel when the doctor said it was an ulcer?")**

★　　　**See if there is partial acceptance. ("Are there times when you feel it may be more serious than an ulcer?")**

★　　　**Challenge inconsistencies. ("You have told me your illness is due to your fall in the bedroom. Do you think all this illness could be due to a fall?")**

★　　　**Avoid giving unrequested information.**

★　　　**Check level of acceptance at each visit. ("How do you feel things are going at the moment?")**

A patient who denies his illness with one person may not do so with another. John Hinton interviewed 80 married patients dying of cancer and found that 69% spoke about their illness to their spouse, 35% to the staff and 85% to the interviewer.

Inadequate denial can also cause anxiety. Occasionally patients confront the facts relentlessly and allow themselves little relief from their fears. Most people have sad or morbid thoughts intermittently, but there are some patients who seem unable to think of anything else. Sometimes it is a form of self-punishment (guilt, depression) or a way of punishing others (anger). Cognitive approaches, which give the person insight into the connection between thoughts and feelings, can be helpful. (see Anxiety)

DEPRESSION

★   **Sadness is natural in dying patients.**

Reactive depression often responds to good symptom control and improved family communications. **Endogenous depression** is not common, and can be difficult to diagnose in terminally ill patients. The usual indicators of depression (disturbed sleep, anorexia, weariness, constipation, reduced libido, emotional lability) are also seen in advanced illness.

The best clues to true depression are:

- Past history of depression
- Expressionless face (unable to greet family)
- Unable to enjoy favorite things
- Low self-esteem
- Persistent guilt feelings
- Delusions ("My cancer is contagious.")

Comments about suicide are not necessarily depressive. They may be the patient's way of saying "I want to stay in control ", or "I want you to understand what I am going through." Chronic pain for months on end (associated particularly with carcinomas of the rectum and tail of the pancreas) can cause depression.

Anti-depressants usually take 2 to 3 weeks to take effect, although a response can occur in 7 to 10 days. They should be started at low dosage and increased quickly to a maximum tolerated dose (usually the dry mouth is the limiting factor). Even in very ill patients large doses can be well tolerated, and it is important to use as high a dose as possible. In frail elderly patients tricyclics may cause confusion. 20% of patients will not respond to tricyclics. Amitriptyline 25mg to 150mg at bedtime also has sedative properties. Imipramine 25mg to 150mg at bedtime is less sedating. (*see Anti-depressants*)

A useful guide to the speed of increase in daily doses is:

Day 1	10mg to 25mg
Day 3	25mg to 50mg
Day 7	50mg to 100mg
Day 10	100mg to 150mg

Note: Elderly or frail patients need lower doses. Side-effects often limit the tolerated dose.

DIABETES

About 5% of patients with advanced cancer have diabetes mellitus.

The patient is usually known to have pre-existing diabetes, but occasionally it occurs secondary to carcinoma of the pancreas or to high dose steroids (or rarely, to ectopic ACTH). Diabetes should be suspected if there is **thirst**, **drowsiness** or **increasing weakness**.

Patients with diabetes generally feel better if blood glucose levels are controlled. Strict control to avoid long-term vascular damage is no longer appropriate, but hyperglycemia should still be avoided.

★ **Aim to keep pre-prandial blood glucose levels below 170mg/dL.**

Patients who have carefully controlled their own diabetes (sometimes for many years) feel psychologically better if strict control is maintained. It is one of the things they can still be positive about, and it helps to give them a feeling that they remain in control.

Mild hyperglycemia may be controllable with an **oral hypoglycemic**.

Patients with advanced illness **starting on insulin** should initially have a safe starting dose of 10 units of insulin 2 times a day, preferably using Mixtard or Novolin 70/30 biphasic insulins (which are more convenient to use at home). Adjust the dose daily until pre-prandial capillary blood glucose levels are around 170mg/dL. At first, monitor capillary blood glucose levels 4 times a day (before meals and at bedtime) for in-patients, and at least 2 times a day if the patient is at home. (An increasing number of diabetic patients are successfully using portable glucometers at home, enabling closer monitoring and increased independence.) Once controlled, monitor capillary blood glucose levels once every few days unless hypoglycemia is suspected.

A diabetic patient starting insulin needs specialist education and advice.

The goal of **diet** is to spread carbohydrate intake over the whole day and to have it covered by insulin. Patients with a short prognosis can relax dietary restrictions on cakes and candy, increasing insulin dosage as necessary.

Patients started on insulin should be warned about **hypoglycemia** in the usual way, and should carry sugar. Hypoglycemia is commonest after a missed meal and should be suspected if the patient has headaches, confusion, sweating or tremor.

If the patient is vomiting it is better to use regular insulin 3 times a day, adjusting the dose according to capillary blood glucose levels as follows:

Blood Glucose	Units of Insulin
< 170mg/dL [*10mmol/L*]	0
170-260mg/dL [*10-15mmol/L*]	10
260-340mg/dL [*15-20mmol/L*]	20

When changing back to a 2 times a day insulin regime, give the same total number of units per day.

Insulin requirements in advancing disease may **decrease** due to weight loss and anorexia.

During the **terminal phase**, insulin may still be needed. Even if the patient is not eating, the liver continues to produce glucose. The basal requirement is usually about 10 units 2 times a day (more in a large or obese patient). If the patient becomes unconscious during the terminal phase, insulin should be stopped.

DIARRHEA

Diarrhea (frequent or fluid bowel movements), occurs in about 5% of hospice patients.

Oral **loperamide** 2mg to 4mg every 6 hours acts locally on the gut and is usually more useful than the centrally acting opioids (morphine, codeine, diphenoxylate) because the patient is often already taking opioids. Loperamide should also be available if drugs that can cause diarrhea are prescribed.

The most common causes of diarrhea are:
1. Fecal impaction
2. Steatorrhea
3. Malignant intestinal obstruction (dysfunction)
4. Laxative imbalance or drugs
5. Rectal tumor (discharge plus blood)
6. Fecal incontinence
7. Carcinoid tumor

1. **Fecal impaction** is commonly seen in patients on opioids who have been given laxatives either too late or in too low a dosage. It can often be diagnosed from the history. There are no bowel movements for several days, and then there is passage of small amounts of liquid feces, sometimes without control. Rectal examination reveals a large, clay-like lump of feces which usually has to be removed by manual evacuation under sedation. Occasionally the rectum is ballooned and empty, and the impaction has occurred higher up (palpable abdominally or visible on plain abdominal x-ray). The patient may require in-patient admission to clear this sort of constipation. (see Constipation)

2. **Steatorrhea** means loose, pale, foul-smelling feces. (Relatives sometimes fear they contain cancer.) Steatorrhea can be missed without a good history. The patient usually complains simply of diarrhea, but steatorrhea does not respond to anti-diarrheal drugs. It is due to malabsorption of fat, and is most commonly seen in patients with carcinoma of the pancreas. The patient usually has bowel movements four or five times a day, with large quantities of feces that tend to float, and are difficult to flush away in the toilet. Steatorrhea responds to pancreatic enzyme replacement tablets containing all major pancreatic enzymes: lipase, protease and amylase.

The enzymes are destroyed by gastric acid and therefore tablets are best taken immediately before a meal or a snack, or with milk. (The required dose may be 2 to 10 tablets or more, depending on the strength of the pancreatic replacement used.) The dosage is adjusted according to the frequency of bowel movements. Excessive dosage may irritate the skin around the anus. Resistant steatorrhea may further respond by giving cimetidine 200mg, 30 minutes before the meal, to reduce gastric acid secretion. Measurement of fecal fats by the laboratory is unnecessary: the clinical picture is usually obvious once considered.

3. **Malignant intestinal obstruction** is usually seen with carcinoma of the ovary (25% develop obstruction) or carcinoma of the colon or rectum. In reality, it is often malignant intestinal "dysfunction" rather than "obstruction" because bowel disturbances are often intermittent and can either cause constipation or diarrhea. (see Intestinal Obstruction)

Diarrhea in this situation is best treated with loperamide 2mg to 4mg every 6 hours (care being taken to stop it after the diarrhea has settled, to avoid constipation). Diarrhea due to malignant intestinal dysfunction can respond to high dose steroids (dexamethasone 8mg per day).

Occasionally a malignant ileo-colic fistula causes a short circuit of the bowel. Diarrhea can then be worsened by retrograde bacterial overgrowth in the small intestine (which is normally sterile) with deconjugation of bile salts and malabsorption of fat. This can respond to oral tetracycline 500mg every 6 hours.

4. **Laxative imbalance** — The incorrect use of laxatives can cause diarrhea. If the patient is on opioid analgesics it is essential to take laxatives daily. Usually there has been under-use of laxatives in a patient on opioids which has allowed constipation to develop. Excessive laxatives are then taken to clear the constipation and hard feces are finally passed, followed (sometimes explosively) by soft feces.

Other drugs that can cause diarrhea include antibiotics, antacids with magnesium salts, NSAIDs and anti-fibrinolytic drugs. Oral phosphate used to treat hypercalcemia causes severe diarrhea. Chemotherapy (especially with mitomycin or fluorouracil) can cause diarrhea.

5. **Rectal tumor** — Mucous discharge or bleeding from carcinoma of the rectum can be treated by radiotherapy. A palliative colostomy does not relieve these local symptoms. Hydrocortisone foam, one applicator-full 2 times a day, can be helpful, as can oral steroids (dexamethasone 8mg 2 times a day). Profuse mucous diarrhea can cause hypokalemia. Laser therapy via an endoscope can be very successful in reducing bleeding and discharge from carcinoma of the rectum, and it can also improve the patency of the lumen and prevent obstruction. It usually needs to be repeated. The discharge can be foul-smelling and metronidazole (500mg every 8 hours) usually reduces the smell. (see *Lasers*)

Bulk-forming drugs (methylcellulose tablets or granules) can help control diarrhea due to rectal tumors, by establishing a bowel routine. They take 2 or 3 days to take effect, and dose is tailored to effect.

6. **Fecal incontinence due to loss of sphincter control** — There may be perineal numbness, usually as part of spinal cord compression syndrome with paraplegia. It is usually best managed by reducing or stopping laxatives and giving daily or alternate-day manual evacuations. (see *Spinal Cord Compression*)

Fecal incontinence may be due to a recto-vaginal fistula, and the patient may be too embarrassed to complain that feces are leaking from her vagina. A palliative colostomy should always be considered for this distressing condition. (see *Fistulas*)

7. **Carcinoid tumors** are slow-growing tumors of the small intestine (less commonly bronchus, large bowel or pancreas) which can secrete 5HT (serotonin) causing:

- Diarrhea
- Wheeze
- Flushing

These symptoms do not occur if blood from the tumor passes through a normal liver, so these tumors only produce symptoms once liver metastases have occurred. (Bronchial carcinoids are often metabolically inactive.) The primary tumor usually remains small but massive hepatomegaly eventually occurs. It is occasionally possible to block the metabolic effects with drugs, but treatment may fail because tumors can produce more than one active agent.

Diarrhea can be profuse (1 liter per day) and may not respond to anti-diarrheals. If the terminal ileum has been resected diarrhea may be due to excess bile salts, and cholestyramine can help. If it is due to 5HT, 5HT antagonists may help, either cyproheptadine 4mg to 8mg 4 times a day, or methysergide 1mg at bedtime increasing to 1mg to 2mg 3 times a day. Bulking of the feces (with methylcellulose) can reduce the frequency of diarrhea and establish a bowel routine.

DIET

(see Anorexia, Nutrition)

Many patients and carers worry about "correct diet". Dietary advice should be available to patients in the same way as physiotherapy, occupational therapy or psychotherapy.

The carer's interest in a patient's food intake carries a message. Even when a patient is unable to enjoy eating, attention to an adequate dietary intake can provide psychological support to both patient and family. There are social and emotional aspects to eating.

Advice from a dietitian is usually welcomed. The dietitian can give advice on:

- Overcoming eating problems
- A balanced diet
- Dietary supplements
- Special diets

When discussing diet it is important to consider any eating problem which includes:

- Poor appetite (*see Anorexia*)
- Taste changes (*see Taste*)
- Sore mouth (*see Mouth Care*)
- Difficult or painful swallowing (*see Dysphagia*)
- Early fullness (*see Small Stomach Syndrome*)
- Nausea (*see Nausea & Vomiting*)
- Weakness or embarrassment
- Boring food

Dietary advice generally includes:

- Encourage fluids
- Encourage fiber (fruit and vegetables)
- Eat little and often
- Eat whatever you enjoy (no foods are harmful)

Fluid and a moderate amount of fiber will help to prevent constipation. Taste changes are common and new food preferences often develop, much to the person's surprise. Long-standing dietary restrictions (for example, low salt or low fat diets) can usually be relaxed if the patient is finding them irksome.

It can be helpful to ask the patient to outline his normal daily food intake. Fortifying a normal diet with increased protein (meat, fish, nuts, beans, eggs, cheese, milk) and increased calories (pasta, bread, jam, cakes, butter) is one way of boosting dietary intake. High dose Vitamin C (500mg 4 times a day) for 6 weeks may improve appetite and well-being.

Dietary supplements are helpful for patients with a reduced appetite. Energy supplements in the form of tasteless glucose polymers (Polycose) are useful. These can be added to drinks, soups, casseroles, custards, tapioca and milk puddings. The aim is to add as much as possible without altering the flavor or texture of food.

Nutritionally complete foods (Ensure Plus, Sustacal, etc.) can replace eating for patients unable to manage normal meals due to weakness, small appetite, nausea or dysphagia. These have disadvantages (they are sometimes seen as "invalid foods", or reduce the appetite for normal meals, or simply become boring), but they can be very helpful for weak patients who want to maintain a normal food intake. Small, frequent sip feedings (50ml per hour) are encouraged. A dietitian should advise on selecting suitable supplements that the patient likes.

Special dietary regimes are often promoted to cancer patients. These diets are usually only one part of a holistic approach to health (complementary to orthodox medicine) which encourages patients to be active in maintaining their own health. There is no evidence that they improve prognosis. The diets are sometimes accompanied by megavitamin therapy and other oral supplements (including selenium, zinc, herbal mixtures, carrot juice, evening primrose oil, glanolin, etc.) some of which are very expensive.

These diets are usually low calorie, vegetarian diets. The high fiber element can make them unmanageable for patients with a colostomy or an esophageal tube. Provided they are not physically harming the patient or causing undue expense, such special diets can on occasion improve patient morale.

DISCOMFORTS

★ **"Minor matters are important to the bedridden."** (Jane Zorza)

In our enthusiasm to control cancer pain, nausea, vomiting, dyspnea, dysphagia, anorexia and other major symptoms, it is sometimes easy to overlook details which can be so important, and can greatly reduce discomfort, improve morale, and raise the pain threshold.

For example:
- Syringing ear wax
- Treating ingrowing toe nails
- Relining loose dentures
- Arranging routine dental work
- Rehydrating dry skin
- Changing eyeglass prescription, adjusting fit

Poor hearing is often due to ear wax. Ear drops (such as warm olive oil) may only need 30 minutes to soften wax sufficiently to allow syringing.

DISTANCING BEHAVIOR

Distancing behavior by professionals discourages patients or family members from disclosing their real concerns.

Some examples of this behavior are:

- Selective attention
- Normalizing
- False reassurance

Selective attention — When a patient mentions both physical and psychological problems, many doctors and nurses will focus on the physical.

Normalizing attempts to reduce the importance of something. ("You're bound to feel upset, everybody does in your position.") This protects the carer from his own emotional responses of anger, sadness or fear.

False reassurance (or premature reassurance), with the excessive use of positive statements or unrealistic promises also blocks the patient from sharing fears. False reassurance destroys trust. (see *Trust, Reassurance*)

Non-verbal distancing behavior — The most powerful messages are given non-verbally. (see *Non-verbal Communication*)

Gestures which may convey your intention of keeping emotional distance include:

- Handshake with palm down
- Poor eye contact
- Looking away or eye closure
- Body turned away
- Feet turned away (if standing)
- Chin down or neck rubbing (conveys criticism)
- Barriers (desk or any object held in front of the body)
- Arms folded across chest (conveys suspiciousness)
- Displacement gestures (picking at clothing)
- Territorial display (leaning on furniture)

Clusters of signals convey attitudes and feelings rather than single gestures. While some gestures are culturally determined, many are nearly universal. Eye contact (normally 60% to 70% of the time) and facial expression can convey openness and acceptance, but the above signals may detract from that impression.

Health care professionals often work under considerable pressure. They fear being overloaded with the problems of patients and families, which can often re-awaken powerful personal emotions, and which can tap their resources, both personal and professional. Thus they sometimes wish to "keep their distance".

Health care professionals (and volunteers) must be encouraged and helped to deliver good care. Careful selection of staff, proper training in communication skills (demonstrations, role play, video feedback), good staff support mechanisms, opportunities for continuing education, and proper structuring of the workload so staff in the front line of caring for the dying and bereaved get time away on a regular basis, all help carers to respond appropriately to the concerns and needs of patients and families. (see Burn Out)

DIURETICS

Diuretics cause diuresis, and the urinary frequency may be more of a burden to the person than the edema.

Prescribing a diuretic is one of the few occasions when a combination drug is helpful. For routine use a combination of a loop diuretic (potassium losing) and a potassium sparing diuretic is useful to avoid the need for potassium supplements.

Loop diuretics act within 60 minutes, and the diuresis lasts 4 to 6 hours.

For resistant edema, the dose may have to be increased to furosemide 80mg 2 times a day, or bumetanide 2mg 2 times a day (which is better absorbed), with spironolactone 200mg 2 times a day. (Amiloride and triamterene are weak diuretics and are not aldosterone antagonists.) Avoid IM injections which are poorly absorbed.

A very useful additional drug for resistant edema is metolazone 10mg to 20mg per day, in addition to high dose furosemide and spironolactone. It can often produce a diuresis when other drugs have ceased to be effective.

Problems with diuretics:
- Urinary frequency
- Disturbed sleep
- Urinary retention (if prostatic)
- Dry mouth
- Nausea (spironolactone)
- Hypokalemia

- Cramps (sodium loss)
- Dizziness (hypovolemia)
- Tinnitus (high dose furosemide)
- Rashes (amiloride, triamterene)

High dose spironolactone may be indicated for ascites. (*see Ascites*)

Leg swelling due to lymphedema responds poorly to diuretics. (*see Lymphedema*)

DROWSINESS

At least 30% of patients with advanced cancer complain of drowsiness at times. A drowsy patient can be less distressing to the carers, but it is a mistake to think that drowsiness is a good thing for ill patients. Most patients dislike feeling drowsy and unable to concentrate.

The main causes are:

1. Morphine
2. Psychotropic drugs
3. Hypercalcemia
4. Uremia
5. Hyponatremia
6. Infection
7. Advancing illness

1. **If the patient is pain-free and drowsy, reduce the dose of morphine.** The correct dose of morphine is the dose that relieves the pain without causing drowsiness. Morphine drowsiness is characteristically reversed by stimulation (conversation, for example). Some patients don't mind this drowsiness. ("I don't get so bored.") If reducing the dose of morphine causes an increase in pain (and other pain-relieving drugs have been tried or considered) then this drowsiness due to morphine may **very rarely** have to be accepted.

If the pain is reduced (following palliative radiotherapy or a nerve block, for example) then the stimulating effect of pain (on general alertness and also on respiration) is lost. Morphine can then cause drowsiness, and in severe cases respiratory depression. (*see Analgesics, Morphine*)

2. Previously acceptable doses of **psychotropic drugs** may become too high, as renal or hepatic function deteriorates, or due to drug interactions. Reduce the dose of the psychotropic drug, and stop any unnecessary drugs.

3. **Hypercalcemia** (calcium above 12.0mg/dL [*3.0mmol/L*]) can cause drowsiness (usually with nausea and thirst). (*see Hypercalcemia*)

4. **Uremia** can cause drowsiness (usually with confusion, nausea, hiccups and tremor). There is no treatment, but knowing the cause of the problem greatly improves management, and enables explanation to patient and family.

5. **Hyponatremia** (plasma sodium below 120mmol/L) can cause drowsiness. It can occur with adrenal metastases or in small (oat) cell carcinoma of the bronchus. It responds to fluid restriction. It is rare. (*see Confusion*)

6. **Bacteremia or septicemia** (from urinary tract infection or pressure sores) can present as drowsiness (sometimes with flushing or tachycardia). Steroids may prevent fever. An antibiotic may be indicated.

7. Increasing drowsiness is a feature of **advanced disease**. Patients sometimes fear that drowsiness means the beginning of the end. It helps to be optimistic as well as honest: "It is part of your illness, but your energy goes up and down when you are ill, and some days you need more rest than others."

If drowsiness is distressing (if a patient wants to be more alert for a special occasion) then oral dextroamphetamine 2.5mg to 5mg per day can sometimes be helpful as a short-term measure. There is risk of agitation.

DYSPHAGIA

Dysphagia means difficult or painful swallowing.

In one study, 12% of 797 cancer patients complained of dysphagia on admission to a hospice, and 60% of the patients with dysphagia responded to medical treatment.

Causes:
- Candidiasis
- Carcinoma (esophagus, oropharynx, stomach)
- Mediastinal nodes (breast, lymphoma)
- Pharyngeal damage (cancer plus radiotherapy)
- Neuromuscular (*see Amyotrophic Lateral Sclerosis*)

Note: Benign peptic stricture is a possibility.

Recurrent cancer of the pharynx (previously treated with radiotherapy) can cause complete dysphagia without any obstruction at post-mortem. This is due to muscular inco-ordination and splinting of the pharynx, and can respond to high dose steroids.

Assessment:

- Observe swallowing
- Liquids or solids?
- Painful?
- Dribbling? (total dysphagia?)
- Coughing after liquids? (fistula?)

The most important first step in managing dysphagia is to watch the patient attempting to swallow — to assess both pain and degree of difficulty. If the patient is managing to swallow saliva (about 500cc per day) he should be able to sip fluids. A patient with a fistula into the bronchus will cough up orange sputum after a drink of orange juice.

★ **If swallowing causes burning or discomfort, assume candidiasis is present.** (see Candidiasis)

Management options:

1. Treat candidiasis (thrush)
2. Liquidize food
3. Consider drug routes
4. Palliative radiotherapy
5. Dilation
6. Esophageal tube
7. Laser
8. High dose steroids
9. Management of a fistula
10. Total dysphagia

Discussion:

1. **Candidiasis** tends to cause pain when swallowing (worse with hot drinks). Severe esophageal candidiasis can occur even with no evidence of oral thrush. A systemic anti-fungal, ketoconazole 200mg 2 times a day, should be used. Swallowing improves within 24 to 48 hours.

2. **Liquidize food**, or use liquid food supplements.

3. **Drugs** may have to be soluble or given by suppository or continuous subcutaneous infusion.

4. **Palliative radiotherapy** can shrink mediastinal nodes. Carcinoma of the esophagus has usually already been treated with radical, maximal dose radiotherapy, and further treatment is not possible.

5. **Endoscopic dilation** of the tumor can bring temporary relief (days to weeks), but there is a risk of perforation. Dilation has a place in the initial management of moderate dysphagia (for solids but not liquids) and can bring improvement. Endoscopy takes 10 to 15 minutes and does not require x-ray screening facilities. If dysphagia recurs quickly, other methods must be used.

6. **Esophageal tubes** are always worth considering in severe dysphagia. Tube insertion is possible in 90% of patients. They are best inserted under general anesthesia and x-ray control, although they may be inserted under sedation. The tumor must first be dilated and this can cause a fatal perforation and mediastinitis. (There is about a 10% mortality with this procedure.)

Previous radiotherapy does not preclude tube insertion.

Intubation of tumors occurring in the lower third, or for recurrent tumor at an anastomosis, can be difficult because the tumor may not hold the tube in place.

The results are good. 30% of patients have normal swallowing and 60% can manage semisolids. The patient is unaware of the tube when it is correctly positioned.

The patient is advised to:

- Chew food well
- Avoid large boluses of meat
- Take fizzy drinks (club soda, tonic water) with and after meals

7. **Endoscopic laser treatment** is becoming increasingly available. In one series of 68 patients 98% had relief of symptoms, and the results are as good as tube insertion. The treatment involves endoscopy under sedation. The malignant stricture is usually dilated first (with the usual risk of perforation) before the laser can be used. The laser destroys all intraluminal tumor. Treatment takes about 20 minutes, and may have to be repeated after about 3 months. It cannot be used for dysphagia due to extrinsic compression or due to circumferential tumors. (*see Lasers*)

8. **High dose steroids** (dexamethasone 8mg to 12mg per day) can be very effective in relieving dysphagia, sometimes for many weeks. This can be effective whether the cause is carcinoma of the esophagus, mediastinal nodes, postoperative stricture or pharyngeal induration due to oropharyngeal carcinomas. It is presumed to work by reducing inflammatory edema. The dexamethasone has to be given by injection (8mg IM per day for the first few days) if dysphagia is severe, or soluble prednisolone 30mg 3 times a

day can be used. There is a risk of causing hunger without improving swallowing, but this rarely occurs and hunger pains can be reduced by a small dose of morphine. (see *Steroids*)

9. If a **broncho-esophageal fistula** develops, the patient complains of coughing after fluids. The cough can sometimes be reduced by taking semisolids (custard, jello) while at an angle of 45 degrees. The insertion of a tube can seal a fistula, and should be considered in a patient with a relatively good prognosis. In most patients aspiration pneumonia supervenes after a few days, and should be treated symptomatically (with morphine and scopolamine).

10. Patients with **total dysphagia** can still enjoy the taste of different drinks even though they have to spit them out. They have to spit out saliva, and reducing saliva with an anti-cholinergic drug can be helpful.

★ **In total dysphagia, nasogastric feeding, parenteral feeding and gastrostomy can have a place in exceptional circumstances for a very few patients, but are usually best avoided as they can prolong a distressing death.** (see *Nutrition*)

DYSPNEA

Dyspnea means a distressing difficulty in breathing. It is a symptom, not a sign. A patient may have difficulty breathing and yet have no abnormal physical signs.

Incidence — Shortness of breath is reported in about 40% of cancer patients on admission to a hospice, (and in 70% of those with lung cancer). Most of these patients have mild shortness of breath on exertion, which is part of the picture of increasing weakness. Only about 5% to 10% of patients have distressing dyspnea that severely limits their mobility.

Sudden onset of dyspnea suggests arrythmia, embolus or left ventricular failure due to a myocardial infarction. Onset over hours or days suggests infection or effusion. Gradual onset over weeks suggests tumor growth or anemia (or rarely multiple pulmonary emboli).

Episodic shortness of breath is usually due to hyperventilation. Any patient with both dyspnea and cancer is prone to episodes of anxiety or panic. However it can occasionally be due to arrythmias, broncho-esophageal fistula or pulmonary emboli.

Treatable Causes of Dyspnea	Treatment
Anemia	Blood transfusion
Cardiac failure	Diuretics
Pleural effusion	Aspiration
Pericardial effusion	Aspiration
Pneumothorax	Chest drain
Bronchospasm	Bronchodilators
Lung infection	Antibiotics
Lobar collapse	Radiotherapy
Superior Vena Cava (SVC) obstruction	Radiotherapy
Ascites	Paracentesis
Pulmonary emboli	Anti-coagulants

Management options:

1. Morphine
2. Bronchodilators
3. Theophylline, aminophylline
4. Nebulized local anesthetic
5. High dose steroids
6. Physiotherapy
7. Reassurance
8. Breathing exercises
9. Relaxation therapy
10. Anxiolytics
11. (Oxygen)
12. (Nabilone)

1. **Morphine** reduces the inappropriate and excessive respiratory drive which is a feature of dyspnea. A low dose is often sufficient in a patient who is not already taking morphine. A starting dose for treating dyspnea should be 2.5mg to 5mg of oral morphine every 4 hours. It reduces inappropriate tachypnea (rapid breathing) and over-ventilation of the large airways (dead space). It does not cause CO_2 retention used in this way, and it can even reduce cyanosis by slowing ventilation and making breathing more efficient. Doses above 10mg to 20mg every 4 hours are unlikely to give further benefit. Morphine can be given via a nebulizer.

2. **Bronchodilators** are very important because many patients have an unexpected airways obstruction that can

be reversed, improving if not abolishing dyspnea. Nebu-lized adrenergic drugs and/or anti-cholinergic broncho-dilators every 4 hours may be much more effective for weak patients than metered-dose aerosols, and should always be considered for a patient with dyspnea which is not responding to other measures, even if expiratory wheeze is not clinically obvious.

3. **Theophylline and aminophylline** can reduce dyspnea in COPD, not just as a bronchodilator (having an additive effect with adrenergic stimulants), but also by improving ventricular function by peripheral vasodilation. The slow-release oral preparations should be used.

4. **Nebulized local anesthetic** can reduce dyspnea (and cough) in some patients, particularly those with bilateral diffuse disease or lymphangitis carcinomatosa. It can be effective as a single night-time dose, or used every 4 hours if necessary. (An ultrasound or jet nebulizer can be used, but a mouthpiece should be used rather than a mask.) It causes pharyngeal numbness, and the patient should be warned not to eat or drink for 30 minutes after treatment, to avoid choking. It is a technique still being evaluated and the patient should be closely observed during treatment. (see Cough)

5. **High dose steroids** (dexamethasone 8mg per day) can improve breathing if there is airways obstruction and some-times if there is lymphangitis carcinomatosa (when there may be no abnormal physical signs). SVC obstruction may respond, but radiotherapy should always be considered. A week's trial of high dose steroids is also considered if dysp-nea has not responded to other measures.

6. **Appropriate therapies** by a skilled physiotherapist, respiratory therapist and/or relaxation therapist are usually the key elements in managing patients with dyspnea, and can transform the life of these patients, enabling them to cope psychologically and to extend their range of day-to-day activities. Breathing exercises, relaxation techniques and teaching the patient (and family) how to clear secre-tions by gentle shaking of the chest wall may all be involved. (Most patients are too ill for a full program of postural drainage to be appropriate.) Nebulized saline can be help-ful to loosen secretions prior to therapy. (see Physical Therapy)

7. **Reassurance** is effective if the patient feels trust (partly induced by a detailed assessment and examination prior to reassuring). Explanations from all team members need to be the same, so good communication is essential. Reassu-

rance usually needs to be repeated. Common fears are of suffocating or choking to death, and these usually need to be discussed in detail.

The nurse and doctor must examine, explain and reassure. ("You are noticing your breathing, a bit like after running very hard, but parts of your lungs are working well, and the air is going out and in normally. The medicines will help the breathing.") This sort of explanation usually needs to be repeated many times over. Most patients with dyspnea fear that their breathing will get worse and worse, but a peaceful end can be guaranteed, even though in extremely severe cases it has to be by heavy sedation.

8. **Breathing exercises** focus on exhaling completely, lowering the shoulders, and inhaling by moving lower ribs as well as breathing abdominally with the diaphragm. Performed correctly they slow respiration, making it more efficient. The patient often feels more in control by having something he can do about the situation during episodes of breathlessness.

9. **Relaxation therapy** is an essential part of management. Most patients with dyspnea have episodes of panic which tend to cause hyperventilation and worsening dyspnea. Relaxation therapy can reduce the incidence of hyperventilation. It is also helpful during episodes. One patient who was markedly improved said, "Now, when I feel breathless, I know what to think." (see *Relaxation*)

10. **Anxiolytics** can be very helpful, but should be used in conjunction with relaxation therapy and breathing exercises. Diazepam 2mg 3 times a day is often helpful without causing excessive sedation. If the patient already feels drowsy, consider haloperidol 3mg to 5mg 2 times a day.

11. **Oxygen therapy is rarely helpful in chronic dyspnea.** Blood gases are often normal, and relatively few patients are breathless due to hypoxia (end-stage fibrosing alveolitis and COPD can be exceptions). If the patient wants oxygen for psychological reasons, nasal prongs are definitely preferable to a mask which makes talking and eating difficult and cuts the patient off from others (and severely dries out the mouth if not humidified). **Most patients should be weaned off oxygen once other methods are instituted.**

12. **Nabilone** is a synthetic derivative of cannabis with both bronchodilator and sedative properties, which has been used as a second-line drug to morphine for control of chronic dyspnea. It has to be started at low doses (0.1mg 2 times a day) and gradually increased. There is a risk of arrythmias. It remains experimental.

Severe dyspnea — In severe dyspnea even at rest, the patient needs to know that he will not be left alone. An electric fan or humidifier at the bed is often psychologically helpful. Nursing care involves careful positioning (45 degrees usually feels most comfortable), and helping the patient to achieve as much independence as is compatible with his dyspnea. The patient usually prefers people not to crowd round. If the patient remains very distressed despite all possible measures, it may be necessary to give morphine and diazepam in high enough doses to relieve distress, even if this causes drowsiness or unconsciousness.

Terminal bubbling — Secretions in the large airways are occasionally distressing to the patient. More commonly the patient is unconscious and the bubbling "death rattle" distresses the family. Scopolamine 0.4mg IM every 3 to 4 hours, or by continuous subcutaneous infusion, often helps. Sucking out secretions is effective only for a short time. Turning the patient sometimes reduces the bubbling noise. (see *Terminal Phase*)

Note on nebulizer therapy — The **jet nebulizer** works by a stream of compressed air or oxygen which draws the liquid up through a capillary by the venturi effect and then atomizes it into an aerosol of tiny droplets of variable size. 4ml to 6ml of drug solution should be combined with an oxygen flow rate of 6L to 8L/min. During nebulization the solution cools by about 12°C which can cause bronchospasm in some individuals.

The **ultrasonic nebulizer** depends on the high frequency vibration of a piezo-electrical crystal (which vibrates when an electric current is passed across it). The crystal is focused on the surface of the liquid to create a fountain of droplets. Particle size tends to be larger (4 to 10 microns) than with jet nebulizers. Some of the energy from the crystal is converted into heat so that the aerosol is warmer.

Droplets between 1 to 5 microns in diameter reach all parts of the lung right down to the alveoli in normal individuals. Most particles above 8 microns are deposited in the oropharynx. (Droplet size can be measured by collecting the nebulized mist on a thin film of oil on a microscope slide.)

About 12% of the nebulized drug actually reaches the lungs; the rest is either exhaled or stays in the apparatus. In a metered dose inhaler, about 9% of the drug reaches the lungs.

EDEMA

About 20% of terminally ill patients develop ankle edema (excess fluid in tissue spaces).

Ankle swelling reduces mobility, due to:
- Weight gain
- Heavy legs
- Ill-fitting shoes.

There are usually several causes acting together:
- Fluid retention (steroids, NSAIDs)
- Immobility (gravitational)
- Abdominal pressure (hepatomegaly)
- Protein deficiency (low serum albumin)

Other causes include:
- Unilateral deep vein thrombosis
- IVC obstruction (renal cancer)
- Heart failure (raised jugular venous pressure)

Management options:
1. Stop or change drugs if possible
2. Exercise
3. Compression stockings
4. Leg elevation
5. Diuretics
6. Improved nutrition

1. Consider **stopping or changing drugs** that cause fluid retention (steroids, NSAIDs, estrogens).

2. **Exercise** reduces edema because the calf muscle acts as a pump ("the second heart"), improves circulation and reduces venous back-pressure. Walking is best but exercises can help. If a patient is either walking or has his legs well-elevated, edema does not occur. Sitting still for long periods worsens edema.

3. **Compression stockings** will reduce edema. They are worn all day and removed at night. They must be full length to the top of the thigh. (Below-knee stockings cause discomfort and pressure behind the knee.) Compression stockings can be helpful for active patients, especially if diuretics cannot be used (prostatism or frequency due to

bladder tumor, for example). They are difficult to put on, however, and should not be used by weak patients or where edema is unimportant.

4. **Leg elevation** is often recommended, but it is ineffective if it involves "putting your feet up on a stool". This can worsen gravitational edema by discouraging activity. Leg elevation is effective only when the legs are raised to the level of the right atrium (ankle edema is always improved after sleeping in bed). It can be effective if the patient lies down from 30 to 60 minutes with pillows under his legs.

5. **Diuretics** are the mainstay of treatment, but diuretics cause a diuresis and for very ill, weak patients the urinary frequency may be very troublesome. ("I'd rather have the swollen ankles.") Diuretics should be given early in the day to avoid frequency at night, and should be used cautiously in men with prostatic symptoms (poor stream, difficulty starting). (see *Diuretics*)

6. **Increased dietary protein** is helpful only if serum albumin levels are low, if the diet has been poor, and if the patient still has a good appetite.

EMERGENCIES

1. Severe pain
2. Spinal cord compression
3. Superior Vena Cava (SVC) obstruction
4. Seizures
5. Hemorrhage
6. Acute urinary retention
7. Pathological fracture
8. Hypercalcemia
9. Panic attacks
10. Psychosis

1. **Severe pain is a medical emergency**, which requires an immediate response from the hospice or palliative care team. Hopefully the doctor has written orders allowing nurses to immediately increase the dose of morphine when necessary, and will promptly re-assess the patient and write new orders for analgesia at a higher range of doses. (see *Introduction, Morphine, Pain*)

2. **Spinal cord compression** requires immediate high dose steroids and same day radiotherapy (which have a

chance of reversing symptoms if started within 24 hours of onset). (*see Spinal Cord Compression*)

3. **SVC obstruction** can occasionally occur suddenly, with dyspnea and extended neck veins. Urgent radiotherapy may be indicated, but sudden onset suggests that thrombosis has caused complete obstruction, and if the patient is very weak it should be managed as a terminal event. (*see Superior Vena Cava Obstruction*)

4. **Seizures** are best managed by diazepam enemas 10mg which can be repeated until the seizure is controlled. (The rectal route works as quickly as intravenous diazepam.) (*see Seizures*)

5. **Hemorrhage** heavy enough to be called an emergency is thankfully rare. Sometimes the patient dies before drugs can be given. Rapid sedation is difficult because the patient is shocked, veins are difficult to find and peripheral circulation is poor (so IM injections are less effective). Give diazepam enemas as for seizures and a combination of morphine, chlorpromazine and scopolamine IV or IM. Resuscitation and blood transfusion are considered only if the bleeding site can be controlled — otherwise it is dealt with as a terminal event. (*see Bleeding*)

6. **Acute retention of urine** is very distressing. There can be no justification for the upheaval of in-patient admission or a trip to the emergency ward merely for catheterization. A good hospice nurse or doctor carries a supply of catheters!

7. **Pathological fracture** of a vertebra, arm or leg is frightening and can be painful (especially the fracture of a vertebra). First aid involves stabilization and analgesia and then orthopedic fixation whenever possible. Internal fixation of a limb bone is important even if the patient is bed-bound and has a prognosis of only a few weeks, because such fractures are demoralizing and painful, and make comfortable nursing care very difficult.

For a fractured shaft of femur, if the patient is too ill for surgery, apply skin traction with a 5lb to 8lb weight (a catheter bag full of water) and consider an injection of 10ml 0.5% bupivacaine with 80mg (2ml) methylprednisolone into the fracture site using a long needle. (*see Fractures*)

8. **Hypercalcemia** can occasionally present suddenly with confusion, weakness and polyuria occurring over 24 to 48 hours. When this happens the blood calcium level is usually above 16.0mg/dL [4.0mmol/L], and the patient needs intravenous fluids and IV etidronate disodium to bring the calcium levels down. Maintenance therapy with oral phosphate will then be needed. (*see Hypercalcemia*)

9. **Panic attacks** are the commonest emergency situation. Whatever precipitates the panic, the underlying problem is fear. Company from a close relative or a trusted nurse usually helps more than anything else. Sedation may be necessary, and options include IV or rectal diazepam 10mg, or IM haloperidol 5mg to 10mg.

If severe panic and feelings of terror occur in a patient who is near death (for example, with broncho-pneumonia present) the patient needs sedation with a combination of morphine, chlorpromazine and scopolamine. (see *Terminal Phase*)

10. **Psychotic symptoms** are surprisingly rare. If a depression develops into agitation and obsessive rumination there can be, **on rare occasions**, a place for electro-convulsive therapy.

EUTHANASIA

★   **"Euthanasia would be a negative answer to a problem that can be solved by positive action."** (Cicely Saunders)

In advanced disease the patient's interests and rights mainly concern how he lives his remaining days and how he dies. The doctor's duty is to care for the patient in good faith and in the patient's best interests. In the case of a patient near death, stopping certain treatment (but **never** treatment to relieve pain and other distressing symptoms) may be appropriate to the patient's best interests.

The well known medical aphorism still applies:

> *"Thou shalt not kill,*
> *but shalt not strive,*
> *officiously to keep alive."*

This brief discussion focuses on the issue of voluntary euthanasia (when a patient requests death and someone else kills him). A conscious competent patient has the right to refuse life-sustaining treatment, but does not have the right to be killed.

The timely withdrawal of life support machines is a separate issue, and is **not** "passive euthanasia", as it is too often mis-labelled by those who advocate voluntary euthanasia. Advocates of voluntary euthanasia occasionally even argue that adequate pain control somehow constitutes "passive euthanasia" because use of morphine allegedly "shortens life". There is simply no credible medical evidence for this assertion. (The appropriate use of morphine in titrated doses to reduce or abolish pain can on occasion **extend** life by releasing a patient from his physical suffering.)

Patients facing death or dependence sometimes ask "Can't you put an end to it all?" It is often a question asked by those who most fear dying. On further discussion it rarely means "Please kill me", but rather "Will I get pain?" or "Do you understand how awful it is to be dependent on others?" or "Am I being a burden?" Sometimes it is a way of introducing a specific fear that the patient finds difficult to discuss, or a plea for some control over his situation, or for some understanding. **Very rarely is it a request to be killed.**

Euthanasia is illegal. Those in favor of legalizing voluntary euthanasia argue that individuals have the right to self-determination and a right to make choices about how and when they die. Hospice care also emphasizes giving control back to patients and allowing them (and helping them) to make their own decisions. **A person's right to die cannot be translated into a right to be killed, nor into a duty upon someone to kill him.** Euthanasia may sometimes appear a helpful way to put an end to everyone's suffering. In fact, legalized euthanasia would increase suffering.

The main arguments against euthanasia are:

1. It is morally wrong to kill. Any other rule or law in a society is open to abuse.

2. Legalized euthanasia would put pressure on the elderly, the disabled and the dependent. ("I'm such a burden, maybe I ought to ask for it.") A human being is infinitely precious. None of us can judge our own or other people's lives as worthless.

3. Legalized voluntary euthansia would be open to abuse. In theory the person would repeatedly and voluntarily request death, but pressure could be brought to bear on that person in many subtle ways to consider doing this, both by family members and professionals.

4. Legalized euthanasia would promote the attitude that an illness may get so bad that "I may end up asking to be killed." With genuinely compassionate and competent care that need never be the case.

5. Killing a patient would become a therapeutic option. The basic principle of the medical profession is as a servant of life, and the public has a right to absolute trust in that assumption.

6. No one has pure motives (and some people have bad intentions). Even caring family members sometimes say

"We just can't cope", when with a bit of extra support they cope very well and (on looking back) are proud of their achievement. Persuading a person to request euthanasia might appear a tidy solution to an emotionally painful or practically inconvenient situation, but it would bring great guilt to the family, just as a suicide in a family brings guilt and suffering, because any act of killing is wrong.

7. Patients are vulnerable and open to persuasion by a doctor they trust. Doctors who practiced euthanasia could bring considerable non-verbal pressure to bear on patients by their attitudes, and unscrupulous doctors might deliberately put pressure on patients to consider this option.

8. If actively killing a patient became a therapeutic option, the unthinkable would become all too thinkable. There already have been very occasional incidents where health professionals (singly or jointly) have taken it upon themselves to end the lives of elderly or comatose patients (without consent), in effect to relieve their own suffering.

9. Who would do it? Most doctors and nurses would not want to be involved with active killing. Indeed, nurses often feel very guilty if a terminally ill patient dies shortly after a perfectly appropriate injection of drugs given to relieve suffering.

10. We do not know the future. Important things can happen to a person in the last few days of his life, and important things can happen to the whole family, too. It is often a time of reconciliation, reaffirmation and growth. For those who work in hospice and palliative care this is one of the strongest arguments against euthanasia.

Extracts of a letter from a nurse:

"I'd like to share with you my experience of dealing with physicians at the hospital where Sandra P. was admitted (after requesting euthanasia), having attempted suicide. She was in mental torment, curled up in the fetal position, not communicating. The resident physician said he did not feel it was worth getting psychiatric help. I asked to see the attending physician who told me, (quote) 'We don't usually refer these people to a psychiatrist'. I asked what he meant by "these people" and he said 'She's got cancer'. I kept insisting Sandra needed some kind of help, and she was finally transferred to the hospice. I went there to see her before she died. She was very pleased to see me . . . She was smiling, relaxed and more at peace than I had seen her for a long time . . . "

In the secure environment of an in-patient hospice Sandra was encouraged to express her fears and anguish, and her sense of worthlessness. A combination of good physical care and counselling helped her regain her self-control. She was visited and taken out for walks in a wheelchair by her son (whom she had previously refused to see). She died peacefully and naturally about a week later.

EXPLANATION

The original meaning of the word doctor was teacher. At one time the main role of the physician was to explain disease processes to patients and families.

"During my illness I was struck by the great need for information that both patients and their families had . . . they often needed explanation again and again." (Vicky Clement-Jones, a doctor and cancer patient)

★ **Explanation is an essential part of good hospice and palliative care.**

The aims of explanation are:

- To convey information
- To reduce uncertainty
- To increase trust

Clear explanation can be analgesic. For example, abdominal pains are more bearable when it is explained that they are due to constipation and not the spread of cancer. Any new symptom can be very frightening when you have cancer. Even explaining that it is part of the same disease process can make the situation feel more manageable.

In explaining, the following points are important:

1. Ask questions first
2. Categorize
3. Be simple and specific
4. Avoid jargon and euphemisms
5. Repeat (and get the patient to repeat)
6. Use diagrams
7. Use booklets and pamphlets

★ **Information is not retained if the patient is anxious, frightened or naked.**

★ **Facts alone do not reduce fears. Explanation is only one part of reassurance. Fears have to be expressed before they can be worked through.** (see Reassurance)

1. **Ask questions first.** The first step in explaining anything is to **find out what the person already knows**. This highlights misunderstandings and areas of ignorance, and also gives some ideas about a person's belief system. Explanations have to take into account (and "fit") a person's deeply held beliefs.

Questions also help to clarify whether in fact the person wants any further information at all. Do not give unrequested information. It may cause anxiety or anger and is rarely helpful.

2. **Explicit characterization** ("I'm going to tell you two things. First, . . .") provides a helpful framework and improves retention of the information.

3. It is important to be **clear and simple**. A person can rarely retain more than two to three new pieces of information at once. First words are remembered best.

4. **Avoid jargon.** Even words that become commonplace to the professional (catheter, injection, suppository) can be jargon. Assume nothing. We tend to make assumptions all the time about another person's knowledge. It is safest to assume a person does not understand your words and you do not understand his.

5. **Repeat important information.** Repetition helps the memory but it is also a message that you think this information is particularly important. It helps to allow the patient to repeat the information if he wishes, to help confirm that your message was clear.

6. **Diagrams** can be very helpful in explanation. Drawings and pictures (for example, a diagram of where the tumor is inside him and what it is pressing on) can be given to the person to keep, and this can sometimes help a person to feel more in control of the situation.

7. **Booklets and pamphlets** giving concise explanations or general information can be very helpful. These can reinforce a discussion, improve compliance, and increase patient satisfaction. (*see Prescribing*)

★   **Find out what the patient wants to know.**

★   **Avoid giving unrequested information.** (*see Advice*)

★   **Explanation of important information may need to be given to the whole family.** (*see Breaking Bad News, Communication Problems*)

EYE PROBLEMS

Orbital metastases occur most commonly in carcinoma of the breast and malignant melanoma.

They cause:

- Pain
- Proptosis (protrusion of the eyeball)
- Double vision

Visual loss occurs only if a choroidal deposit bleeds into the eye. Early radiotherapy, usually 3,000cGy over 10 days, is indicated to prevent permanent visual loss in patients with carcinoma of the breast who have a reasonable prognosis.

Double vision (diplopia) can occur with raised intracranial pressure (due to pressure on the sixth cranial nerve) or with metastases to the base of the skull (most commonly seen with carcinoma of the breast). High dose steroids and/or radiotherapy to the base of the skull can be helpful. Meanwhile, wearing a patch over one eye relieves the double vision.

Field defects are caused by tumor damage to the optical pathways in the optic nerves or brain. The defect is most often hemianopsia (loss of peripheral vision on one side only). The patient's central vision is normal but loss of peripheral vision can reduce independence and mobility. The patient may fail to notice the defect for some time. Some patients need reassurance that they will not go blind.

Blurred vision can be due to anti-cholinergic drugs (tricyclics, scopolamine, atropine). Occasionally patients on morphine notice intermittent blurring — consider reducing the dose.

Poor vision can add to a patient's problems.

Consider:

- New prescription for eyeglasses
- Stronger lighting
- Magnifier
- Large print books
- Talking books

Dry eyes can occur if the eyelids do not close properly (for example, due to a seventh nerve lesion). Use artifical tears (hypomellose drops) or close the eyelid with hypoallergenic paper tape or even a tarsorrhaphy.

FAMILY MEETINGS

(see Family Therapy, Talking with Families)

Definition — A family meeting is a discussion with involved family members and the caring team to exchange information and improve communications. The patient can be included.

★ **There is often no better way of caring for a patient than demonstrating that the professionals are also concerned about the family.**

What is the aim? — The first aim of a family meeting is to meet some of the needs of each member of the family — needs for information, explanation and the opportunity to safely express and share feelings.

The second important aim is to emphasize that care is family-centered, and that members of a family cope best in a crisis when they support each other.

Discussion — A family meeting is a valuable, and in the long term often a time-saving, method of improving communications among professionals and within the family. It is an essential component of care, and is probably the most neglected aspect of patient care in hospitals (and occasionally in home care settings, too).

Ideally, it should be part of the normal intake procedure to offer to meet the patient with any family members or close friends he would like to have with him. A specific invitation is important. ("We would like to meet with you and your family.") All families benefit from this approach, but it is especially important for families with young children.

★ **Families brought together talk together. They are the experts in the details of their own problems. A single family meeting convened at a time of crisis is often enough to enable a family to solve problems and find new energy for the future.**

Most patients welcome the opportunity to be drawn back into their family circle. Often illness has stripped the person of established family roles and responsibilities. Relationships are often strained through fear or embarrassment at discussing sensitive topics like cancer or dying. ("We didn't want to upset him.") Professionals sometimes unwittingly worsen communication by the incompetent breaking of bad news. ("The doctor told us not to tell him.")

Illness and death can isolate family members as they withdraw into their own particular worries or grief. Meeting a patient alone, and meeting family members without the patient's presence, tends to further split relationships and emphasizes the isolation of the patient. A brief family meeting can strengthen relationships and encourage feelings of shared security. Just sitting down together to talk (free of TV and interruptions!) may be an unusual and strengthening experience. As painful subjects are shared, tension is released.

Patients commonly worry about their families, but many worries and fears go unspoken. A family meeting usually brings relief to patient and family members as these issues are discussed together. For caring relatives, the family meeting emphasizes their strengths. ("You have coped so well up to now.") It can boost their confidence to see that they are in **partnership** with a team of professionals.

Even if the offer of a family meeting is initially refused, the invitation itself is a significant message. It should be gently repeated because resistance and denial are often overcome in time, and the results are almost always beneficial. The visits of family members or close friends who live far away provide useful opportunities for a renewed invitation.

The idea of meeting a whole family (including a very ill person who may be near death) is a frightening prospect for many doctors and nurses. It usually requires experience and learning-by-apprenticeship to feel comfortable with this approach. Psycho-social professionals **who have training and experience in working with families** should involve doctors and nurses whenever possible to demonstrate the many benefits of meeting a family together.

It is important to document the event of the meeting in the clinical notes to maintain communication among professionals. Record who attended, and summarize significant conversations or problems. Note any decisions or conclusions.

FAMILY THERAPY

(see *Communication Problems, Talking with Families*)

Some current concepts of family therapy are very helpful when working alongside families in crisis. In simple terms any attempt to help a family adjust to problems could be called family therapy. In fact, family therapy is evolving as a specialized and effective form of counseling which enables

families to adjust in healthy ways to problems and difficulties, often long-term ones.

**The knowledge and skills of a family therapist are appli-
cable to helping families in crisis.** More work is needed to
define useful interventions in terms of family counseling
around the time of a death. Some basic concepts from
family therapy are outlined here.

There are many different types of families, each with
particular problems and needs, including single parent,
divorced, separated by distance, extended, fostered, com-
munal, step-families and others. Although all families have
certain characteristics in common, it is important not to
assume that one family is like another, or like our own
family.

**When talking to families and when helping them to com-
municate together it is helpful to remember the characteristics of a family, which are:**

1. An interdependent system
2. A life-cycle of development
3. A common history
4. A future together

1. **A family is an interdependent system.** Changes in one
person affect all the family members. It can be very helpful
to say to a family "This problem is affecting all of you ", or
"This cancer is really here in the middle of you all." It can
be important to know who is part of the system, and to ask
"Who is missing from this family?" For example, grandpar-
ents often wish to be included (even once) in a family
meeting and can bring vital new understanding.

Communication within a family often follows a pattern.
Disputes tend to be settled in similar ways. As a family
develops it must be able to change these patterns from time
to time — by open communication and willingness to
change. Failure to adapt results in conflict. Pathological
ways of coping with conflict usually involve blaming other
family members, either by labeling one member (usually a
child) as "sick", or by creating coalitions (the basis of prolonged family feuds which commonly date from a major
crisis such as a death). These pathological patterns can be
prevented around the time of a crisis by encouraging a
family to share their feelings and to **witness each other's
distress**. ("Can you tell us all what it has been like for you to
be a daughter with a very ill mother?") The family counselor
must avoid singling out individuals for responsibility or
blame. **Problems belong to the whole family.**

131

2. **A family has a life cycle.** A normal family develops and changes. Periods of transition occur (a new school or new job, adolescence, marriage, new in-laws, a new baby, retirement) when a family must negotiate new roles and new boundaries. **A major crisis such as a terminal illness in the family may occur during an already stressful transitional phase.** For example, a particular conflict occurs for adolescent children with a seriously ill parent. The normal role of adolescents is to move away from the family, but the illness will tend to draw them back. This can result in powerful feelings of confusion and resentment.

Another difficult situation occurs when parents return to help nurse a married child, become possessive, and exclude the spouse. Parents will normally have stepped back years before to allow the independent couple to make their own decisions. Yet now they may also feel powerfully drawn to nurse their sick child. The counselor needs to ask "What are the pressures and priorities for this family apart from the obvious major crisis?"

3. **A family has a history.** Attitudes and feelings within a family are partly inherited from the past. An impending loss will re-awaken memories of previous losses. **Responses to a loss are more easily understood when previous losses are explored.** Drawing a family tree can be a good way of starting a useful discussion. (see Family Tree)

Family myths and beliefs may be difficult to challenge. Myths and secrets in a family are intended to be protective, but can also put considerable pressure on individuals to behave in certain ways. A family can be helped to re-experience the past and feel less burdened by it. Unresolved grief is the cause of many long-standing family problems. **A death of another family member is an opportunity to re-explore these events from the past.**

> A delinquent boy (and his family) were seen at the time of the death of his grandfather. The family was asked about previous experiences of loss. The boy's father recounted how his own brother had died in an accident at the age of 11. He felt blamed for the accident and a poor substitute for his dead brother ("who was so clever"). The father retold the story for the first time in the presence of his family. Witnessing this grief helped to release his own son from the family myth that the "boys in our family are dumb".

4. **A family has a future.** Even though one member is dying, the family will live on. A crisis is also an opportunity. **"We are not only dealing with present problems ... we are**

modeling a way of coping with future living." (Elisabeth Earnshaw-Smith)

One reason why a cancer death is usually less traumatic to a family than a sudden death is because there is time for anticipatory grief work. The events around the time of a death will powerfully affect the future of individual family members. **It is mutually strengthening when a family (including the dying member) can be helped to discuss the future.** The dying person can retain some control, for example, by discussing the future care of the children, or by teaching a spouse to take over roles and skills.

Anticipatory grief work is often sad, but it can be rewarding. The patient's common worry is "How will they cope without me?" Discussion helps to reduce the isolation of the dying person and is of considerable benefit to the rest of the family in their future adjustment and grief.

> *Mrs. L.T., 12 months after her husband had died from cancer, said "We were very close. For a long time we didn't talk about it. We wanted to protect each other. Then the doctor talked to both of us. I felt angry at the time, but my daughter said, 'It's not the doctor, Mom. It's the fact that Dad's ill.' But by the end he came to accept it. Before he died he said to me 'I have to leave you now and I want you to let me go.' Those words are a great comfort to me now."*

FAMILY TREE (GENOGRAM)

The family tree (genogram) is a simple and very useful tool to promote discussion at a family meeting, or with an individual patient. It also serves as a useful record in the clinical notes.

Drawing a genogram should be a routine part of the initial assessment of a patient. It focuses the attention of the carers on the family as the unit of care, and can remind a patient of the family support available.

Important and relevant information almost always emerges when a family tree is used.

This may include:
- Fears (Who died of cancer?)
- Hopes (Whom do you want to see?)
- Unfinished business (Whom do you feel close to?)

FAMILY TREE

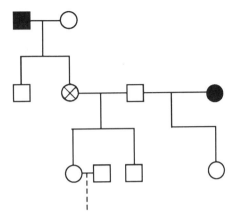

This relatively simple family tree might lead to consideration and discussion of the following information and issues:

- Father died of cancer (Does it "run in the family"?)
- Mother is frail ("Should we tell her?")
- Brother lives abroad ("When should he come home?")
- Husband's first wife died of cancer ("She was in terrible pain.")
- First grandchild expected in four months ("Will I live?")
- Son is "never at home these days"
- Step-daughter is estranged

— KEY FOR DRAWING A FAMILY TREE —

Keep each generation on its own line.

☐	Man (■ Dead)
○	Woman (● Dead)
⊗	Patient (Woman)
⊠	Patient (Man)
○——☐	Married
○—/—☐	Separated

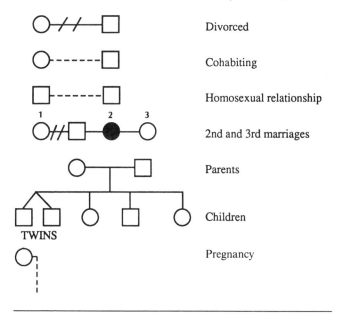

Divorced

Cohabiting

Homosexual relationship

2nd and 3rd marriages

Parents

Children

Pregnancy

TWINS

FECAL INCONTINENCE

Fecal incontinence is a dreaded symptom.

The main causes are:

1. Diarrhea
2. Impacted feces
3. Rectal carcinoma
4. Recto-vaginal fistula
5. Malignant spinal cord compression

1. **Acute diarrhea** can cause incontinence in the elderly, or if disability and weakness prevent quick access to the toilet. Exclude possible fecal impaction and treat with loperamide 2mg to 4mg 4 times a day. (*see Diarrhea*)

2. **Impacted feces** results in small amounts of liquid feces, often with loss of control, after a period of constipation. (*see Constipation*)

3. **Rectal carcinoma** (either untreatable primary carcinoma or anastomotic recurrence) can cause fecal incontinence due to sphincter damage, together with blood, discharge and smell. Palliative colostomy can divert feces but will not reduce blood and discharge. Local treatments such as transanal laser therapy can be helpful. Smell is reduced by metronidazole 250mg to 500mg 3 times a day, and regular changes of pads. (*see Lasers*)

4. **Recto-vaginal fistula** occurs as a complication of pelvic malignancies, or following radiation damage. The patient may be too embarrassed to describe the true situation. A palliative colostomy should be performed whenever possible.

5. Loss of anal sphincter tone is a late complication of **malignant spinal cord compression**. It is usually best managed by inducing constipation with codeine phosphate 30mg to 60mg every 4 hours (or simply by stopping laxatives if the patient is already taking morphine), and clearing the rectum with enemas or manually every third day. (see *Spinal Cord Compression*)

FISTULAS

Fistulas occur in about 1% of patients with advanced cancer. They may be due to malignancy or to a complication of radiotherapy (particularly to the pelvic organs).

Palliative colostomy should be considered whenever possible for a **recto-vaginal fistula** (which causes a distressing continuous leakage of feces from the vagina).

If the patient is too ill to consider surgery management involves:
- Regular cleaning (saline douches)
- Regular change of pads (large pads at night)
- Metronidazole to reduce smell (see *Smells*)
- Anti-fungal pessaries if thrush develops
- Barrier creams (to prevent skin soreness)
- Bowel regulation

Bowel regulation means **avoiding** oral fecal softening agents and emptying the rectum every third day by using oral stimulant laxatives such as senna tablets at bedtime, or suppositories.

A **vesico-vaginal fistula** causes a continuous dribble of urine from the vagina. Urinary diversion procedures (ileal conduit, ureterosigmoidostomy) should be considered if the patient is fit enough. If not, management involves either pads and pants or a urinary catheter. A vaginal tampon is only helpful if the leakage is minimal.

High bowel fistulas contain digestive enzymes. Use barrier creams to prevent skin excoriation.

A **leakage of bile** onto the skin surface can be very difficult to contain. Bile tends to leak through dressings and seals. A useful technique is to apply a colostomy bag that contains absorption flakes. These expand into a gel and "pull" the bile down into the bag, reducing leakage.

A colostomy bag (which must be drainable) can be applied over fistulas to collect fluid. This is a very useful technique to reduce discomfort and smell.

FRACTURES (PATHOLOGICAL)

Almost any malignant tumor can occasionally metastasize to bone, but osteolytic deposits most prone to collapse or fracture are from carcinomas of:

- Breast
- Lung
- Kidney
- Thyroid

Bone metastases are usually painful but pathological fractures can occur when there has been no preceding pain. The axial skeleton and proximal long bones are most commonly affected. (see *Bone Metastases, Bone Pain*)

The aims of treatment are:

- Pain relief
- To preserve mobility whenever possible
- To facilitate nursing care

Assessment — There is pain, deformity and bony crepitus on movement. In a fractured neck of femur the leg is shortened and externally rotated.

X-ray is important to confirm the diagnosis, to plan treatment and to assess the texture of surrounding bone.

First aid — Straighten the limb immediately if there is a marked deformity. Give analgesia as required. The patient is usually frightened and needs reassurance.

Conservative treatment includes analgesia, external splinting, skin traction, and local injection.

Analgesics are only required if there is pain at rest. Pain on movement will not respond to analgesics and is managed by stabilizing the fracture.

★ **If the patient is too ill to consider surgical fixation, the aim of management is to stabilize the fracture and reduce pain enough for the patient to be nursed in comfort.**

Skin traction can very effectively reduce pain, sometimes with a muscle relaxant such as diazepam to reduce muscle spasm. In a patient with a poor prognosis this may be all that is required to relieve pain. A weight of about 5lb to 8lb (a catheter bag filled with water) is usually sufficient.

Local injection into the fracture site using a long needle can sometimes abolish pain for several days. Use 10ml 0.5% bupivacaine with 80mg (2ml) methylprednisolone.

Surgery — Internal fixation is the treatment of choice whenever possible. Immediate referral to an orthopedist is indicated, with a view to prompt treatment and early discharge of the patient.

Radiotherapy — The presence of metal or cement does not interfere with subsequent palliative radiotherapy, which will result in healing of the fracture eventually in about 50% of cases (although pain relief is achieved even in the absence of healing). The usual dose is 2,500cGy in 5 treatments over 2 weeks.

FUNGATING TUMORS

Fungating of cancer onto the skin surface occurs most commonly with carcinoma of the breast, but occurs occasionally at other sites (vulva, rectum). The lesion may be a small dry crusted area needing only a gauze pad, or a large ulcerated area with profuse exudate and capillary bleeding needing dressings 2 times a day. Radiotherapy, chemotherapy or hormone therapy can sometimes produce skin healing.

★ **Fungating lesions are disfiguring, distressing and isolating. The way in which the dressing is done is as important as the dressing itself.**

One method of dressing a large fungating breast carcinoma is as follows:

- Soak off dressing with warm water or in the bath.
- Hold gauze soaked in 1:1,000 adrenaline over any bleeding points until they stop.
- Irrigate with warm saline. Antiseptics are only necessary if there is a heavy infected exudate.

- A small lyofoam dressing may control a persistent bleeding point.
- Irrigate with metronidazole solution or apply sterile metronidazole gel. (The gel is better. It is soothing and stays on the chest wall, and reduces infection and smell. The gel should shortly be available in the United States.) A cheaper alternative is natural yogurt, which is soothing and also reduces anaerobic infection. (Wash off any antiseptic before applying yogurt.)
- Apply a non-adherent dressing. Cavities should be loosely packed with an absorbent non-adherent dressing (such as an alginate dressing).
- Apply foam or other absorbent dressing to soak up exudate.
- Hold dressings in place with tubular elastic netting, which is better than the repeated use of adhesive strapping.
- Place charcoal pads under the netting to absorb smell — these are very effective.

If smell is severe give oral metronidazole 500mg 3 times a day. A broad spectrum antibiotic may be necessary in addition. Smell is very difficult to control if the wound contains black necrotic tissue. This should be removed by painting with streptokinase (an enzymatic desloughing agent) which dissolves the slough. Large areas may need surgical debridement. Avoid chemical desloughing agents which can cause soreness. (see *Pressure Sores*)

GRIEF

Grief is the normal psychological reaction to loss.

Bereavement is the reaction to loss of a loved person.

Mourning is the social expression of grief.

★ **"Dying involves the gradual adjusting to a whole series of losses and disappointments. Each loss causes grief. Very often the earlier losses are harder to cope with than dying itself."** (Colin Murray Parkes)

★ **"The loss of a loved person is one of the most intensely painful experiences any human being can suffer."** (John Bowlby)

Grief is the usual reaction to loss. Understanding the process of grief is important because it affects both the dying person and the bereaved. An understanding of the process, and how it can be facilitated, helps us to draw alongside the dying.

In *Grief Counseling & Grief Therapy*, William Worden writes of the "tasks of mourning", and of grief as a healing process that requires effort. He emphasizes that unresolved grief is a common cause of psychiatric and psychosomatic illness. Where a death is predictable there is time for antici-patory grief to occur. This can be a healing process for both the dying person and for the future of the family. (*see Communication Problems, Family Therapy*)

It is difficult to predict how a person will respond to loss. Every loss is different. The grieving person must have time and space to adjust in his own way. There is no "correct" reaction. The intensity of grief depends on personality, the nature of the relationship, concurrent life crises, and avail-ability of social supports.

Bereavement care starts before the death occurs. The quality of medical and nursing care and support that the patient receives creates powerful memories and affects the bereavement of those who are left. In particular, the way bad news is first communicated will be vividly remem-bered. (*see Breaking Bad News*)

Both the dying patient and the family can and do grieve before the death, which explains why an anticipated death is usually less traumatic than a sudden death. Helping fami-lies to realize this can reduce the alienation that can occur at this time. Sensitive encouragement from professionals can help the family say things that need to be said (often simply "I love you and I will miss you"), which helps con-siderably after the death.

★ **One good memory can replace years of bad memories.**

The events around the time of the death will affect the family in their grief and in future life crises. Anticipatory guidance reduces subsequent problems. Accurate infor-mation, encouragement to express emotions and helping communication between the family and the dying person all help the process of grief. Encourage family members to be present at the time of death and to say good-bye after-wards to the body. This helps to make the loss a reality which can enable the process of grieving to begin.

The tasks of grieving (with thanks to William Worden):

1. To make it real
2. To feel the pain
3. To adjust to the loss

1. **To make it real** — Initial **numbness** is natural, but within a few weeks the person has to **accept** that the deceased has gone. Prolonged denial means the other tasks of grieving cannot be worked through.

Being present at the death, seeing the dead body, saying good-bye, attending the funeral service and talking repeatedly about the event of the death and the feelings about it can help a person to accept the reality of the death.

2. **To feel the pain** — An initial **anxiety state** can occur which is somewhat analogous to the restless searching behavior seen in animals separated from an attachment object. Bereaved persons may be distracted, unable to concentrate, and preoccupied with the deceased. They may become overactive or withdrawn from society. Over 50% of bereaved persons have hallucinations of the deceased.

Physical manifestations (breathlessness, tiredness, tightness in the chest, insomnia) are common. An anxiolytic such as diazepam or lorazepam is helpful only **as a short-term measure** for severe anxiety symptoms or insomnia.

★　　　**Grief itself cannot be suppressed or resolved with drugs.**

Some common feelings are still not generally recognized as part of normal grief, especially **guilt, anger and fatigue**.

Guilt is universal in grief. ("If only . . . ") It may be irrational, or occasionally justified. It needs to be reality-tested. ("How would you have felt if it happened to you?" "If she were here now what would she say?")

Anger is common. ("Look at the mess he's left me in.") Most people feel guilty about feeling angry at the deceased, and displace it on others (threatening to sue the doctor or nurse, for example) or on themselves (causing depression).

All human relationships involve both positive and negative feelings, and it is important that these be brought into balance in grief. Ask "What do you miss about him?" Emphasize positive memories, but give permission to express the negative. Later in grief it can become possible to ask "What don't you miss about him?"

Physical and mental fatigue can be compelling. Simple tiredness occurs from weeks or months of caring for an increasingly ill person, and from making funeral and numerous other necessary arrangements around the time of death. Numbness, restlessness and crying make it difficult to function normally.

3. **To adjust to the loss** — Bereaved persons may need extra support and gentle help in making even simple decisions. A **problem-solving approach** to everyday decisions must be encouraged as they are helped to develop new skills. (see *Support*)

Most bereaved persons can eventually **form new attachments** without feeling they are somehow dishonoring the memory of the deceased. They can think of the deceased without pain, and can start to enjoy their memories. This signals a healthy end of grieving. This stage is sometimes reached within a year but usually takes two or three years, and is sometimes never reached.

If a bereaved person forms a new relationship too soon after losing a spouse, it usually ends in frustration that the replacement person is not a perfect match for the lost partner.

Principles of bereavement support:

- **Grieving takes time.** The person may need extra support in critical periods for at least a year. Critical periods include three months and twelve months after the death, anniversaries and holidays, and religious festivals. Offer continuing support.

- **After visiting, set a specific time to return.** It can be hard for bereaved persons to take the initiative in asking for help.

- **The normal symptoms of grief (restlessness, forgetfulness, poor appetite, insomnia, visions of the deceased) can be frightening.** A bereaved person may fear he is going mad. Just understanding the common symptoms of acute grief, and acknowledging the pain of grief, can help a bereaved person to cope.

- **Avoid platitudes.** ("I know how you feel.") Avoid describing your own losses in detail. This is not helpful. Encourage the bereaved person to talk about the events surrounding the death, and ask about his feelings. This helps him to accept the reality of the loss and to experience the pain of grief.

- A simple **pamphlet** can be very helpful, briefly explaining the normal intense feelings of grief and including information about support groups.

Be aware of those persons who may be particularly at risk of an abnormal grief reaction. They include those who:
- Were over-dependent on the deceased
- Had negative feelings about the deceased
- Are unable to express feelings
- Have concurrent life crises
- Have a history of depression
- Have had difficult reactions to previous losses
- Lack social or family support

About 1 of every 3 persons who suffer a major loss (the death of a child or a spouse, for example) may require special help. Persons who are isolated or severely affected can benefit greatly from regular support given by a competent counselor, from a support group or by trained volunteers.

Pathological grief — If a person fails to work through the tasks of grief, it can become prolonged ("stuck") or exaggerated or may simply present as depression. Pathological grief may require skilled psychotherapy rather than straightforward support and counselling.

Clues to a pathological grief reaction may be:
- Intense grief over two years after the death
- A minor event which triggers intense grief
- Preserving the environment of the deceased
- Showing the same symptoms as the deceased suffered
- Breaking off social contacts
- Phobias about illness or dying
- Prolonged helplessness
- Loss of self-esteem
- Exaggerated anger or guilt
- Changed behavior
- Threats of suicide

Pathological grief can cause years of misery. If it is suspected as a cause of depression a useful first question is "What is the worst thing that has ever happened to you?" Talking about the deceased encourages expression of feelings.

Pathological grief can be due to unfinished business with the deceased person, with whom there was often an ambivalent relationship. The expression of repressed feelings of anger or guilt may need several specialist **sessions of psy-**

chotherapy or psycho-drama, in which these feelings are re-experienced and reality-tested.

Prolonged avoidance of grief can sometimes be overcome by techniques of forced mourning, using "linking objects" (personal possessions or photographs of the dead person) to provoke renewed grief work.

Chronic grief may call for work to improve personal self-esteem. Permission to stop grieving may be needed. The person's purpose in prolonging grief should be explored. (What will this person lose in giving up his grief?)

The psychotherapist often substitutes in part for the deceased, to give comfort and additional support. The psychotherapist must skillfully prepare the grieving person to say good-bye at the end of the therapy.

Grief and the family — Bereavement usually affects a whole family. Therapy for the family unit can be a very effective way of facilitating grief work. Any loss resonates with previous losses, which are often reawakened. Responses to loss are more easily understood in the light of previous losses. Families vary in their ability to express and tolerate feelings and to support each other emotionally. Where grief is not acknowledged it can damage family relations in a number of ways. The role of the deceased in the family may be given inappropriately to a child ("replacement child"). The anger of grief may be displaced onto a family member ("scapegoat") who becomes the target of all wrath. Allowing a family to witness emotional distress in one member can release them to talk about their own feelings. (see *Family Therapy*)

Grieving children can develop psychological disorders. Children most at risk are those bereaved at 3 to 5 years, and in early adolescence. Instinctive protectiveness often leads families to exclude children from bad news. Yet children need to find their own answers to loss and death.

The impact of death depends on the strength of the attachment, which may be as strong to a grandparent as to a parent.

Children often see bereavement in terms of desertion. ("Daddy left me.") They also commonly see death as somehow their fault. These fantasies need to be brought into the open and clarified. Ask the child what he thinks. Children often fear that one death may herald another, particularly if someone else in the family becomes ill. They need reassurance and explanation.

Children cope best when they are included and allowed to witness the sadness of other family members. Children should be gently encouraged to attend the funeral. If they do not, they benefit from an alternative ritual of some kind. One study showed that children who attended funerals had less deviant behavior and increased crying, and that children who cried more (and talked about the lost person) had fewer behavioral and emotional problems.

Children's fears and feelings lie near the surface. Grief is incorporated into play. Playing at "funerals" may seem macabre to adults, but children express their feelings through play. Children also express their concern in practical ways. One child shocked her family by asking "Will the funeral be expensive?" only minutes after her father had died. It sounded callous, yet her immediate concern was the future support of her mother.

Anger may be acted out at school and be mistaken for naughtiness. The parents should be encouraged to stay in close touch with the child's teachers.

Children usually need to ask a lot of questions and need a lot of explanation. Explanation must use the words and concepts of the family's own belief system, which must first be explored. Explanations need to be clear and simple. ("Death means a person stops moving and breathing and is still and peaceful.") **Children can cope well with bereavement provided they are supported and encouraged to grieve. Children do not cope well with the mystification of death. Secrecy is not protective — it causes confusion and isolation.**

> *Mrs. C.M., a 42-year old woman with a glioma, died in an in-patient hospice. She denied her illness, but at a family meeting two weeks before her death one son, Darren (age 6), shocked his parents by suddenly announcing "Mommy is dying, she will be dead before Christmas." Two months later Darren's father phoned the hospice asking for help because Darren's behavior was disturbing. A meeting was arranged with the doctor and social worker. (The room was equipped with ice cream, and paper and pencils for drawing.) As they came into the room, Tommy (age 4), suddenly asked "Can we see the bed where Mommy died?" The boys were taken there, but their father refused to go. When they returned, Tommy announced he "wanted to pee" so his father took him to the toilet. On the way back, Tommy led his father to the room where his mother had died, and showed him the bed.*

The boys had their ice cream, chatted and drew pictures. Darren brought the conversation round to his mother by telling a joke he had made up, about a snowman who wanted a wife. (It emerged that his mother had given him a large poster of a snowman before she died, which hung above his bed.) The father, a quiet man, suddenly said he had recently taken Tommy, the younger boy, to see his mother's grave. The doctor asked why Darren had not gone. The father explained that the grave was in the village churchyard across a busy road, and he was worried Darren might try to go there by himself. The social worker asked Darren if he would like to visit his mother's grave and Darren said he would.

Young children need to mourn. Parents often say "The child is too young to understand" because they need to protect themselves from the idea of their child's sadness and grief. (see *Children, Talking with Children*)

HALITOSIS

Halitosis means foul smelling breath. The usual cause is either **poor oral hygiene** or a **lung abscess**, which still produces halitosis when the patient exhales through the nose.

Metronidazole 250mg to 500mg 3 times a day is active against anerobes and is useful in reducing halitosis due to gingivitis or lung abscess.

Increase **routine oral hygiene** to every hour if necessary. Treat oral thrush. Dentures should be removed at night. Obtain dental treatment as required for caries, gingivitis, etc. (see *Candidiasis, Mouth Care*)

Gentle mouthwashes and oral rinses are useful if there is **oropharyngeal malignancy**. Sodium bicarbonate applied with swabs will remove debris and is less unpleasant than hydrogen peroxide mouthwash.

Oral deodorants (chlorophyll tablets) can be helpful but are short-acting.

HALLUCINATIONS

A hallucination is the illusion of perception when there has been no sensory input. Some patients are very distressed by hallucinations, others are not and may only mention them if asked. ("Have you seen anything strange or unusual lately?")

Hypnogogic hallucinations occur when falling asleep or waking. These are **normal**, and occur in about 50% of people in acute grief. They can be visual or auditory.

Morphine can very occasionally cause hallucinations. If the dose of morphine becomes too high, most patients feel drowsy, a few develop nausea, and a small number hallucinate. **Hallucinations are most common when morphine is started in too high a dosage.** They stop as soon as the dose of morphine is reduced.

Toxic confusional states make patients see things. These are not hallucinations but misperceptions of visual stimuli (patterned wallpaper becomes snakes). The patient is rambling, behaving inappropriately and easily startled. (see *Confusion*)

Brain secondaries very rarely cause hallucinations. Occasionally temporal lobe seizures can cause hallucinations (of smell, taste or hearing), with stereotyped motor behavior (sucking, grimacing, repeated head movements), and, commonly, a feeling of epigastric discomfort. This can be controlled with carbamazepine.

Psychosis can cause hallucinations — usually voices. (Ask "Do you hear voices? What do they say?") There may be a history of psychosis. There is disordered thought with delusions (bizarre beliefs) and paranoia. High doses of haloperidol or chlorpromazine may be needed. (see *Paranoia*)

HEROIN

Should heroin be legalized for pain control in the U.S.A.?

No. As far as the body is concerned, morphine and heroin (diamorphine) are the same drug. Heroin is diacetylmorphine. It is the same molecule as morphine, but with two acetyl (C_2H_5) groups added. It is rapidly metabolized to monoacetylmorphine, then to morphine, in the body. Heroin and morphine have identical effects. Heroin is slightly better absorbed from the gut, so a lower dose (in a ratio of 3:2) is needed to be equi-analgesic. (A patient who is pain-controlled on 30mg oral morphine every 4 hours would be pain-controlled on 20mg oral heroin every 4 hours.)

Clinically, the only advantage of heroin is that it is more soluble than morphine. (500mg of heroin dissolves in 0.8ml of water, as compared to 10ml of water to dissolve 500mg morphine sulfate.) Heroin injections can therefore be of a smaller volume.

HERPES

Both shingles (herpes zoster) and cold sores (herpes simplex) occur with increased frequency in patients with malignancy, especially those who are immuno-suppressed during or after chemotherapy. Shingles is also more common in the elderly due to a natural decline in cell-mediated immunity. Shingles causes a painful eruption of vesicles in one dermatome (a section of skin supplied by one cutaneous nerve).

Persisting pain in the skin after the rash has healed (post-herpetic neuralgia) is more common in the elderly. It occurs in about 10% of patients under 60 and about 40% of those over 60. In about half of these it lasts over a year. It is a nerve pain (burning, stabbing pain which fluctuates in severity and which can be worsened by emotional tension). About 2% of shingles affects the eye. The nasociliary nerve (supplying the tip of the nose and the cornea) is affected. Keratitis and uveitis can occur and can cause loss of vision.

Oral acyclovir in high dosage (800mg 5 times a day for 5 days), started within 48 hours of the rash appearing, can reduce the severity and pain of the rash and will reduce the severity of eye complications. It does not reduce the likelihood of post-herpetic neuralgia. Acyclovir has few side effects because it is activated by an enzyme specific to the herpes virus.

There is no firm evidence that steroids (commonly used) or amantadine (occasionally used) at the time of the rash reduces the incidence or severity of neuralgia.

Post-herpetic neuralgia is difficult to treat and may require a combined approach. (see Nerve Pain)

HICCUP

Intractable hiccups is a rare but distressing problem. It may be due to phrenic nerve irritation (in the neck or mediastinum), gross hepatomegaly elevating the diaphragm, gastric distention (gas or food), or uremia.

Gas may be relieved by peppermint water (which relaxes the lower esophageal sphincter) or by Mylanta, which has an anti-foaming action.

Metoclopramide 10mg to 20mg 4 times a day is often effective. Chlorpromazine 25mg 2 or 3 times a day is also an effective drug, particularly in uremia. For severe hiccups try chlorpromazine IV 25mg.

Radiotherapy to a large mediastinal tumor may be indicated.

Phrenic nerve interruption is a last resort. The nerve can be crushed in the neck under local anesthetic, or a 5% phenol injection can be given into the neck.

HOARSENESS

The common causes of a hoarse voice are:

- Laryngeal thrush (*see Candidiasis*)
- Recurrent laryngeal nerve palsy

Patients often fear that the voice will be lost completely. They can be reassured that this will not occur.

Hoarseness due to laryngeal palsy is usually seen in cancer of the bronchus. It can be treated with a **teflon injection** lateral to the paralyzed cord. This pushes the cord medially so it opposes with the functioning cord, restoring the voice.

HOME CARE

The following issues are important:

1. Choosing the place of care
2. The place of death
3. Symptom control at home
4. Team communication
5. Family communication
6. The burdens on carers
7. Visitors
8. Practical suggestions
9. The terminal phase at home
10. After a home death

1. **Place of care:**

★   **Home can be the very best or the very worst place to die.**

The advantages of home care include:

- Feeling secure
- Flexible routines
- Reduced medical intervention
- The patient remains part of the family
- Control (professionals become the visitors)

On the other hand, isolation and physical suffering can be extreme if patients at home are neglected, if physical symptom control is inadequate, and if family carers (or neighbors and friends) cannot obtain adequate assistance and support.

Even if a patient lives alone, it is still possible to offer home care. Neighbors, friends and community volunteers can sometimes agree to a roster of daily responsibilities. It is best for one person (a neighbor or friend) to assume primary responsibility for liaison with the home care team, and for scheduling.

The prime factor in deciding where a terminally ill patient should be cared for is the patient's own wishes. Some patients feel that a hospital is no place for a person who is seriously ill. Other patients feel more secure in an in-patient setting. Some may fear "becoming a burden to their family" if they choose to stay at home. **It is important to listen carefully to the patient.** While every effort should be made to comply, the patient's wishes have to be considered in light of practical issues such as the availability of professional and volunteer support, and the attitudes and abilities of family members.

Hospice involvement needs to occur early, when patient and family members have time to build trusting relationships with team members. The home care team needs time to make sensible plans.

2. **Place of death:**

★ **Death is a social event, not a medical event.**

One of the most important and difficult questions that professional carers need to ask patients — gently and at the right time — is "If the time comes for you to die, where would you like to be?" One way of raising this issue might be through a discussion about a living will. (see *Living Will*)

The terminal phase in the home is usually straightforward if the family has been well prepared. The family may or may not want a member of the home care team present. This preference should be respected.

As the disease advances, many families are unsure of whether they can continue to cope at home. Appropriate encouragement and support may enable them to do so.

Some families find they simply cannot manage (because of carers' ages, work schedules, traveling distance, or other practical or psychological problems). A planned, timely admission to an appropriate in-patient facility may be necessary. It is essential at this time to encourage discussion between the patient and family to avoid feelings of resentment or guilt.

★ **The precipitate transfer of a patient from home simply to die elsewhere a few hours later can rarely be justified. It is too often the mark of a family poorly supported by professionals.**

3. **Symptom control at home** — Excellent symptom control is almost always possible in the home, given willing carers and a competent home care team.

The most difficult condition to manage at home is **confusion**. (see *Confusion*)

Other difficult problems are **severe diarrhea**, **heavy bleeding** or **seizures**, although even these situations can be managed in the home.

Intestinal obstruction can be managed medically in the home with a continuous subcutaneous infusion of appropriate drugs. **Terminal dehydration** rarely causes thirst, but if thirst becomes a problem in a patient with dysphagia, it can be simply managed in the home by giving a tap water enema using a urinary catheter.

Procedures such as aspiration of pleural effusions or ascites, and some nerve blocks, can all be performed in the home. **There is no justification for sending patients to the hospital for simple procedures like insertion of a urinary catheter.** Even if a brief out-patient visit to the hospital is occasionally needed (for example, for a single dose of radiotherapy for bone pain) the appointment can be precisely scheduled to cause the least possible inconvenience to patient and family.

It is sometimes assumed that some treatments are not suitable for home care, but we need to question whether these beliefs are related to tradition or to practicality. Home care team members must be prepared to act on occasion as advocates not only for their patients, but for home care itself.

4. Team communication:

★ **Communication between the home care team and family members (to explain and reassure) is usually the single most important element in enabling care to take place at home. Home care arrangements can break down if simple reassurance is lacking at a critical moment.**

★ **Family members are part of the caring team.**

Family members are often uncertain about whether they will cope. An encouraging comment from a member of the home care team ("We think with our help you will manage very well.") can give a family enough confidence to continue.

The home care team must communicate together. Care must be coordinated to be effective. **Conflicting advice (especially about prescribing) destroys trust.** Failure of home care team members to keep their promises to patient and family (about the date and time of the next visit, for example), or to respond promptly and courteously to telephone calls, destroys trust.

The home care team must help the family to anticipate problems. Anticipation saves time and energy. For example, if a patient is becoming incontinent, it is wise to cover the mattress with a plastic sheet before it is soiled.

The prepared family will have fully discussed their worries before the terminal phase:

- What will happen?
- Will we cope?
- What about the children?
- How will we know he's dead?
- Whom do we contact if we need to?
- What do we have to do afterwards?

5. Family communication — Many families need help in communicating together when one member is dying.

Poor communication is a common reason for breakdown of home care arrangements. Communication problems often cause tension and irritability. The patient too often becomes isolated by a "conspiracy of silence". No one talks of the illness or of dying, for fear of upsetting the others. A skilled professional or volunteer can often bring great relief to a family simply by **seeing them together**, asking what each understands about the illness, and encouraging them to share their feelings together. ("How is your husband's illness affecting you?") (see *Communication Problems, Family Meetings*)

Children of all ages cope very well with death provided they are included in the event, encouraged to ask questions, allowed to help from time to time, and later encouraged to express their grief (through drawings and play). (see *Children, Grief*)

6. **The burdens of carers** — It is essential for families to organize their own schedule of caregiving. **Carers need to rest**, and to leave the house from time to time.

Carers are often expected to cope with complicated problems, such as:

- Giving medications
- Monitoring symptoms
- Nursing tasks
- Learning new skills (such as lifting and moving the patient)
- Living on a reduced income
- Adapting the home
- Adopting new roles (highly stressful)
- Emotional pressures
- Explaining to others
- Allowing anticipatory grieving

Physical exhaustion leaves less energy for emotional problems. Family carers suffer from emotional exhaustion ("burn out") as well as professionals. (As one daughter said, "Nobody ever asks how I am. I could scream every time the phone rings!") **Hospice day care** and brief in-patient **respite care** can be important in helping fatigued family carers. (see *Burn Out, Day Hospice, Respite Care*)

7. **Visitors** — Too often visitors exhaust both patient and carers. A schedule of visiting times is helpful, and can be organized by a firm, tactful family member or friend. It can bring great relief to ask whether visitors are proving tiring, and for a restriction on times and numbers of visitors to be "prescribed" by the nurse or doctor. (see *Visitors*)

8. **Practical suggestions** — The **ideal sick room** is light and airy, with a comfortable bed, a high armchair, a pleasant view, a convenient telephone, a remote-control TV and an adjacent bathroom. A V-shaped pillow and a light, colorful quilt can make life in bed more bearable. In hot weather, air-conditioning (or at least an electric fan) can be helpful. Most important of all, **the sick room should be one in which the patient feels at ease**, and which is not isolated from the rest of the house.

Home care of terminally ill patients can be made considerably easier by the use of **simple aids and appliances**. Rental is usually preferred to purchase, as different equipment may be needed at different stages. (Some hospices and home health organizations maintain an "equipment closet" for free borrowing.) The use of complicated (and often expensive) medical equipment requiring frequent professional interventions **should be avoided**.

Aids to mobility:

- Appropriate footwear (if feet are swollen)
- Cane or tripod cane
- Zimmer walker
- Raised toilet seat
- Wheelchair
- Bathing aids (bath seat, non-slip mat)
- Adaptations to living area (handrails, ramps)

Aids for bedbound patients:

- Easily removable bedding
- Bedside light, handbell
- Tissues and basin (for mouth rinses)
- Backrest or V-shaped pillow
- Trapeze bar
- Legrest or cradle
- Hoyer lift
- Bed table, book stand
- Fire-resistant apron (for smoking in bed)

Equipment for symptom control:

- Drug card
- Portable subcutaneous infusion pump
- Compression sleeve (for lymphedema)
- Nebulizer
- TENS machine
- Heating pad

Equipment for skin care:

- Sheepskins
- Heel and elbow pads
- Spenco mattresses and cushions
- Ring cushion

Incontinence aids:
- Bedpan or urinal
- Portable commode
- Disposable underwear and pads
- Protective undersheet
- Urinary condom or catheter

Eating aids:
- Insulated carafe (for cool drinks)
- Ice-maker
- Blender (for dysphagic patients)
- Microwave oven
- Flexible straws

9. **The terminal phase at home** — As death approaches, it is important for home care team members to remember the following:

- Maintain analgesia (morphine can be given by suppository or continuous subcutaneous infusion).
- A continuous subcutaneous infusion can be very useful; methotrimeprazine will control agitation and scopolamine will dry up secretions and control bubbling.
- Patients may require an indwelling urinary catheter or urinary condom in the last few days, but only if necessary.
- A schedule of caregiving continues to be important, as an expected 24-hour vigil can turn into a long week of waiting.
- Rehearse emotions and procedures. ("How will you feel?" "What will you do?")
- Teach the family to recognize the signs of death, while explaining that even nurses and doctors are not always sure of the moment death occurs. Explain that the body need not be removed immediately, and can safely remain at home for several hours following death.
- Encourage the family to include children. Explain to them. ("Grandma will stop breathing soon and get very still, and then she will have died.") Give them jobs to do to be useful.
- A 24-hour telephone contact to the home care team is very important, and is very rarely abused.

- Advise family members not to dial 911 as death nears, to preclude the likelihood of resuscitation efforts or ambulance transportation to the hospital emergency ward.

- Arrange with the attending physician to come to the home to certify the death, in states where nurses are not yet authorized to do so.

10. **After a home death, families often have a sense of achievement.** ("We are so glad we were able to keep him at home.") This is usually a comfort in their grief, and facilitates the normal grieving process. **A death at home can be a sad but profoundly moving experience which paves the way to eventual healing and growth for the family.**

"I was dreading this last part, but every day has been a memory to treasure — I wouldn't have missed it for the world." Mrs. G.T. (whose husband was dying at home)

HYPERCALCEMIA

Definition — A corrected blood calcium level above 10.5mg/dL [2.6mmol/L] is defined as hypercalcemia. In fact, in the hypercalcemia of malignancy, symptoms are unusual until blood calcium levels are above 12.0mg/dL [3.0mmol/L].

Mechanism of hypercalcemia — Although hypercalcemia is associated with extensive bone metastases in diseases such as carcinoma of the breast, it has been recognized for 30 years that hypercalcemia can occur in malignancies without bone involvement.

Increased tumor mass leads to greater production of parathyroid hormone related protein which acts on the kidneys to increase calcium reabsorption. Osteolytic cytokines probably cause hypercalcemia only if the first mechanism is also operating.

Incidence — Hypercalcemia occurs in about 8.5% of patients with cancer. It is more common in advanced disease (80% of cancer patients with hypercalcemia die within one year), but it can occur at any stage and can be self-limiting. In one study, checking calcium levels of patients with breast cancer on admission to the hospital showed 5.3% had hypercalcemia, but checking levels every 6 weeks showed that 43% had hypercalcemia at some stage. Most cases were mild (levels below 12.0mg/dL [3.0mmol/L]) and severe cases (levels above 16.0mg/dL [4.0mmol/L]) were rare, occurring only in about 4% of cases.

156

Tumors causing hypercalcemia — It is particularly associated with **squamous carcinomas** and **hematological malignancies (myeloma, lymphoma, leukemia)**.

It is commonest in carcinomas of:

- Breast
- Bronchus

It occurs in about 25% of patients with squamous carcinoma of the bronchus but it is rare in small (oat) cell and adenocarcinomas.

It can occur in a wide variety of tumors, including:

- Kidney
- Head and neck
- Esophagus
- Cervix
- Ovary
- Uterus

It is very rare in adenocarcinomas of the:

- Stomach
- Pancreas
- Colon
- Prostate

Symptoms — **The most important symptoms suggestive of hypercalcemia in patients with malignant disease are:**

- Drowsiness
- Nausea
- Thirst
- Polyuria

The combination of these symptoms makes hypercalcemia very likely.

Hypercalcemia also causes other symptoms: lethargy, anorexia, dry mouth, muscular weakness, constipation, confusion and anxiety.

These are all common symptoms in any patient with advanced malignancy and therefore hypercalcemia can easily be missed.

Management options — Even if the patient has a short prognosis of only a few weeks, it is worthwhile to treat hypercalcemia to relieve symptoms. Untreated the patient will die in a few days if calcium levels rise above 16.0mg/dL [4.0mmol/L]. (It may occasionally be decided that the hypercalcemia is a terminal event and should not be treated.)

Levels above 14.0mg/dL [*3.5mmol/L*] require IV rehydration with 2 to 3 liters normal saline per day with potassium supplements (monitor serum electrolytes) combined with daily IV infusions of etidronate disodium (7.5mg/kg/day) for 3 days. This regime is simple and effective.

After rehydration calcitonin SC (by subcutaneous injection, 200 units 2 times a day) is often used, but has only modest, short-lived effect (2 to 3 days). It can have a place in treating moderate hypercalcemia (12.0mg/dL to 14.0mg/dL [*3.0mmol/L to 3.5mmol/L*]). It commonly causes nausea and vomiting. It is expensive.

Once calcium levels have returned to normal, patients should maintain good fluid intake, and calcium levels should be monitored regularly, weekly at first and then monthly. **Maintenance therapy is usually required.**

The options include:
- Oral phosphate
- Oral steroids (for myeloma, lymphoma, leukemia)
- Hormone therapy (breast cancer)
- Oral etidronate disodium

Oral phosphate 500mg 1 or 2 times a day effectively maintains normal calcium levels. Start gradually to avoid nausea. Almost all patients develop diarrhea (even if on morphine) and require loperamide. Renal damage due to renal calcification is a long term risk, but not significant in patients with a prognosis of 6 months or less.

Steroids are often given for hypercalcemia, but are usually effective only in hematological malignancies.

In breast cancer (for patients with hormone-sensitive tumors) **hormone therapy** can effectively prevent hypercalcemia recurring.

Biphosphonates — Etidronate disodium IV is effective and is the current drug treatment of choice for severe hypercalcemia. Oral etidronate disodium is available for maintenance therapy but current evidence suggests it is effective in fewer than 50% of patients. A newer generation of biphosphonates (now available only for investigational use) is effective both orally and IV. These can be used for long periods and are relatively non-toxic. These include aminopropilidine biphosphonate (APD), and dichloromethylene-biphosphonate. When available, these drugs will offer greater efficacy in the maintenance treatment of hypercalcemia of malignancy.

INSOMNIA

Insomnia lowers the patient's pain threshold, exhausts carers and is a common cause of breakdown in home care arrangements.

Insomnia may be due to **symptoms** (pain, sweats, incontinence, cough, itch) or **anxiety** or **depression**. The cause usually becomes clearer if a careful history is taken from the patient and family of time of sleeping, time of waking, reasons for waking and also previous sleep pattern.

Sometimes simple remedies such as lighter blankets or a night-light can help.

Fear and loneliness are worst at night. Recurrent nightmares can make patients fear sleep. It is important to discuss nightmares with patients (without attempting interpretation) because it allows them to express fear without having to relate it directly to their real situation.

Some patients fear dying in their sleep, and the comment "You will pass away peacefully in your sleep." can unwittingly cause insomnia. Anxieties about dying may need to be discussed.

Boredom or lack of activity during the day may worsen insomnia, and the answer may be referral to a skilled occupational or recreational therapist.

The hospital routine can often disturb sleep (waking patients to take sleeping pills, for example).

"Sleep when it comes is an uncommon blessing and is not to be wantonly interrupted." (Norman Cousins, *Anatomy of an Illness*)

Drug treatment — If the patient is depressed, prescribe a sedative anti-depressant such as oral amitriptyline 25mg to 150mg nightly 2 hours before bedtime.

Hypnotics should be short-acting (temazepam 15mg to 60mg). The maximum dose should be tried before changing to another hypnotic. (*see Benzodiazepines*)

If anxiety is the main problem, oral chlorpromazine is very effective for some patients. An initial dose (10mg to 25mg) around 5:00 p.m. followed by a second dose (25mg to 50mg) at bedtime is often successful.

If the patient is waking to take 4-hourly morphine in the night, it is usually possible to achieve longer lasting analgesia by doubling the dose at bedtime. Alternatively, change from 4-hourly morphine to 12-hourly MS-Contin.

For patients who are very distressed by lack of sleep, an IM injection of morphine (half the day-time 4-hourly oral dose), chlorpromazine 50mg and scopolamine 0.4mg is very effective and can be safely repeated after 4 hours.

★ **By using these three groups of drugs (hypnotics, anxiolytics and opioids) and making detailed adjustments (to doses and times given) it is usually possible to achieve a good night's sleep in even the most intractable insomnia.**

INTERVENTIONAL RADIOLOGY

Symptoms can occasionally be relieved by techniques of interventional radiology without the need for surgery.

The techniques include:

1. Biliary drainage
2. Nephrostomy
3. Percutaneous gastrostomy
4. Tumor embolization
5. Percutaneous abscess drainage
6. Celiac plexus block

1. The best intervention for **obstructive jaundice** that is causing severe itching is the **insertion of a biliary endoprosthesis** either endoscopically or by a percutaneous transhepatic approach (external drainage of bile into a colostomy bag is to be avoided whenever possible as bile leakage is always troublesome).

2. **Percutaneous nephrostomy** to relieve **bilateral ureteric obstruction** should be followed by the insertion of ureteric stents whenever possible (so the patient does not have the problems of external drainage).

3. **Percutaneous gastrostomy** can be performed under local anesthetic. Its main value is in patients with neuromuscular dysphagia.

4. **Embolization of the vascular supply** to tumors has been used mainly in hepatoma, hepatic metastases, renal carcinoma and head and neck cancers. A variety of embolic agents have been used, including gelfoam, alcohol, stainless steel coils, autologous clots and polyvinyl particles. The main indication is usually pain control, but the procedure itself can cause severe post-infarction pain and the results are often disappointing.

5. Virtually any **intra-thoracic or intra-abdominal abscess** can be successfully **drained by a percutaneous catheter**. A needle is directed by either fluoroscopy, ultrasound or CT, a guidewire introduced and then a catheter with multiple side holes is placed into the cavity. It is the treatment of choice for abscess drainage in the terminally ill.

6. (see Celiac Plexus Block)

INTESTINAL OBSTRUCTION

Bowel obstruction occurs in about 3% of patients with advanced cancer, most commonly with cancers of the ovary (25%) and colo-rectal cancer (10%), but occasionally with endometrial, prostate, bladder and stomach cancers, and lymphomas.

In cancer patients who develop intestinal obstruction it is often assumed that recurrent tumor is responsible. However, **severe constipation can mimic obstruction**.

Assessment — Symptoms can include:

- Continuous pain
- Colicky pain
- Nausea
- Vomiting
- Constipation
- Diarrhea
- Abdominal distention

Colic causes episodic severe pain (i.e., the severity of the pain fluctuates) and it can be associated with bubbling bowel noises (borborygmi) and also nausea. It does not respond to opioids, but responds to an anti-spasmodic such as scopolamine.

Diarrhea can occur as well as constipation — intestinal **dysfunction** is often a more correct term than "obstruction", because the **obstruction can be intermittent** and bowel function can return spontaneously after a few days.

Make the distinction between **nausea** (a very unpleasant symptom, albeit invisible) and **vomiting** (which the patient may not find too distressing if it is intermittent).

Assess **distention**. Is it gaseous, or is it in fact ascites which could be relieved by paracentesis? Large tumor masses preclude surgery. Lack of distention suggests extensive fixation of bowel by tumor deposits and means surgery is unlikely to help. Perform a rectal examination to exclude constipation.

Plain abdominal x-rays may show fluid levels. Barium studies are useful and can usually delineate a large bowel obstruction.

Management options:

1. Surgery
2. Suction and rehydration ("conservative management")
3. Continuous subcutaneous infusion of drugs ("symptomatic management")

1. It is important to **consider surgery** in a cancer patient who develops obstruction for the first time, because:

- 10% have a benign cause
- 10% have a new primary cancer
- A majority will not re-obstruct

Carefully selected patients can get useful palliation for several months. On the other hand, operative morality is high (14% to 32%).

If obstruction recurs, medical management focusing on symptom control is usually a better option for the patient than further surgery.

2. In **conservative management**, naso-gastric suction and IV rehydration are important if surgery is planned, but they should not be used to control symptoms, since they are rarely effective and only add to the discomfort of terminally ill patients. They usually involve hospitalization, immobility and discomfort and **should be avoided**. In terms of symptom control, most studies show a poor response rate (1% to 14%) for conservative management.

3. **Symptomatic management** with drugs (usually via continuous **subcutaneous** infusion using a small, portable battery-operated pump) can effectively control symptoms and has several advantages:

- Patient can eat and drink
- Patient can be mobile
- Home care is possible

In a study of 40 hospice patients with intestinal obstruction treated medically it was possible to abolish symptoms in the majority of cases. (Only 30% of patients continued to have mild symptoms of visceral pain, colic or nausea. 76% of patients continued to have mild vomiting — not more than one episode per day with little or no nausea.)

Controlling symptoms — A continuous **subcutaneous** infusion using a small, portable battery-operated pump is usually the best route for drug administration, although mild or intermittent pain can be controlled using other routes (sublingual, rectal, IM injection).

The drugs commonly used (mixed together) in a continuous subcutaneous infusion are:

- Morphine or hydromorphone — for visceral pain
- Scopolamine — for colicky pain (0.8mg to 2.4mg per 24 hours)
- Haloperidol — for nausea (5mg to 10mg per 24 hours)

The dose of opioid analgesic needs to be carefully titrated to the pain, and will depend on the dose of opioid analgesic that previously controlled the pain.

If nausea persists then stronger anti-emetics are required instead of haloperidol. Use cyclizine 100mg to 150mg per 24 hours, or methotrimeprazine 50mg to 100mg per 24 hours. (see *Subcutaneous Infusions*)

The aim of symptomatic management is to **control pain and nausea**, and to **allow fluids and a soft diet**. Some food is absorbed in the upper small bowel above the obstruction. Occasional short episodes of vomiting once or twice a day may have to be accepted. Patients usually tolerate vomiting well, provided they are free of nausea and receive appropriate explanation.

A fecal softener (docusate sodium syrup 100mg to 200mg every 8 hours) is given so that if bowel function is restored (which it can be) constipation is not an additional problem. Stimulant laxatives should be **avoided** as they worsen the colic.

★ **This regime can keep patients well hydrated and virtually free of symptoms for many weeks.**

ITCHING

Itching (pruritis) is a rare but distressing symptom. Intense itch is a form of pain.

Causes include:

1. Eczema or allergy
2. Candidiasis
3. Drug reactions

    4. Cholestasis

    5. Malignant skin infiltration

    6. Generalized non-specific

★   **Itching is made worse by anxiety or boredom.**

1. **Eczema** or **skin allergies** can still occur in terminally ill patients, and respond to topical steroids. There is usually a past history.

2. **Candidiasis** causes soreness as well as itch. Damp macerated skin (in groin, gluteal cleft, under breasts) can become infected with candida because maceration (excessive water in the keratin layer of the skin) breaks the protective barrier of keratin and allows infection to enter. Treat with an antifungal lotion, miconazole nitrate 2%, to allow evaporation and drying of the skin.

3. **Drug reactions** are usually obvious, with rash or urticaria. Some drugs (chlorpromazine, for example) cause cholestasis. Epidural morphine can cause itching which can respond to antihistamines.

4. **Cholestasis** causes itching due to bile-salt retention in the skin. In the early stages jaundice may not be obvious. (see Jaundice)

Management options include:

- Cholestyramine 4g every 6 to 8 hours
- Aluminum hydroxide 1.5ml every 6 hours
- Antihistamines
- Biliary stent (see Jaundice)
- Radiotherapy to nodes at the porta hepatis
- High dose steroids to relieve biliary pressure

Cholestyramine binds to bile-salts and reduces absorption. It is unpleasant to take. Aluminum hydroxide also reduces bile-salt absorption but is less effective. Antihistamines will reduce bile-salt itching in some patients. The non-specific measures discussed below can also help.

4. **Malignant skin infiltration** around a breast cancer sometimes causes pricking pain and itch which can respond to an anti-prostaglandin such as naproxen 250mg to 500mg 2 times a day.

6. **Non-specific itch** may be reduced by one or more of the following measures:

- Avoid heat
- Treat dry skin

- Apply calamine lotion
- Apply 10% crotamiton cream
- Antihistamines
- Night sedation
- Methyltestosterone
- Apply topical steroids
- Plasma exchange

Overheating increases itching. Avoid hot baths and use cotton clothes to reduce sweating.

Dry skin can contribute to all forms of itching. Skin hydration often reduces itch. In normal skin a layer of grease (from the sebaceous glands) keeps the keratin layer hydrated and firm. With dry skin, keratin flakes off and exposes deeper layers causing inflammation and itch. Generous use of aqueous cream as a soap substitute and bland bath oils can restore skin hydration.

Calamine lotion is soothing. It cools by evaporation and leaves a fine coating of powder.

10% crotamiton cream has an anti-pruritic action, but avoid the eyes.

Antihistamines can reduce all forms of itch. They are successful for some patients but not for others. Terfenadine 60mg 2 times a day is useful because it is not sedating. A sedative antihistamine (oral promethazine 75mg, for example) can be useful at bedtime.

Methyltestosterone 25mg 3 times a day occasionally reduces severe itching, despite its known tendency to cause cholestasis. The mode of action is unknown. It takes 7 to 10 days for maximum effect. It is **contraindicated** in cancers of the prostate or male breasts.

Topical steroid cream may be necessary if there is secondary inflammation from scratching.

Plasma exchange has been used as a last resort to relieve intense itch.

JAUNDICE

Jaundice is usually due to obstruction of bile flow (from liver to bowels). Bilirubin pigment stains the skin and eyes yellow. Urine becomes dark (bile pigment). Bowel motions are pale (lack of bile pigment).

The main problems are:

Fear — The patient commonly fears that jaundice means the disease is advancing rapidly. It can be helpful to explain that jaundice in itself is relatively harmless (some people with liver diseases such as chronic hepatitis can be jaundiced for years). The dark urine is sometimes mis-diagnosed as dehydration.

Itch is the main physical symptom. Some patients have severe itching, others have very little. When itch is trouble-some (particularly if it is disturbing sleep) and the patient is relatively well and expected to live more than a month, then a **bile drainage procedure** should be considered. An ultrasound scan will demonstrate dilated bile ducts, and confirm that the jaundice is caused by obstruction of the common bile duct (and is not due to another cause such as drug-induced cholestasis). The best technique is to insert a biliary prosthesis (stent) by a retrograde approach via endoscopy. A guide wire is passed through the tumor and the stent then pushed over it. This is usually simpler for the patient than the percutaneous trans-hepatic approach to the bile duct used by interventional radiologists (although this technique may be necessary for high obstruction). (see Itching)

The **external drainage of bile should be avoided** whenever possible, because bile seeps through all known dressings and appliances to stain clothing and cause skin soreness.

Jaundice due to tumors of the Papilla of Vater can be relieved by simple diathermy sphincterotomy. Surgical by-pass procedures such as cholecystojejunostomy should be performed prophylactically at laparotomy for inoperable carcinomas of the pancreas or biliary duct.

LASERS

Laser treatment can bring immediate symptom relief without the side effects of chemotherapy and radiotherapy. Lasers have been used since 1982 for endoscopic palliation of inoperable tumors of the bronchus and esophagus.

The Nd YAG laser can re-canalize or de-bulk advanced tumors of the bronchus, esophagus or rectum, and can be transmitted by flexible fibers via a fiberoptic endoscope. It vaporizes tumor cells and coagulates blood vessels up to 1mm in diameter. It can relieve local symptoms — dyspha-gia, dyspnea, hemoptysis, rectal bleeding and obstruction. It usually needs to be repeated. (see Bleeding)

Only exophytic tumors are suitable for laser resection.

Laser therapy (photo-resection) is indicated for **dyspnea or recurrent hemoptysis in patients with bronchial cancers** which have a significant intraluminal component. It can reduce the size of the obstructing tumor and improve breathing in 75% of patients, and controls bleeding in 60%. It can be used under local anesthetic, but smoke is generated, which causes coughing. Most physicians prefer to use a rigid bronchoscope under general anesthetic. It is useful for the urgent treatment of severe stridor due to tracheal tumors. Laser has the advantages of immediate response, no systemic toxicity, and the ability to repeat treatment when required.

Dysphagia due to esophageal cancers can be relieved by laser therapy. Preliminary dilation of the tumor is necessary when using a no-touch laser. New sapphire probes now allow direct contact and thus can treat tumors when obstruction is complete and even a guide wire cannot be passed. The technique is effective and over 90% of patients have improved swallowing. (The perforation rate is about 4%.) Once the patency of the lumen is restored, treatment can be repeated every 4 to 6 weeks. Laser therapy can be used to treat overgrowth of a prosthetic tube.

Further study is needed to compare laser treatment alone, and in combination with intracavity radiation and prosthetic intubation.

Laser can control **obstruction, bleeding and discharge from rectal cancers**. Pain relief can be provided by tumor de-bulking only, but not if the lesion has invaded the sacrum or sacral plexus. Incontinence due to the spread of the tumor into the anal margin cannot be relieved. Laser provides palliation that is as good as (or better than) radiotherapy, electro-coagulation or cryotherapy. A rectal wash-out is required before treatment, which is usually under general anesthetic, because the heating effect can be painful. The perforation rate is low. The treatment can be repeated every 4 to 6 weeks. In occasional patients, the benefits last several months.

With superficial **bladder tumors** there is a small body of evidence that laser therapy produces a lower recurrence rate than resection or electro-coagulation. Laser therapy for deep penetrating bladder tumors may have a place in patients unfit for radical treatment, to de-bulk tumors or control bleeding.

LAXATIVES

(see Constipation)

About 80% of hospice patients eventually need a regular laxative. Almost all patients on regular opioids need daily laxatives. As analgesic doses increase, laxative doses need to increase.

Classification of laxatives:

- Bulking agents (bran, or fiber laxatives)
- Fecal softeners (docusate sodium)
- Colonic stimulants (senna, bisacodyl, casanthrol)
- Small bowel (osmotic) flushers (weak: lactulose, strong: magnesium sulfate)

The action of all these drugs is complex and poorly understood.

Most patients require a **fecal softener plus a colonic stimulant laxative**. A good regime for most patients taking opioids is Senokot-S (senna concentrate and docusate sodium) or Peri-Colace (casanthrol and docusate sodium) 1 to 3 tablets 2 times a day. A suppository or micro-enema should be given on the third day if the bowels have not moved, and the dose of oral laxatives increased.

If the motions are soft but remain infrequent, give additional stimulant laxatives. If motions remain hard add a small bowel flusher (lactulose syrup 10ml to 30ml 3 times a day or magnesium sulfate 5ml to 10ml with plenty of water, in the morning).

★ **Abdominal cramps can occur with stimulant or osmotic laxatives and are dose dependent.**

Bran, taken with food or fruit juice, is an effective high fiber preparation. The full effect may take some days to develop. 60% of the bran is excreted (increasing the bulk by holding water). Stools also hold more water because fecal transit time is shortened. The other 40% of the bran is degraded by bacteria which stimulates bacterial growth (and bacteria make a substantial contribution to fecal mass). Many ill patients, however, cannot tolerate a high fiber diet.

Bulking agents are useful in the management of colostomy, ileostomy, hemorrhoids and anal fissure. They can help to encourage formed motions in patients with rectal discharge or bleeding. They increase fecal mass and each dose should be taken with plenty of water. They should be avoided if there is an intestinal stricture. They can take several days to produce an effect and are less useful than the stimulant or osmotic laxatives for bowel regulation.

Docusate sodium (Colace) is only a mild laxative. It is a surface wetting agent that lowers surface tension and allows water to penetrate hard feces. It also promotes secretion of fluid in both the small and large bowel. It has a weak effect on gut motility. It acts within 1 to 2 days, and should be started at the maximum dose of 500mg per day in divided doses.

Lactulose (Chronulac Syrup) is a semi-synthetic disaccharide (galactose-fructose) which is not absorbed by the GI tract, and is therefore **safe for diabetics**. It has an osmotic effect so water and electrolytes are retained in the bowel lumen. It is estimated that 30ml of lactulose increases colonic fecal volume by about 500ml and this stimulates peristalsis in both the large and small intestine. Lactulose is metabolized by gut bacteria to acetic and lactic acids which prevent bacterial conversion of urea to ammonia and is therefore useful in hepatic encephalopathy. Lactulose 10ml to 30ml 3 times a day, plus a stimulant laxative, is usually necessary if the patient is taking opioids. It is effective within 2 days. It causes nausea in some patients. Higher doses can cause abdominal distention and gas. Tolerance may develop. The sweet taste of lactulose can be masked by mixing it with fruit juice.

Magnesium sulfate is a harsh small bowel (osmotic) flusher which also has peristaltic action, and is usually reserved for severe constipation resistant to other laxative regimes.

LISTENING

★   **There is more to listening than waiting to speak.**

★   **Listening is the most important (and most difficult) of all the skills needed to help patients and families. It is the foundation of good care.**

True listening is a form of hospitality. It is making space in our schedule for the concerns of others. It demands energy and commitment. It does not need to be unduly time-consuming.

A doctor with advanced cancer said to a group of medical students, "Give me just 10 minutes of interested, uninterrupted listening, and I'll tell you all you need to know to help me."

Energetic listening is ideally preceded by a period of solitude and reflection, however brief, so we can be entirely present for the other person. We listen best to others if we have already listened to ourselves. (*see Burn Out*)

Sit down. We listen with our whole body. Our non-verbal communication (eye contact, facial expression, posture, hand movements) will signal our true depth of listening. (*see Non-verbal Communication*)

Set aside time for listening. It is possible to spend a lot of time with a person and never listen properly.

Set clear boundaries. ("We can talk together for 20 minutes now and if necessary we can meet again tomorrow afternoon.") Be realistic about your own time limitations, but always keep a promise to return.

Basic listening skills include:
1. Reflecting
2. Tracking
3. Repeating
4. Exploring
5. Clarifying
6. Linking
7. Silence
8. Noticing

1. **Reflecting** is an important technique early in a conversation. ("Why do you ask that?") It encourages a person to keep talking, and helps the listener to tune in to a person's belief system and focus of concern. It avoids assumptions about what is being asked.

2. **Tracking** is listening for key words or phrases, then turning the word or phrase into a question. This is more likely to lead to relevant discussion than asking random questions.

3. **Repeating** a phrase or sentence shows you are listening, and draws the speaker's attention back to what he said. Getting the person to repeat or to summarize can help him to analyze his own feelings.

4. **Exploring** is gently seeking more information. ("Could you say a bit more about . . . ?") By listening carefully, you may notice a word or phrase used but quickly dropped. This sometimes points to a sensitive subject that requires

gentle probing. A great deal of constructive discussion can take place when a subject like this is "incised".

5. **Clarifying** may be for your benefit as a listener. ("Could you explain that again, please?") It is very important that you understand what is being said. Clarifying is also a useful technique to help the speaker take another look at something.

6. **Linking** demonstrates careful listening. ("You said your wife had been more irritable, and earlier you said your daughter had not been coming home so much. Do you think those things are connected?") Linking can draw things together and can sometimes bring new insights.

7. **Silence** allows a person to analyze his feelings. Silence must be friendly and relaxed, and the listener should signal that the silence is comfortable to him. Sometimes after a period of silence the question "What are you thinking about?" brings up a relevant topic for discussion.

8. **Noticing** when a person's behavior conflicts with what he is saying, and kindly pointing out the discrepancy, can result in real emotions being expressed. (This works only when the person trusts you and feels you like him.)

Changes of subject, illogical or seemingly irrelevant comments are motivated by something. Sometimes it is evasion due to fear or embarrassment. It can be helpful to say "It seems difficult for you to talk about this." Sometimes it is an important clue that should be picked up. For example, during a conversation about symptoms a person may say "No never, well not since I was in the army." It is easy to pass quickly over additional information when it doesn't fit the scheme we are using, but a response like "Oh, you were in the army, tell me about that " may well reveal vital information.

You are not listening when:
- You are in a hurry
- You think about yourself
- You interrupt
- You ask the same question twice
- You don't ask any questions
- You change the subject
- You assume you know what I'm going to say
- You over-react to certain words
- You feel critical of me

LIVER METASTASES

The liver is the commonest site for metastases. 40% of all cancers develop liver metastases.

Tumors which frequently develop liver metastases include:

- Pancreas (about 75%)
- Stomach (about 50%)
- Colo-rectal
- Breast
- Bronchus
- Unknown primary site
- Melanoma
- Carcinoid tumors

Tumors that can occasionally spread to the liver include thyroid, renal and choriocarcinoma.

The symptoms of liver metastases are:

- Weight loss
- Pain
- Swelling

Rarer symptoms include jaundice, fever, hypoglycemia and liver failure (and, in carcinoid tumors, flushing or wheezing).

The usual **prognosis** for patients with liver metastases, from the time of symptoms, is about 18 months for a solitary metastasis, but only 3 months with widespread liver involvement. There have been recorded cases of patients with histologically proven liver metastases living more than 5 years. (The prognosis with carcinoid tumors can be 10 to 15 years.)

Surgery — Resection of hepatic metastases is only feasible with colo-rectal tumors, and only about 10% of these patients are suitable for surgery. The primary tumor must have been completely removed, and there must be no extrahepatic metastases. CT scan must show that the liver metastasis is resectable with a clear margin. In selecting patients for surgery the size of the metastasis, and the time it developed, do not affect the results. Some surgeons are now operating on patients with 2, 3 or 4 metastases.

The surgeon must be practiced in the technique of segmentectomy using an ultrasound cutting device (which destroys liver tissue and skeletonizes the blood vessels for ligation). One or more of the 8 anatomical segments of the liver is excised. Segmentectomy is technically easier than local excision of a metastasis. Removal of a single liver segment requires a post-operative recovery time similar to cholecystectomy.

There is an 80% 1-year survival, and in a series of 800 cases 25% were disease-free at 5 years. Hepatic artery ligation or embolization do not improve survival.

Chemotherapy — There is no place for systemic chemotherapy. Single agents (such as fluorouracil) produce a partial response (some reduction in tumor volume) in 20% of patients, but have no effect on survival. (Very toxic combination chemotherapy only improves the partial response rate to 30%.)

Intrahepatic cytotoxic infusions using implanted pumps are being evaluated at many centers, but there is no evidence yet that these prolong survival. The indications (as for surgery) are a patient with total excision of a colo-rectal tumor, and the liver as the sole site of metastases.

LIVER PAIN

Liver pain is a visceral pain (dull, heavy, deep continuous aching pain). It is due to stretching of the liver capsule. It is usually felt in the epigastrium or right side, but is sometimes presents as "backache" and in 2% of patients as groin pain. Pain can also be referred to the chest wall or right shoulder, and this referred element can be opioid insensitive. In any severe visceral pain there can be an autonomic component (pallor, sweats, tachycardia) but such severe pain is always preventable.

Management options include:

1. Morphine
2. Celiac plexus block
3. High dose steroids
4. Liver embolization
5. (Radiotherapy)

1. Liver pain usually responds well to a correctly titrated dose of **morphine**. (*see Morphine*)

2. **Celiac plexus block** is a good technique which gives complete or partial pain relief in 90% of patients. It should be considered as soon as opioids fail to give complete pain relief or are causing unacceptable side effects. (*see Celiac Plexus Block*)

3. **High dose steroids** (dexamethasone 8mg per day) may reduce peri-tumor edema and capsule tension and can sometimes reduce pain. They are an **adjuvant** treatment and should be used in this way if analgesics and celiac plexus blocks have failed to give complete pain relief.

4. **Liver embolization** can be performed by an interventional radiologist. The hepatic artery is cannulated (via a percutaneous, transhepatic approach) and the branch supplying the involved segment of liver is embolized (with gelfoam or thrombin). This causes a liver infarction which can be extremely painful for several days (with fever and leucocytosis).

The technique is sometimes used to reduce liver pain in vascular tumors (primary hepatoma, or metastases from some tumors — thyroid, renal or choriocarcinomas — that only rarely spread to the liver). **It has no place in routine pain control of liver metastases**.

Liver embolization has also been used in carcinoid tumors (to reduce hormone secretion), and as a method of delivering cytotoxics attached to lipoidol which accumulates in the tumor deposits.

5. **Radiotherapy** can sometimes shrink liver metastases and reduce liver pain, but radiotherapy to the liver causes nausea and vomiting, and should not be considered for pain control.

LIVING WILL

A "Living Will" is an advance directive expressing a person's wishes about life-sustaining treatment should he or she become incapable of taking responsibility for his or her own health care. The preparation of Living Wills is becoming increasingly common in the United States.

The purpose of the Living Will is to protect individuals from the indignity and suffering of treatments which attempt to extend life inappropriately. A Living Will cannot be used to request euthanasia ("mercy killing"). The right to a dignified death must not be mis-translated into a right to be killed. (see Euthanasia)

The Living Will is intended to protect the rights of the individual. It has the additional benefit of encouraging discussion among patient, family and professional carers about the most appropriate care for that individual. A copy of the Living Will should be kept in a person's medical records, and should be reviewed from time to time.

A Living Will is a signed, dated and witnessed document. A Living Will can include a Durable Power of Attorney for health care, which appoints a trusted "attorney-in-fact" to make medical treatment decisions if the person is unable to do so.

A Living Will should state clear preferences about use of life-sustaining treatments (like cardiopulmonary resuscitation, mechanical ventilation, kidney dialysis), or invasive measures for providing nutrition and hydration. It may also state a preference for dying at home.

At present the following states have enacted "Living Will statutes": Alabama, Alaska, Arizona, Arkansas, California, Colorado, Connecticut, Delaware, Florida, Georgia, Hawaii, Idaho, Illinois, Indiana, Iowa, Kansas, Louisiana, Maine, Maryland, Minnesota, Mississippi, Missouri, Montana, Nevada, New Hampshire, New Mexico, North Carolina, North Dakota, Oklahoma, Oregon, South Carolina, Tennessee, Texas, Utah, Vermont, Virginia, Washington, West Virginia, Wisconsin, Wyoming and the District of Columbia.

In a state which has not yet enacted such a statute, a Living Will may still be executed, and may serve as evidence of seriousness of purpose and intent.

For additional information about the general purposes and specific wording of a Living Will, please contact:

> CONCERN FOR DYING
> 250 West 57th Street, Room 831
> New York, NY 10107
> (Telephone: 212-246-6962)

LUNG METASTASES

Lung metastases develop in about 30% of patients with advanced malignant disease. Lung metastases only rarely cause symptoms.

Excision is usually undertaken only when attempting cure, most commonly in primary cancers of colon, kidney, sarcomas and testicular teratomas. The 5-year survival after resection of lung metastases is around 20% to 30%.

CT scan assessment is essential before excision is undertaken.

The usual indications are:

- Primary tumor controlled
- No extra-thoracic metastases
- Relatively fit patient with good lung function

Radiotherapy can be helpful for:

- Hemoptysis
- Chest pain (invasion of pleura or chest wall)
- Dyspnea due to lung collapse
- Pleural effusion (in lymphoma)

In these cases radiotherapy is given to a localized area of affected lung, the usual dose being 2,000cGy in 1 week, or 3,000cGy in 2 weeks, depending on the volume of lung to be irradiated.

Whole lung irradiation is sometimes used to treat metastases from sarcomas, or testicular tumors, when chemotherapy has failed. There is a risk of pulmonary fibrosis following lung irradiation.

LYMPHEDEMA

Lymphedema is a subcutaneous accumulation of protein-rich fluid due to damaged or blocked lymphatic vessels.

Causes — It is most commonly seen in the arms of post-mastectomy patients, or following radiotherapy to the axilla (and this can occur 10 years after treatment, even when there is no evidence of recurrence of cancer). Pelvic malignancy can cause lymphedema in one or both legs. Initially the edema is pitting, but the subcutaneous tissues eventually become thickened, fibrosed and leathery. Recurrent cellulitis can occur, causing further damage to lymphatics.

Management options — A daily regime of medical management can give good results, sometimes even with long-standing lymphedema. The effect of treatment is monitored by measuring limb circumference (at fixed points) and recording the data.

Diuretics are seldom helpful.

Reducing the size of a heavy, aching, disfiguring arm or leg almost always improves the patient's morale.

Ms. E. MacT., 48, with advanced melanoma and a lymphedematous leg, had compression therapy which reduced the above-knee circumference by 5 inches over 2 weeks. She said, "This treatment has helped me more than anything I've had done."

Medical management involves:

1. Bandaging
2. Compression stockings and sleeves
3. Sequential compression pump
4. Massage and exercise
5. Skin care advice
6. Prophylactic antibiotics

1. **Bandaging is necessary:**

- To reduce swelling
- To treat swollen fingers
- If there is lymph leakage
- If there is pain in the arm

A good method is to:

- Apply a full-length non-elastic cotton sleeve (to avoid skin creases when bandaging).
- Apply a narrow bandage to each finger (starting distally) and back to the wrist (leaving the palm free).
- Pad arm creases with cotton wool (especially elbow crease and back of the hand)
- Pad whole arm with foam sheet or Webril
- Bandage the arm with an elastic bandage.
- Apply a second (wider) cotton sleeve over the elastic bandage (so it does not catch on clothing).

It takes about an hour to teach the technique to a willing family carer. The bandages should ideally be re-applied every day over a 2-week period to gradually reduce swelling. Careful measurement of the arm is important to monitor reduction of swelling.

After a regime of bandaging, maintenance therapy with a support sleeve and daily use of a compression pump at home will be sufficient for several weeks. Bandaging may have to be repeated (perhaps for 2 weeks every 6 weeks).

2. Light surgical **compression stockings and sleeves** can be used to maintain a good fit and keep pace with reduction in limb size. Proper fitting is necessary. In severe cases these have to be worn continuously and only removed for bathing, and will need to be worn indefinitely. If it is best to

use garments designed to apply a pressure of about 25mm Hg. Finger swelling can be made worse by a compression sleeve and requires time-consuming finger bandaging. Satisfactory elastic gloves are not yet available.

3. **Compression pump** — Only a minority of patients need pneumatic compression, which can speed the initial rate of improvement, but does not necessarily lead to a better outcome. It can be useful as maintenance therapy between bandaging programs.

The compression pump stimulates lymphatic flow. The Jobst single chamber system has been superseded by multi-chambered intermittent sequential machines. The usual recommended pressure is 50mm Hg, but some patients need to start around 30mm Hg and build up to 50mm Hg over 2 to 3 days. The limb may require 4 to 6 hours per day if it has become hardened (usually in 1 to 2 hour treatment periods). Smaller pumps are available for home use.

Compression is unlikely to be effective if there is swelling beyond the root of the limb (in the chest wall or lower abdomen).

4. **Massage and exercises** — Normal lymph flow depends on body movements and can be encouraged by skin massage to increase the flow in proximal skin lymphatics. Daily self-massage of the skin of the chest and abdomen for 15 minutes can help to reduce swelling. Daily limb exercises will improve circulation and reduce joint stiffness. Massage and exercise should be routinely used in conjunction with bandaging and compression garments.

5. **Skin care** — Daily skin hydration (with aqueous cream as a soap substitute) is important. With gross swelling sensation is reduced and skin damage and ulceration can easily occur, so the limb should be kept away from excessive heat, detergents or hard objects. (Patients should be advised to use oven, washing-up and gardening gloves if an arm or hand is affected, and to avoid carrying heavy objects.)

6. **Prophylactic antibiotics** are indicated if cellulitis has occurred more than once. Fungal infections in skin creases also require treatment with anti-fungal cream. Avoid venipuncture or using a blood pressure cuff on an affected arm.

Diuretics — In gross lymphedema there can be a secondary venous component with some of the edema due to immobility and loss of muscle pumping. A diuretic may slightly reduce tissue tension but is rarely helpful.

High dose steroids can occasionally relieve early edema due to recurrent pelvic malignancy, but in most cases are ineffective.

LYMPH NODES METASTASES

Palpable lymph nodes metastases occur in the neck, axilla and groin.

Lymphatic spread is a common feature of many cancers, the cancer spreading from the area drained by the lymph nodes. Usually the enlarged nodes are recognized during follow-up of a patient with cancer. Sometimes node involvement is the first feature of disease (typical in papillary tumors of the thyroid, nasopharyngeal carcinomas and occasionally in melanoma). Sometimes the primary remains undetected. (see *Unknown Primary Cancer*)

Recurrent tumor following treatment usually occurs within 12 months. Mobile nodes will usually be excised surgically by a block dissection. Fixed nodes may be treated with radiotherapy or chemotherapy.

Problems include:
- Large lumps
- Ulceration (infection, bleeding)
- Lymphedema
- Skin necrosis
- Arterial occlusion

Radiotherapy can shrink **nodal deposits** and can sometimes heal **ulceration**. Patients who have previously had radiotherapy risk skin damage, but implants of radioactive gold grains or iridium wire can still be used. In the neck it is possible to resect recurrent disease, remove radiation-damaged skin, repair with a myocutaneous flap (usually from the pectoral region) and irradiate through the graft.

Lymphedema needs to be treated early with compression therapy. (see *Lymphedema*)

Skin necrosis can occur after block dissection and may require excision and grafting. Small areas of necrosis may be removed with salicylic acid ointment and may heal spontaneously.

Arterial occlusion can occur after radiotherapy. It causes ischemic changes in the arm or leg, or, if in the neck, dizziness and fainting. Occasionally an arterial bypass may be necessary.

MENINGEAL METASTASES

Meningeal metastases (carcinomatous meningitis) are strongly suggested by neurological problems at several levels, and a myelogram may show tumor nodules.

These cause:
- Headache (with or without neck stiffness)
- Pain in the lower back and buttocks
- Cauda equina damage
- Malignant cells in CSF (raised protein, low glucose)

(*see Cauda Equina Damage*)

MEPERIDINE

Meperidine is a short-acting synthetic opioid. It is possible **but not advisable** to use it as an alternative to morphine for moderate pain.

It has three disadvantages:
- Erratic oral absorption
- It is short-acting (1 to 3 hours only)
- It cannot be used above 300mg because of a toxic metabolite which causes tremor, twitching, agitation and seizures.

When converting to morphine, the oral equivalents are:

2-3 hourly meperidine	4-hourly morphine
100mg	10mg
200mg	20mg
300mg	30mg

Meperidine is stronger by injection. 100mg IM meperidine is equivalent to 15mg IM morphine. Meperidine is too irritant for use in continuous subcutaneous infusions.

METHADONE

Methadone is a synthetic opioid that acts on CNS morphine receptors and peripherally on the gut.

Methadone is too long-acting for clinical use and should be avoided.

Given repeatedly methadone has a half-life of 1 to 3 days, and cumulates. At a given dose, a steady plasma level may not be reached for 1 to 2 weeks. A small increase in dose can produce a massive increase in plasma level 1 to 2 weeks later. Severe drowsiness and even respiratory depression may therefore occur some days after starting, especially in elderly patients, or in patients taking cimetidine (which inhibits metabolism).

Like morphine, methadone has no ceiling, and the oral dose needed to control severe pain varies from 20mg to 900mg per day. It is 2 times as potent by injection (give half the oral dose). Regular oral doses are 4 times more potent than morphine. If it is used, it should be prescribed on a 12-hourly dosage.

Methadone is too inflexible for routine use, and increasing the dose is difficult because the patient has to be carefully monitored for some time.

Methadone is occasionally useful to control **cough** in patients already on morphine. The addition of methadone linctus (2mg in 5ml) 5ml to 10ml every 8 hours can sometimes help suppress a dry cough resistant to morphine.

MORPHINE

★   **Morphine is the strong opioid of choice.**

★   **Some pains (visceral and soft tissue) respond well to morphine and some (bone, nerve and colic) do not.** (see Pain)

Oral morphine should usually be started in a dose of 5mg to 10mg every 4 hours when moderate analgesics are no longer effective. Never prescribe PRN. A laxative and an anti-emetic must be started at the same time.

In titrated doses morphine is an analgesic and does not cause euphoria. Mild drowsiness may occur for the first 2 to 3 days of treatment. The principle is to **increase the dose in steps until the patient is pain-free but still alert**.

If a patient who is pain-free becomes **drowsy**, the dose should be **reduced**. When morphine is used carefully by finding the correct dose for a particular patient's pain, there are no dangers of needing escalating doses, or of causing respiratory depression.

The **myths of tolerance, addiction, and respiratory depression** have contributed to the poor management of cancer pain. These myths are based on single-dose studies in animals and humans without pain. **Chronic pain prevents these side effects.** (*see below*)

MS-Contin (morphine sulfate controlled-release) is a very useful drug in terminal care (particularly for home care) when properly administered on a **12-hourly schedule.** It is ordinary morphine in a slow release form. Its bio-availability is excellent. (Absorption of MS-Contin may be delayed by a fatty meal.)

It is usually safe to start MS-Contin 30mg every 12 hours for pain, unless the patient is debilitated or elderly. A starting dose of MS-Contin 15mg every 12 hours is recommended for elderly or debilitated patients. (Start MS-Contin 10mg every 12 hours for these patients in countries where 10mg tablets are available.) Start haloperidol 1.5mg at bedtime simultaneously to prevent nausea. Start a laxative (Peri-Colace or Senokot-S) immediately.

It is usually best to titrate the dose using 4-hourly oral morphine. Once the patient is pain-controlled on a regular 4-hourly dose, **then** change to the equivalent dose of MS-Contin given every 12 hours. The total dose of MS-Contin over 24 hours is the same as the total dose of 4-hourly morphine. (4-hourly dose of morphine x 3 = 12-hourly dose of MS-Contin.)

4-hourly dose of oral morphine	12-hourly dose of MS-Contin
5	15
10	30
20	60
30	90
60	180
90	270

In the United States, MS-Contin is available in 100mg, 60mg, 30mg and 15mg strengths.

Always prescribe MS-Contin on a 12-hourly regime. Increase the dose if pain occurs. A 6-hourly or 8-hourly regime should be avoided, as it can cause episodes of drowsiness due to peaks of absorption. When increasing the dose, it is safe to use the MS-Contin increments shown above. If the patient is pain-free and drowsy, reduce the dose.

In a study of 38 patients switched from oral MS-Contin to the same dose rectally, pain control was maintained in all the patients. The dose range (using 30mg tablets) was between 2 and 10 tablets every 12 hours. The duration of use ranged from 1 to 30 days (mean 11.5 days). None of the patients experienced any local rectal side-effects such as irritation or burning. (Rectal administration of MS-Contin is not approved by the FDA.)

Beware of patients on MS-Contin who have their pain controlled by other means, such as nerve block. The sudden reduction in pain can mean that the patient is getting too much morphine, and this has caused severe respiratory depression. Change to an equivalent dose of 4-hourly morphine **before** such procedures, and observe the patient carefully afterwards.

When is it wrong to use morphine? It is wrong to use morphine without proper assessment of the pain. Intermittent pains (bone pain, nerve pain, colic) respond poorly or not at all to morphine. Many pains (15%) are not related to the cancer (heartburn, peptic ulcer, anal fissure, etc.) and will not respond to morphine.

Can morphine be started too early? No. A common fear of doctors is this: "If morphine is started now the patient's body will develop tolerance. Higher and higher doses will be needed. When pain worsens later, it will no longer be effective." This does not occur. **Used properly in chronic pain, morphine is an analgesic with no properties of tolerance.** If the pain is constant the correct dose (the one that controls the pain without causing drowsiness) can remain constant — for weeks, for months, or even for years in some cases. If the pain is reduced, the dose of morphine will need to be reduced. If the pain increases, the dose will need to be increased.

What is the correct dose? The correct dose of morphine is the dose that relieves the pain without causing drowsiness. To find the correct dose, the principle is to titrate — to start with a low dose and then promptly increase it until the pain is relieved.

Mr. J.P. has carcinoma of the larynx with metastases in the right cervical nodes. He enjoys going to the pub for a drink in the evenings, but finds that his neck and right shoulder ache. Codeine 60mg every 4 hours has previously relieved the pain, but the ache is getting worse. Mr. J.P. is frightened of starting morphine, saying "It's only an ache, if it turns into pain I'll let you know." Before long, even wearing his heavy tweed jacket makes his shoulder ache, and an alert home care nurse observes that he has stopped going to the pub. He is persuaded to try oral morphine, 10mg every 4 hours. His ache is better, and he is able to go out again in the evenings. In fact, although he is much better, the ache returns about 3½ hours after each dose, and he has about ½ hour of increasing pain before each dose. The dose of morphine is therefore increased to 20mg every 4 hours, and he is completely free of the ache. He is changed to MS-Contin 60mg every 12 hours for the sake of convenience. Mr. J.P. is delighted, and so is the owner of the pub he frequents!

What if the patient gets drowsy? In any patient on morphine the rule is this: if pain-free and drowsy, reduce the dose. Be sure to exclude other causes of drowsiness (hypercalcemia, for example). (*see Drowsiness*)

Remember, **some pains respond poorly to morphine**. Neuralgias, bone pains, incidental pains like tension headaches, anal fissures, abscesses, colics (gut, renal and biliary), and distention pains like gastric distention and tenesmus are among those. Increasing the dose of morphine for those pains will make the patient drowsy without relieving the pain.

Is there a maximum safe dose of morphine? No. The principle is this: if 4-hourly morphine relieved the pain a bit, increase the dose in steps until the pain is relieved, using the increments of 5mg, 10mg, 20mg, 30mg, 45mg, 60mg, etc. The dose should be increased every four hours if there is still pain. 90% of patients with morphine-responsive pains will have relief within that 5mg to 60mg range, but occasionally, as the case history below shows, the dose may need to be 500mg or higher.

Mr. N.C. is 27, a computer programmer, with a hepatoma. A previous embolization for liver pain had little effect, and his family doctor prescribed oral morphine 10mg every 4 hours. He found that taking a double dose every 2 hours was helping but not abolishing the pain. He was seen at the hospice outpatient clinic, and the dose was increased to 60mg every 4 hours. This abolished the pain, and he returned to work. A week later he was still pain-free, and was changed to MS-Contin 180mg every 12 hours — to make it easier to take as a twice-a-day regime. Three weeks later he again had severe right-sided pain, and was admitted to the hospice. Morphine was re-started at a dose of 90mg every 4 hours and was increased after one dose to 150mg every 4 hours. He was then pain-free, and after 36 hours returned home and went back to work. A week later in the clinic he was complaining of breakthrough pain between doses. The dose of morphine was increased to 300mg every 4 hours, with a double dose (600mg) at bedtime to allow him 8 hours of sleep. On this regime he remained pain-free for 8 weeks, working full time, driving his car, and not feeling drowsy.

★ **At higher doses of morphine the incremental increases have to be bigger.** (For example, increase straight from 150mg to 300mg 4-hourly. The dose has been doubled, as when increasing from 5mg to 10mg, or from 10mg to 20mg.)

What dose of morphine should you use for the patient with severe pain, when you are unsure of the analgesic history? The principle is to start with a low dose and observe frequently.

Mr. A.U. is 67, is known to have advanced carcinoma of the bronchus, and presents with severe continuous lateral chest pain. He is unable to give a detailed history. His wife says he has been taking a lot of analgesics of various kinds recently, but has never had morphine. We start with a low dose — morphine 5mg IM — and observe. (In severe pain the IM route is initially better than oral medication as it works faster.) After 20 minutes Mr. A.U. still complains of severe pain — give morphine 10mg IM and observe. After another 20 minutes, the pain is easing but still troublesome — another 10mg morphine IM. Mr. A.U. is now pain-free and drowsy. (He may be drowsy at this stage because of previous lack of sleep and exhaustion.) We re-assess the patient 4 hours after the first injection and he is pain-free. He has had 25mg morphine IM, so we prescribe morphine 25mg IM every 4 hours. (If he remains pain-free but drowsy, we reduce the dose.) Mr. A.U. is able to swallow and is not feeling sick (nausea causes gastric stasis and prevents absorption) so we promptly change to oral medication — 50mg morphine orally every 4 hours (twice the IM dose!) and observe.

Which is the best route for morphine? Morphine is effective by all routes: oral, rectal, sublingual, subcutaneous, intramuscular, intravenous. The sublingual dose is equivalent to the oral or rectal dose. When changing from the oral or rectal route to one of the other systemic routes (subcutaneous, IM or IV), cut the dose in half.

IV infusions of morphine are often used if a patient has a permanent indwelling intravenous catheter. This route can be effective (although it may well not be ideal from the patient's point of view and is rarely used for analgesia in Britain). It has one major **disadvantage**: tolerance sometimes develops to morphine administered by the IV route (either infusion or bolus). The patient needs higher and higher doses every 1 to 2 hours, and pain can escape control. Transferring such patients to oral morphine, or to morphine by continuous **subcutaneous** infusion, gives better pain control with lower doses. The reason why tolerance can develop rapidly to IV morphine, **but not by other routes**, remains unknown.

Morphine Myths

I. Tolerance

II. Addiction

III. Respiratory depression

I.   **What about tolerance?**

Patients commonly fear that tolerance will occur. ("I didn't take the pain medication in case it doesn't work later when I'll need it more.") **This misconception needs to be explained. Tolerance (needing higher and higher doses with diminishing analgesic effect) does not occur** when oral, rectal, sublingual, subcutaneous or intramuscular morphine is used to control visceral or soft tissue cancer pain. (As explained above, it may occur in IV use.) The fear of tolerance is based on the clinical mis-use of morphine in pains poorly responsive to morphine, such as nerve pain, bone pain or colicky pain. (Morphine is ineffective for these pains, and the tendency is to give higher and higher doses, which are also ineffective.) In fact, 90% of patients never need more than 60mg of oral morphine every 4 hours, irrespective of duration of use.

The dose of morphine may increase for the first few weeks as the dosage is titrated (starting with a low dose, then increasing). Dose increase is usually of the order of 30% over two weeks. **Once a pain is controlled by morphine, the patient can stay on the same dose for weeks or months.** The longer a patient is on morphine, the more likely he is to have a **decrease** in dosage.

Mr. J.M., age 55, with hepatic liposarcoma and liver pain, was well controlled on oral morphine 150mg every 4 hours. On this dose he was pain-free and mentally alert (demonstrated by his ability to complete The Times crossword puzzle each day). After some weeks he noticed some drowsiness, and he had one hallucination (he thought he saw someone sitting on his bed). The dose of oral morphine was decreased to 120mg every 4 hours, and after a few days (because he still felt a bit drowsy) to 90mg every 4 hours. He remained pain-free on this dose until he died 2 months later.

II.   What about addiction?

★   **Patients often fear addiction. Patients with chronic pain do not and cannot get addicted to morphine.** This is proved clinically by seeing patients whose pain is abolished (with a nerve block, for example) when even high doses of morphine used for several months can be stopped immediately with no withdrawal effects. Patients who are terminally ill still often fear that they may become addicted to morphine. They and their families can be reassured. This cannot happen when morphine is correctly used to control their pain.

Mr. N.C., who was well controlled on 300mg morphine every 4 hours (see case history earlier), had increasingly severe pain. For three weeks he was pain-free on 600mg morphine every 4 hours, but he then needed a further dose increase to 1000mg morphine every 4 hours. At this point a celiac plexus nerve block was performed for pain control and this abolished his pain. He stopped all morphine the same day and he suffered no withdrawal effects (proving he was not addicted despite the high doses).

A month later he suffered a different pain, this time due to an ileofemoral thrombosis in his left leg. Morphine was started while he was in the hospital for monitoring of anti-coagulant therapy, and the dose was gradually increased to 60mg every 4 hours. This dose controlled the pain for 2 to 3 hours, and he was told (wrongly) that higher doses could not be given. On returning to hospice care his morphine dose was increased to 150mg every 4 hours, and his pain was controlled. After a week his pain decreased as the thrombosis resolved and he became drowsy. Morphine was decreased to 100mg every 4 hours. He remained pain-free and alert until his death 10 days later. Mr. N. C. had not developed tolerance to morphine. A different pain required a different dose.

What about narcotic addicts? Known narcotic addicts with cancer pain respond normally to morphine. The dose is titrated, and the pain is controlled. The regular use of oral morphine to control pain does not have any euphoric effects (which usually occur only after an IV bolus of a relatively high dose).

Morphine should never be withheld from a patient with proven cancer "in case the patient is a narcotic addict". If the patient is pretending to have pain in order to get morphine for his addiction, then oral doses every 4 hours will bring no satisfaction, which will be clinically obvious.

III.   **What about respiratory depression?**

★   **Respiratory depression does not occur when morphine is correctly used to control pain.**

In one study of 20 cancer patients (12 with COPD) taking at least 100mg of morphine per day for at least 7 days, only one had an elevated pCO_2 level. As long as morphine is titrated, and the dose is reduced if drowsiness occurs, there is no danger of respiratory depression. **Following pain-relieving procedures** (such as a nerve block), morphine should be stopped. If pain persists morphine should be promptly restarted in low dosage and titrated.

What about drug interactions? Morphine can be safely prescribed with all other drugs **except monoamine oxidase (MAO) inhibitors**, which are occasionally used as anti-depressants. Hypertensive crisis or mental excitation can occur.

What about morphine and alcohol? It is safe to have an alcoholic drink. Many patients taking morphine enjoy their accustomed cocktail each evening. In fact, most British in-patient hospices have a small bar or a drinks trolley for just that purpose!

MOUTH CARE

Mouth care is important. Debilitated patients commonly develop a sore, dry mouth and **70% of patients with advanced cancer develop oral thrush**.

Routine mouth care involves:

- Rinsing with diluted mild mouthwash (every 12 hours)
- Brushing of teeth (every 12 hours)
- Soaking of dentures overnight
- Cleaning with Toothette (every 2 to 4 hours)
- Applying Vaseline to dry lips

Cleaning with a foam-stick applicator (Toothette) dipped in water or sodium. bicarbonate (or impregnated with lemon glycerin) needs to be done after every meal and more frequently in patients who are mouth-breathing (consider using a room humidifier).

Patients should be encouraged to do their own mouth care to maintain their independence. For weak patients the nurse or family carer can use a Toothette, or put on a disposable glove and wrap gauze around a finger. If there is difficulty opening the mouth (in oropharyngeal cancers) irrigate regularly with a gentle mouthwash using a syringe and very soft mouth brush.

Radiotherapy to the mouth can cause extreme dryness and soreness. A mucilage of lemon syrup, water and methylcellulose (1:1:2) with soluble aspirin dissolved in it is soothing. The mouth should be rinsed regularly with diluted Peridex mouthwash to prevent **gingivitis**.

Three Common Problems
I. Dry mouth

II. Sore mouth

III. Coated tongue

I.   **Dry mouth** — At least 50% of patients suffer from dryness of the mouth due to thrush (candidiasis), dehydration, effects of anti-cholinergic drugs, diuretics, or morphine.

Management options:
- 2-hourly mouth care
- Stop unnecessary drugs
- Treat for thrush
- Artificial saliva
- Suck ice

Mouth care needs to be performed every 2 hours for a dry mouth.

Drugs can cause dryness of the mouth (especially tricyclics, phenothiazines, diuretics). Stop unnecessary drugs or use ones with the least anti-cholinergic side-effects.

Thrush often presents as dryness, before soreness and the typical signs develop. **All patients with advanced illness complaining of a dry mouth should be treated for thrush.** Angular stomatitis is usually due to thrush (very rarely is it due to vitamin deficiency). The patient's mouth should be gently inspected daily with a padded spatula and flashlight. (see Candidiasis)

Artificial saliva can be helpful, especially for the very dry mouth following radiotherapy. Drinks that stimulate the flow of saliva (mild lemon juice, grapefruit juice, tonic water, club soda) can be encouraged.

Crushed ice on a teaspoon is all that many patients need, particularly in the terminal phase.

II.   **Sore mouth may be due to:**
- Thrush
- Loose dentures
- Gingivitis
- Mouth ulcers

Management options:
- Always **treat for thrush**. (see Candidiasis)
- Dentures become loose and rub (because of weight loss and loss of oral tissue). It is a simple matter to **reline dentures**, and a visit to the dentist for that purpose can actually produce a disproportionate boost to morale.
- Gingivitis usually causes halitosis as well as soreness and should be treated with **metronidazole**.
- Mouth ulcers can be helped by **triamcinolone acetonide dental paste** applied 2 or 3 times a day, and at bedtime.
- Soreness of the mouth and throat can be treated symptomatically with **viscous lidocaine mouth rinse**.

III.   **Coated tongue** is unpleasant, can cause halitosis, and predisposes to oral thrush.

Management options:
- **Effervescent Vitamin C tablets** (where available), placed on the tongue and dissolved, 4 times a day.
- **Fresh pineapple** (which contains proteolytic enzyme, ananase). It can cause stinging which is reduced by freezing the slices and dipping them in powdered sugar.
- **Hydrogen peroxide mouthwash** froths and removes surface debris (in a mix of 2% hydrogen peroxide with water). Some patients find it unpleasant to use.
- **Clotrimazole lozenges** dissolved slowly in the mouth, for resistant thrush.

MUSCLE SPASMS

There are 5 types of muscle spasms:

1. Spasticity
2. Secondary to bone pain or fracture
3. Myofascial
4. Night cramps
5. Tetany

1. **Spasticity** is due to spinal cord damage (paraplegia) or stroke (hemiplegia). Painful flexor spasms can occur. Diazepam 5mg to 10mg at bedtime is the drug of choice. Baclofen 5mg to 30mg 3 times a day (after food) is less sedating and acts centrally at the spinal level. The dose should be built up slowly to avoid nausea and drowsiness. Physiotherapy, using passive movements, is important to prevent flexion contraction.

2. **Bone pain** can precipitate muscle spasm. Muscle spasm round a **fracture** can be relieved by skin traction. (see Bone Pain, Fractures)

3. **Myofascial pain** (or myofibrosis) occurs especially in the shoulders and neck. It is worse on movement, and there is an area of muscular tenderness (trigger point). The possibility of bone metastases must be considered and excluded. Myofascial pain often responds to local heat and massage. A local injection of 5ml 0.25% bupivacaine with 2ml methylprednisolone into the tender spot can bring dramatic and long-lasting relief. Simpler and often very effective is ethyl chloride spray which causes evaporative cooling.

4. **Night cramps** usually respond to quinine sulfate 260mg at bedtime.

5. **Tetany** causes muscular cramps in the hands with tingling (especially peri-oral). It is usually due to hyperventilation secondary to anxiety (respiratory alkalosis increases calcium binding to albumin). It is prevented by teaching breathing exercises and relaxation techniques. (see Dyspnea, Relaxation)

NAUSEA & VOMITING

Nausea and vomiting occur in 60% of terminal cancer patients at some stage but tend to be intermittent (in one study 21% of patients reported nausea and vomiting at each evaluation).

The plan of management is:

1. History and examination
2. Consider causes
3. Choose anti-emetic(s)
4. Choose route
5. Change anti-emetic regime
6. Consider steroids
7. Consider ranitidine
8. Change or reduce opioid
9. Remember anxiety
10. Celiac plexus block (very rarely indicated)

There are usually several causes contributing to nausea (for example, anxiety, a new NSAID, constipation, and the strong smell of cooking all playing a part).

It can be helpful to think in terms of a **nausea threshold** (analogous to a pain threshold) and to consider several approaches to raising the nausea threshold.

1. History and examination — A past history of peptic ulcer may be relevant — a peptic ulcer may cause nausea with little pain (masked by steroids or analgesics).

Try to discover if there is a pattern to the nausea:

- After certain drugs
- After meals (if so, try metoclopramide)
- On movement (try cyclizine)
- In certain situations (anxiety-related)
- With certain smells

Ask about:

- Epigastric pain (?gastritis)
- Pain on swallowing (?oral thrush)
- Pain on standing (?mesenteric traction)
- Thirst (?hypercalcemia)
- Hiccup (?uremia)

- Heartburn (?small stomach syndrome)
- Dysuria (?urinary tract infection)
- Constipation (?constipation!)

★   **Nausea can become a conditioned response.**

The most dramatic example of a conditioned response is nausea after chemotherapy, then nausea on arriving at the chemotherapy clinic, then finally on seeing the appointment card for the chemotherapy clinic. For this reason, to abolish prolonged nausea may require high doses of anti-emetics for a few days to break the association of events and surroundings with nausea.

★   **Palliative radiotherapy rarely causes nausea unless the field includes the celiac plexus (anterior to L1).**

Examination:

- Mouth (?oral thrush)
- Speech, arms, legs (?brain metastases)
- Abdomen (?hepatomegaly ?obstruction)
- Rectal (?constipation)
- Bloods (urea, calcium, drug levels)
- Mid-stream clean catch urine specimen

★   **Neurological signs are usually obvious if nausea or vomiting are due to brain metastases. Papilledema is an unreliable sign of raised intracranial pressure.**

2. **Causes of nausea (which may respond to treatment other than anti-emetics):**

- Drugs
- Oral thrush
- Brain metastases
- Anxiety
- Gastric irritation
- Small stomach syndrome
- Intestinal obstruction
- Constipation
- Hypercalcemia
- Uremia
- Low grade urinary tract or pulmonary infection

It is useful to remember this list and apply it when nausea is a problem in advanced disease. Reversible causes are often found, but **it is important to abolish nausea as quickly as possible and to use anti-emetics with other treatments initially**.

Drugs that can cause nausea include:

- Opioids
- NSAIDs
- Antibiotics (metronidazole, erythromycin)
- Digoxin (consider drug level)
- Estrogens
- Cytotoxics
- Many others!

Stop as many drugs as possible. Remember, metronidazole and alcohol together will cause headaches and nausea.

It can be important to discover whether uremia is the cause (even though it is untreatable) because it means you can stop looking for other causes, you can explain to the patient and family why nausea and vomiting are present ("Is the cancer spreading, doctor?"), and because chlorpromazine is usually the best drug.

3. Choose an appropriate **anti-emetic**. Haloperidol is effective as a twice-a-day regime. Chlorpromazine may be more suitable if sedation is needed, or if hiccups are troublesome. Metoclopramide is useful if poor gastric emptying is a problem. (*see Phenothiazines*)

Cyclizine is particularly useful if there is an element of motion sickness or as a logical addition to a drug acting at the CTZ. Methotrimeprazine as a continuous subcutaneous infusion is the most powerful anti-emetic but can cause drowsiness. (*see Anti-emetics*)

4. **Choose the appropriate route:**

- Oral
- Suppository
- IM injection
- Subcutaneous

The **oral route** is best for prophylaxis. If a patient is feeling nauseated or vomiting more than two or three times a day, oral absorption is reduced and **suppositories** or **injections are needed for at least 24 hours before trying oral anti-emetics again**.

Some patients are well-controlled on suppositories, others dislike them or cannot use them.

A **continuous subcutaneous infusion** is useful for severe nausea and vomiting to avoid repeated injections. (*see Subcutaneous Infusions*)

★   **In nausea there is a reflux of duodenal contents into a relaxed stomach, therefore there is poor absorption of oral drugs.**

5. **Change anti-emetic regime** — Try full doses of one anti-emetic before changing to another. Sometimes the patient needs two (and rarely three) anti-emetics for good control. It is logical to combine anti-emetics that act at different sites, for example, haloperidol (CTZ) with cyclizine (vomiting center). (The combination of haloperidol with metoclopramide is likely to result in dystonia and stiffness, and should be **avoided**.)

6. **Consider steroids** — A trial of high dose steroids is considered in three situations which can cause nausea and vomiting:

• Raised intracranial pressure

• Hypercalcemia

• Malignant pyloric stenosis

Apart from these, steroids can have a direct anti-emetic effect. The mechanism of action is unknown but the usefulness of steroids in cytotoxic-induced sickness is documented. It is common for steroids to reduce or abolish nausea in advanced malignancy, and they should be tried for severe nausea resistant to anti-emetics. (see *Steroids*)

7. **Consider an H$_2$ receptor antagonist** — Gastric irritation can occur with NSAIDs. Epigastric discomfort may be masked by steroids and analgesics. H$_2$ receptor antagonists should be considered for nausea especially if there is a history of peptic ulceration or if nausea is associated with heartburn. The usual dose is ranitidine 150mg 2 times a day. A trial of ranitidine may be indicated in nausea resistant to anti-emetics.

8. **Consider changing or reducing the opioid drug** — Nausea related to morphine can occur because the patient is taking more morphine than required. A reduction in pain occurs (either spontaneously, or following radiotherapy or a nerve block) and the previous dose of morphine is now too high, commonly causing drowsiness, but also occasionally nausea.

30% of patients experience mild nausea for a few days after starting morphine. An anti-emetic (such as thiethylperazine 10mg 2 to 3 times a day, prochlorperazine 5mg 3 times a day, or haloperidol 0.5mg to 1.5mg at bedtime) can be prescribed to prevent this nausea.

About 1% of patients are intolerant of morphine, which causes severe, persistent nausea and vomiting despite treatment with anti-emetics. These patients require an alternative opioid analgesic (hydromorphone, oxycodone, buprenorphine, methadone).

All these drugs can themselves cause nausea (particularly buprenorphine in about 20% of cases) but true morphine-related nausea can be abolished in an individual by changing to one of these opioids. (see Analgesics)

9. **Nausea and anxiety** — Anxiety can cause nausea. Nausea can cause anxiety. ("Is the cancer spreading?") Some people react to anxiety by feeling nauseated. Relieving anxiety (often by sharing worries and fears) can help to reduce or abolish nausea.

10. **Celiac plexus block** — A celiac plexus nerve block should be considered for intractable nausea resistant to other treatments. It can abolish nausea — possibly because the trunk of the left vagus passes through the plexus. In fact, intractable nausea is extremely rare if the regimes described in this section are applied. (Intractable nausea may very rarely be due to a brainstem metastasis involving the vomiting center.) (see Celiac Plexus Block)

Vomiting with little or no nausea can occur in:

1. Regurgitation
2. High intestinal obstruction
3. Raised intracranial pressure

1. **Regurgitation** is usually seen in carcinoma of the esophagus with total dysphagia. It is usually obvious from the history of food sticking and coming back (the food contains no acid). A pharyngeal pouch can also cause regurgitation.

2. **High intestinal obstruction** — Malignant pyloric stenosis is associated with vomiting of large volumes (300 ml to 600 ml) of undigested food some hours after a meal, with little preceding nausea. The force of the vomit can make it come down the nose. There is no bile in the vomit. Duodenal obstruction (due to carcinoma of the pancreas) produces a similar pattern. A "vomit chart" is occasionally helpful to see the typical pattern if the patient is a poor historian. A palliative gastro-enterostomy can prevent the problem. High dose steroids (dexamethasone 8 mg per day — initially by IM injection) can reduce peri-tumor edema and improve gastric emptying.

3. **Raised intracranial pressure** is classically said to cause early morning headaches and vomiting, with little or no nausea. In fact, in advanced disease due to cerebral primary tumors or cerebral metastases both headache and vomiting are uncommon.

★ **It may not be possible to abolish vomiting, but patients can accept occasional vomiting provided they are free of nausea.**

NERVE BLOCKS

Definition — A nerve block is the insertion of a needle close to a nerve — sometimes requiring fluoroscopic x-ray control — in order to inject a solution to cause a neural blockade (temporary or permanent).

★ **About 7% of hospice in-patients with cancer pains benefit from some kind of nerve-blocking procedure.**

Indications for a nerve block:

- Localized pain
- Pain uncontrolled by drugs plus psychotherapy
- Pain unresponsive to chemotherapy or radiotherapy
- No coagulopathy (stop warfarin!)
- No tumor at site of injection
- Willing patient and family
- Possible side-effects explained
- Benefits explained (so expectations are realistic)

The most useful nerve blocks are:

Nerve Block	Main Indications
1. Celiac plexus block	pancreas, liver pain
2. Paravertebral block	chest wall pain
3. Epidural steroids	root irritation
4. Epidural morphine	morphine side-effects
5. Epidural local anesthetic	pelvic or leg pain
6. Psoas compartment block	hip or lumbar root pain
7. Intrathecal neurolysis	perineal pain

Nerve blocks that are occasionally indicated are:

8. Caudal block	sciatic root pain
9. Local infiltration	fractured humerus, femur
10. Brachial plexus block	arm neuralgia

1. **Celiac plexus block** (see Celiac Plexus Block)

2. The **paravertebral nerve block** is used to control pain from the thoracic spine and chest wall. Although sometimes called a somatic block it also involves the sympathetic supply. It is often more useful than an intercostal block because it covers several segments.

It can be particularly useful for:

- Chest wall pain
- Mesothelioma pain
- Vertebral metastases
- Esophageal pain (T3, 4, 5)
- Rib fractures
- Post-thoracotomy pain
- Post-herpetic neuralgia

X-ray control is used to place the needle (under local anesthetic) in the paravertebral space. Complications are rare.

3. **Epidural steroids** can be given into the epidural space which lies inside the vertebral bone, but outside the dural sac and the cerebrospinal fluid (CSF). A **single injection** of steroids (methylprednisolone 80mg to 120mg) into the epidural space can be useful for root irritation after vertebral collapse. It can be given at any level. It can give pain relief within 48 hours that can last for weeks.

4. **Epidural morphine infusion** can be useful if a patient on high dose morphine has troublesome drowsiness. It is a safe procedure that should normally be considered before other more destructive nerve blocking procedures. The incidence of morphine side-effects is reduced compared to other routes. The starting dose is normally around 25% of the regular oral dose (for example, a patient on 60mg oral morphine every 4 hours would be given 15mg epidurally as a bolus, which may last 8 to 12 hours). In one study of epidural morphine in 37 patients with intractable cancer pain the average daily dose was 24mg of epidural morphine; the duration of epidural use ranged from 2 to 177 days. Visceral and bone pain responded better than nerve pain. If the analgesic effect is lost despite high epidural doses of morphine (over 100mg per day), it is sometimes possible to regain the effect by stopping morphine for 48 hours (to "rest" the receptor), using epidural clonidine in the interim (as a substitute analgesic), then stopping clonidine and re-starting morphine in lower doses than before. Alternatively, continue morphine and consider adding di-

lute (0.125%) bupivacaine (usually 10mls every 2 to 3 hours) which can reduce pain without causing leg weakness or urinary retention. (*see Spinal Opioids*)

5. **Epidural local anesthetic** (widely used in obstetrical practice) has the disadvantage of causing weak, numb legs and urinary retention. It can have a place for severe pelvic pain or painful pressure sores when the patient is already immobile and has a urinary catheter.

6. **Psoas compartment block** is useful for pain due to infiltration of the lumbosacral plexus, or for hip pain (either arthritic or malignant). The psoas compartment lies anterior to the transverse processes of the lumbar vertebrae. It can be identified by injecting dye under x-ray control. Local anesthetic and steroids are injected. Reversible leg weakness sometimes occurs. Pain relief is usually good.

7. **Intrathecal neurolysis** is the injection of a neurolytic agent into the CSF to destroy sensory nerve roots (but motor nerve roots are also at risk). The spread of the neurolytic agent is controlled by gravity. The patient is positioned so that the anterior (motor) roots are rotated **away** from the neurolytic agent. It is usually reserved for patients with perineal pain (for example, a pelvic recurrence following surgical abdomino-perineal resection) who are already immobile and have a permanent urinary catheter, since there is a risk of causing leg weakness or urinary incontinence. Leg weakness may be temporary (for 2 to 3 days) but can be permanent. Some centers use intrathecal neurolysis to treat thoracic or upper lumbar nerve root pain.

8. **Caudal** (sacral) extradural nerve blocks can reduce sciatic or perineal pain. The needle is inserted via the sacral hiatus to gain access to the trans-sacral canal. 0.5% bupivacaine is used initially, and if the effect of the block is acceptable a neurolytic agent can then be used.

In one series of caudal blocks (using a cryoprobe) for sciatic pain, 12 out of 17 patients had pain relief. Although its main use is in the management of acute pain, it has been used with success for patients with cancer pain. It can be repeated.

Cryoanalgesia is the application of a cryoprobe to a peripheral nerve. It blocks nerve conduction and relieves pain. It produces a reversible block for a median duration of 11 days (range up to 224 days).

The cryoprobe is applied under local anesthesia. It contains a nerve stimulator for accurate positioning. The probe releases liquid nitrous oxide which freezes to -60°C. The axon dies but regrows at 1mm/day, giving a more prolonged block than local anesthetic but without the risk of painful neuralgia following neurolytics. Occasionally relief lasts several months, despite early recovery of motor and sensory function.

9. **Local infiltration** (see *Fractures*)

10. **Brachial plexus block** is rarely indicated. A continuous infusion of local anesthetic can occasionally be useful for cancer pain, but it causes a numb, paralyzed arm which the patient may find more unpleasant than the pain. Neurolytic agents are contraindicated, partly because the patient may want the effect reversed, and partly because of high incidence of painful neuritis at this site.

Discussion:

★   **The indication for a nerve block is pain irrespective of prognosis. A nerve block may be worthwhile even in a very ill patient if pain is not otherwise controlled.**

A **graduated approach** to pain control is adopted, so that non-invasive low-risk techniques are used before nerve blocks are considered. A nerve block should never be used as sole therapy. In certain situations, however, if a nerve block is known to be very effective it should be considered early (for example, a celiac plexus block for pancreatic pain not responding to titrated doses of morphine).

★   **Nerve blocks are an adjunct to other treatments. They can reduce pain but rarely abolish pain.**

★   **Anti-coagulant therapy is an absolute contraindication to nerve blocks.**

A **reversible diagnostic block** should be performed with a local anesthetic before neurolytic agents (phenol or absolute alcohol) are used to give long-lasting blockade. (This is best explained to the patient as "a trial run", rather than an "experiment".) **This is to establish distribution of pain and observe side effects.**

A diagnostic somatic block causes decreased sensation to pinprick. If the patient continues to complain of pain despite evidence of a block, or if the patient claims pain relief with no evidence of a block, it is futile to proceed to a therapeutic block. Occasionally a local anesthetic block can last weeks or months, for unknown reasons.

Bupivacaine (0.5%) is the best local anesthetic for nerve blocks. The duration of action is 8 to 12 hours, and there are few side effects up to 2mg/kg.

The dose of morphine should be reduced or stopped following a nerve block, and the patient observed for 24 hours. Morphine requirements may decrease as pain lessens. Drowsiness or even respiratory depression can occur if the patient remains on more morphine than is now required for the pain. One method is to stop morphine and promptly re-titrate (use an initial low dose of morphine if there is still some pain and increase the dose every 4 hours as necessary). (*see Morphine*)

It is essential that the actual nerve block procedure be painless. The object is to relieve suffering. The procedure should normally be carried out under local anesthetic and sedation with IV midazolam, which also causes retrograde amnesia.

Detailed explanation is essential. The terminally ill patient is vulnerable, and needs to have a sense of control over medical intervention. Often the patient has already adjusted to the idea of having no more invasive procedures, and it is therefore psychologically difficult to undergo a nerve block. However "routine" nerve blocks may be to the doctor, if the patient is dubious it is usually better to postpone the procedure. The family should also be clearly told what is being considered, and why.

NERVE PAIN

Definition — Pain which occurs in an area of abnormal or absent sensation, due to lesions in the central or peripheral nervous system is called "nerve pain". It is also called **deafferentation pain** (pain that does not depend on activity in pain receptors).

Discussion — Nerve pain is poorly understood and difficult to treat. Nerve pain often responds poorly to morphine and other opioid drugs.

The clinical picture includes:
- Continuous burning and aching pain
- Stabbing pain superimposed
- May be in distribution of nerve
- Numbness, tingling
- Hyperalgesia (slight pain like pinprick felt as severe)
- Allodynia (light touch feels painful)
- Pain-induced insomnia

The pain is severe and continuous and often disturbs sleep, but it can fluctuate in severity and can be reduced by diversional therapy or elevation of mood. There may be a positional element to the pain (presumably because of pressure on nerve roots).

It typically occurs in the arm when there is involvement of the brachial plexus (from Pancoast's syndrome or axillary nodes) or in the leg when there is involvement of the lumbo-sacral plexus with pelvic tumors.

Brachial plexopathy occurs with tumors in the apex of the lung or direct infiltration of the plexuses due to metastases, usually from breast, lung or lymphoma. Pain typically precedes neurological signs by weeks or months. (see Pancoast's Syndrome)

Involvement of the lower cord of the plexus causes:

- Pain (in shoulder or paraspinal region)
- Tingling and pain (in 4th and 5th fingers)
- Wasting (in small muscles of the hand)
- Sensory loss (in medial hand and forearm)
- Ptosis (in sympathetic fibers near lower cord of plexus)
- Cord compression (epidural invasion)

Tumor in the supraclavicular region involves the **upper cord of the plexus** causing burning pain in the index finger and thumb. A CT scan will usually demonstrate a well-defined mass which may extend down to the apex of the lung, or across the infraclavicular region.

Lumbo-sacral plexopathy occurs with invasion of the sacrum due to pelvic tumors (usually colo-rectal or cervical) but also occurring in breast cancer, lymphoma and sarcomas. It usually suggests advanced disease. CT scan may demonstrate tumor but can appear normal.

The clinical picture (which can be bilateral) includes:

- Sacral pain (aching, pressure-like)
- Weakness in the leg
- Root pain in the leg (burning, stabbing)
- Numbness or tingling:
  - Anterior thigh (L1, 2, 3)
  - Lateral calf (L4)
  - Big toe (L5)
  - Back of the leg (sacral nerves)

Assessment — Diagnosis is often suspected from the description of the pain (burning, stabbing) and confirmed by evidence of reduced or altered sensation in the region of pain.

★ **TENS is rarely helpful for nerve pain, and tends to exacerbate it.**

Management options for nerve pain include:

1. Explanation
2. Trial of morphine
3. Tricyclics
4. Anti-convulsants
5. Membrane stabilizing drugs
6. Trial of high dose steroids
7. Diversional therapy
8. Special techniques (rarely)

1. It is helpful to **explain the nature of the pain** to the patient, emphasizing the following:

- It is nerve damage pain (not tissue or organ damage)
- It responds poorly to analgesics like aspirin and morphine
- Tricyclics should be started to treat pain
- First step is to get a good night's sleep

2. A **trial of morphine** is important because some neuralgic pains respond partially, especially if there is a deep, aching component to the pain. There can also be an element of soft tissue pain superimposed on the neuralgic pain. The correct dose of morphine is the dose that reduces the pain as much as possible without causing drowsiness. (Drowsiness without pain relief means the pain is not morphine-responsive or poorly morphine-responsive.) Start with a low dose and promptly increase in steps. (*see Morphine*)

3. **Tricyclics** — Imipramine is the drug of choice, although other tricyclics are probably equally effective. The aim is to increase the dose as quickly as possible to 100mg to 150mg per day (it is unusual to need more than 100mg).

The speed of increase in dose depends on the severity of pain and the degree of supervision, but a useful guide is:

Day 1	10mg to 25mg
Day 3	25mg to 50mg
Day 7	50mg to 100mg
Day 10	100mg to 150mg

Elderly or frail patients need lower doses. Side-effects (especially a dry mouth) often limit the tolerated dose. Onset of relief is unusual before Day 4 or 5, and unlikely with only 25mg.

4. **Anti-convulsants** can sometimes relieve the severe stabbing (lancinating) pains of neuralgia. They act by inhibiting trans-synaptic discharges and reducing neuronal excitability.

The useful drugs are:

- Clonazepam
- Carbamazepine
- Valproic acid
- Phenytoin

They should be tried in the above order. No one particular pain syndrome responds to a particular drug. These drugs have been studied in non-malignant nerve pain. Controlled studies of their use in nerve pain of malignancy are lacking.

Clonazepam has been the most effective drug in comparative studies (there are no double-blind studies) but it also causes the most drowsiness. About 40% of patients respond. The starting dose is 0.5mg at bedtime for 1 week, increasing gradually to a maximum of 3mg per day in divided doses.

Carbamazepine is effective for trigeminal neuralgia (80% respond within 24 hours), and for painful diabetic neuropathy (in one double blind study 28 out of 30 patients responded). 20% of patients with nerve pain due to malignancy respond. The starting dose is 100mg 2 times a day, increasing gradually (to avoid drowsiness) until a response is achieved, up to a maximum of 400mg 3 times a day.

Valproic acid starting at 200mg 3 times a day or 500mg at bedtime (increasing to 600mg 4 times a day) is commonly chosen as first line treatment for stabbing neuropathic pain, because it causes less drowsiness than clonazepam or carbamazepine. About 20% of patients respond.

Phenytoin is known to be significantly more effective than placebo for painful diabetic neuropathy. The usual starting dose is 300mg at bedtime (increasing to 600mg per day). About 20% of patients respond.

Ideally a trial of each drug should last 4 to 6 weeks, but with severe pain and a short prognosis this period may have to be reduced to 1 to 2 weeks.

5. **Membrane stabilizing drugs** — Flecainide is a membrane stabilizing drug originally used to treat tachyarrythmias. It has been used to treat the pain of malignant infiltration of nerve following a double-blind study which demonstrated that mexiletine (a similar drug) produced significant improvement in painful diabetic neuropathy. The dose of flecainide is 100mg 2 times a day. In one series 6 out of 17 patients with nerve pain had complete analgesia for 1 to 26 weeks.

Clonidine 25 micrograms 3 times a day increasing to 100 micrograms 3 times a day has been successfully used to control nerve pain. Clonidine is an alpha-2 agonist which may work by stimulating the descending pathways. Epidural clonidine has been successfully used for pain control. (see Nerve Blocks, Pain Pathways, Spinal Opioids)

6. A **trial of high dose steroids** can reduce nerve pain, probably by relieving nerve compression. A 10-day trial of dexamethasone 8mg per day may be indicated especially if other drugs have failed. This can occasionally produce a dramatic response.

7. **Diversional therapy** — Pain is a somato-psychic experience. A person is more able to cope with a continuous pain if he feels cheerful, secure and preoccupied with an interest or a project. An imaginative occupational therapist or recreational therapist can sometimes transform the patient's existence.

8. **Special techniques** — In intractable nerve pain special techniques may **very occasionally** be required, including nerve blocks, spinal opioids or cordotomy. (see Cordotomy, Nerve Blocks, Spinal Opioids)

NERVE PALSIES

Weak patients tend to sit for long periods of time, resting their arms on the arms of a chair. This can cause pressure on the **ulnar nerve** on the medial side of the elbow, and the **radial nerve** on the medial side of the humerus.

Ulnar nerve palsy causes tingling and numbness in the 4th and 5th fingers. Only if prolonged will it also cause wasting of the small muscles of the hand. Management involves taking the pressure off the nerve, perhaps using padded arm rests.

Radial nerve palsy causes wrist-drop, often occurring after the patient has fallen asleep with the inside of the upper arm leaning on a hard surface. Management involves a wrist splint to keep the wrist extended so the hand can grip. Wrist extension usually returns within 2 to 3 weeks.

NON-VERBAL COMMUNICATION

We give and receive powerful non-verbal messages about each other. When we say we have "an intuition" or "a feeling about someone" we have usually been reading non-verbal cues. If words and body language are incongruent it is the latter that is believed. ("He said the operation was a success, but I didn't believe him.") Body language is very difficult to control or alter. Some is autonomic and outside conscious control (skin flushes, pupil size).

★ **Body language must be interpreted in context. It is clusters of signals that convey information. There are significant cultural variations in how body language is interpreted.**

Eye contact should ideally occur for 60% to 70% of the time during a conversation (less can seem evasive, more can seem hostile or flirtatious depending on other signals). Poor eye contact may be due to shyness or awkwardness, but tends to suggest dishonesty or coldness. Looking only at the eyes and forehead (instead of the whole face) can convey coldness. **Even brief eye contact with a smile can be supportive behavior in a crisis.** (see *Support*)

Facial expression is very important. Many expressions are universal. For example, the eye-brow is raised for a greeting, or the furrowed brow and tightened muscles around the eyes suggest sadness or tension. (In primates, this latter facial expression often precedes a loud scream.) No other animal has as many superficial facial muscles as man, and we recognize each other not by smell but by facial characteristics. We can detect the most minute changes in facial expression and we are sensitive to their meaning. We become skillful at facial displays, but most people cannot sustain them for long. (Notice how hospitalized patients relax their facial muscles a few seconds after the doctor has visited them and left their bedside.)

Posture conveys attitudes. Sitting down with someone is a powerful message. ("On the level" means honesty.) We tend to turn our body towards what interests us. This can give away our true feelings. When standing we point our feet towards what interests us. We cross our arms or legs when we feel defensive, or want to distance ourselves from someone. Leaning back on a chair can make us appear aggressive or domineering. When two people are in agreement they often mirror each other's posture and unconsciously take up the same position as each other. The distance we stay from others conveys a message. Entering a person's intimate zone (about 12 inches) is often allowed for doctors and nurses in the right context, but can sometimes signal either flirtation or aggression (depending on other cues and on culture). Richard Asher observed that the distance a person sits from the back of a chair often correlates with anxiety levels.

Gestures and mannerisms can easily be misinterpreted. Looking over the top of eyeglasses tilts the chin down which tends to convey disapproval. Fidgeting with the hands may be a habit, but tends to convey irritation or frustration. A palm-downwards handshake signals a dominant attitude, a palm-upwards handshake signals willingness to give control to the other person. Hand-to-face gestures are mostly displaced hand-over-mouth gestures (seen often in lying children) and often indicate that the person is having negative thoughts.

The spoken word has music as well as content. Tone of voice, volume, variation, emphasis, sighs, laughter, pauses — all convey messages. Not discussing a topic can be a powerful communication. Even sad words ("You have got a serious illness which is going to shorten your life ") can be spoken in a depressing, pessimistic way or a kind and supportive way.

Touch is a very powerful form of non-verbal communication. This is emphasized by a psychological experiment in which the feelings of subjects towards a librarian (in fact an actress) were significantly affected by whether or not she touched their hand (very briefly) as she returned their library card. (*see Touch*)

Smell affects communication (and is the basis of the perfume industry). A foul-smelling wound or discharge reduces communication and can be socially isolating.

Non-verbal signs of anxiety, awkwardness or anger include:

- Looking away
- Eye closing (for longer than one second)
- Side glance with furrowed brow
- Chin down
- Displacement gestures (picking at clothes)
- Hand-to-face gestures
- Fingers in the mouth
- Neck rubbing
- Clenched fists
- Tight grip (on objects or self)

When talking to patients ask yourself "What is my body communicating?" Feelings affect body language, and body language affects feelings. Consciously practicing good body language habits may produce positive feelings. (*see Talking with Patients*)

Awareness of non-verbal communication is not new. The following passage was written over 3,000 years ago: "If you have been foolish, exalting yourself, or if you have been devising evil, put your hand on your mouth." (Proverbs 30; verse 32)

NOSE BLEEDS

Nose bleeds can be trivial or very severe.

Management options:

- First aid for **minor bleeds** consists of local pressure maintained for 10 minutes. The patient should sit up (less pressure.)

- In **moderate bleeds**, a toothette swab soaked in topical adrenaline (1 in 1,000) can be pushed firmly up the nostril.

- In **heavy bleeding**, the nose should be packed firmly, under local anesthetic spray. Ribbon vaseline gauze should be packed into the nose using a nasal speculum and angled forceps, and left for 2 to 3 days before being removed.

- For **recurrent nosebleeds**, cauterization of the blood vessels responsible should be considered, except in leukemia.

- In some patients with **thrombocytopenia** a platelet transfusion may be indicated. (*see Leukemia*)

NSAIDs (ANTI-INFLAMMATORIES)

Non-steroidal anti-inflammatory drugs (NSAIDs) are thought to work by inhibiting prostaglandin synthesis (prostaglandin being one of the mediators of the inflammatory response). Bone metastases are thought to release prostaglandins. Single doses of NSAIDs are analgesic, repeated doses are anti-inflammatory.

Indications for NSAIDs:
- Bone pain from metastases
- Arthritis
- Night sweats
- Skin pain (see *Breast Cancer*)

★ **NSAIDs reduce or abolish bone pain in about 80% of cases.**

Which NSAID? — A patient on a mild NSAID such as ibuprofen who still has bone pain should be changed to one of the stronger drugs listed below.

First choice is often naproxen 500mg 2 times a day either by tablet, or suspension. Oral indomethacin 50mg 4 times a day, or two 50mg suppositories 2 times a day, is more potent (but more frequently causes side effects).

The more potent NSAIDs are more effective, but also tend to cause more side effects. Good comparative trials have not been done, so it is difficult to know which are best. If a patient fails to respond to one NSAID (or has adverse reactions) it is sometimes advisable to try a drug from a different group (although there is no evidence to support this idea).

Useful NSAIDs from different groups include:
- Naproxen — a proprionic acid
- Diclofenac — an acetic acid
- Piroxicam — an oxicam
- Indomethacin — an indole
- Choline magnesium trisalicylate — a salicylic acid

NSAID side effects:
- Fluid retention
- Dyspepsia (about 20% of patients)
- Peptic ulceration
- Skin rashes

- Urticaria
- Aplastic anemia
- Headache, dizziness (from indomethacin)
- Renal damage

Dyspepsia can still occur when NSAIDs are given in suppository form, although it may be less severe than with oral NSAIDs. Oral NSAIDs should be taken after food. Concurrent H_2-receptor inhibition (ranitidine 150mg 2 times a day) may be indicated to prevent dyspepsia.

If a patient has a history of peptic ulceration it is still safe to use NSAIDs covered by ranitidine. In most patients the bone pain will be reduced or abolished, without gastric irritation. (If dyspepsia occurs, the NSAID should be stopped.) (see Bone Pain)

NUTRITION

Pathophysiology — About 20% of cancer patients die because of gross wasting (cachexia) and no other obvious cause. The dietary intake of protein and calories is insufficient to meet the needs of the tumor, and the patient may experience profound weight loss despite a reasonable food intake. A tumor approximating 2% of body weight can use over 40% of a person's daily caloric intake. The capacity for a tumor to enlarge while the rest of the body wastes has led some researchers to call a tumor a "nitrogen trap".

**Three Distinct Clinical Situations
In Planning Nutritional Support**

I. Patients undergoing treatment aimed at cure

II. Patients with dysphagia, enjoying general well-being

III. Terminally ill patients who are no longer active

Cancer patients have altered food metabolism, possibly due to tumor hormones such as a cachectin. In starvation the body normally responds by lowering its metabolic rate, but in cancer there is frequently an increased metabolic rate. The pattern of metabolism is changed. A tumor can metabolize large quantities of glucose by the inefficient process of anaerobic glycolysis, which produces lactic acid. The conversion of lactic acid back to glucose in the liver (the Cori cycle) demands energy, as does the breakdown of protein to glucose. These high-energy metabolic processes may account for the raised metabolic rate seen in many cancer patients. Protein metabolism is also affected, and protein breakdown (which slows down after a period of "normal" starvation) continues at a rapid rate in some cancer patients.

I.   In **patients undergoing vigorous treatment aimed at cure** IV hyperalimentation (total parenteral nutrition) is sometimes used in the maintenance of health of patients. It has no advantages over enteral therapy in patients with functioning bowels. Chemotherapy can cause recurrent enteritis. Vigorous nutritional support may help sustain a patient through radical treatment (although firm evidence of this is lacking).

II.   **Patients with dysphagia enjoying good general well-being**, but who are unable to swallow due to cancers of the head and neck, esophagus or stomach, or to neuro-logical conditions such as amyotrophic lateral sclerosis (ALS), can benefit from nutritional support which enables them to ingest enough calories to remain active (and prevents the postural hypotension that under-nutrition can cause).

Management options for this group of patients include:

- Fine bore nasogastric tube
- Gastrostomy
- Jejunostomy
- Pharyngostomy

These procedures may be indicated only in a patient who cannot swallow and who complains of thirst or hunger.

Modern fine bore nasogastric tubes are tolerated quite well. Gastrostomy can be performed percutaneously under endoscopic control. Liquid feeding can be given overnight and disconnected during the day.

IV nutrition is not indicated because it defeats the main aim, which is improved patient activity.

III.   **Terminally ill patients who are no longer active do not need such invasive nutritional support for several important reasons:**

- Intensive feeding does not prolong survival or increase tumor response.
- Intensive feeding cannot reverse weakness or weight loss.

- Intensive feeding does not reduce symptoms or make the patient feel physically stronger.

- Intensive feeding involves medical and nursing procedures (such as tube insertion) which may be unpleasant for a weak patient (and which can create additional problems of leakage and smell).

- Tubes and IV lines tend to increase the emotional distance between patient and family, at a time when emotional closeness is of paramount importance.

For patients who are not active, the more intensive measures are not indicated, but nutritional support continues to be important. Interest in the patient's food intake carries a message from the caregiver. Advice from a dietitian can be invaluable. (see *Diet*)

Management options at this stage include:

- Improving appetite (see *Anorexia*)
- Dietary supplements
- Liquidized food
- Fortifying sip feeds

Dietary supplements containing tasteless glucose polymers can be added to drinks, soups, casseroles or puddings to boost calorie intake.

Sip feedings with nutritionally complete liquid foods can replace eating if the patient is weak. Small frequent amounts (50ml per hour) are encouraged.

★   **Humans can survive for many months on a semi-starvation diet.**

Comment — A reduced diet does not shorten prognosis in advanced disease. For an inactive patient with advanced cancer a low food intake does not cause hunger. Patients may even occasionally notice that a reduced food intake produces a feeling of well-being (as can a prolonged voluntary fast in a healthy person).

Patients' concerns ("I'm losing weight" "I'm not eating enough") often relate to worries about having a serious disease and facing death, and **need to be understood in the context of spiritual anguish**. Patients can usually be helped to come to terms with their true situation by gently explaining their true needs, and allowing them to express their fears. (see *Spiritual Pain*)

Family members need support, because feeding the patient may have been all they could do to help. Since food is essential for life, family members often wrongly assume that more food will prolong life, and need explanation and reassurance. Family members need help to understand the continuing importance of their supportive role even when they can no longer focus on feeding. (Family members should be discouraged from forcing unwanted food on weak patients.)

Professional carers can be tempted to focus on technical methods of nutritional support, rather than on the more difficult issues of spiritual distress. ("I'm wasting away.")

The main problems of reduced food intake are the related psychological concerns of the patient, family members and professional carers.

Measures of nutritional support (such as enteral tubes and IV hyperalimentation) which may be appropriate (ordinary) in patients undergoing treatment aimed at cure or enjoying good general well-being, become inappropriate (extraordinary) in far advanced disease, and should usually be avoided. Such measures do not add to the dying patient's comfort, and may indeed cause unnecessary distress. They may prolong the process of dying by a few days, but do not improve the quality of remaining life.

The decision to remove a tube or IV line is simply one of patient comfort. If the patient wants a tube or IV line removed, it should be removed. If the dying patient is unconscious, professional carers should focus on the real issue, the comfort of the patient, and gently explain to family members that tubes and IV lines do not significantly prolong life.

Removing tubes and IV lines can be difficult if patient, family members or professional carers believe incorrectly that these prolong life, or are needed for comfort. (In Britain, the great majority of patients die with no tubes or IV lines in place, and they die comfortably.)

Teaching professional carers about spiritual support of terminally ill patients and their families gives them skills to help again, and reduces their need to perform technical interventions which have no advantage for the patient, and distract attention from more important spiritual and emotional issues.

OCCUPATIONAL THERAPY

Occupational therapy can be defined as the science of healing by occupation. Humans have a need to engage in occupations and roles, and occupation is a natural means of restoring function. Occupational therapy is traditionally prescribed for patients whose functional abilities are going to improve. However, occupational therapy is also an essential component of hospice and palliative care. Loss of independence and role can result in social death prior to biological death. Occupational therapy can help a person to adopt new and appropriate functions and roles and to maintain self-esteem.

"A person's self-esteem, mastery and adaptation rest in the ability to be purposefully engaged in regular and familiar life experiences." (Kent Tigges)

Occupational therapy aims to improve the quality of remaining life and focuses on **rehabilitation of the whole person**.

Promoting physical independence may involve an assessment of daily living skills, home visits, adapting the home to promote independence and safety and selecting suitable aids and adaptations for disability. (see *Amyotrophic Lateral Sclerosis, Home Care*)

Once symptoms are controlled, **boredom** remains a genuine problem for the many patients who remain restricted by disability or lack of energy. Such patients often find it difficult to be imaginative and to initiate activities. Skillful and enthusiastic occupational therapists can transform the remaining life of these patients. (see *Boredom*)

Patients can become dominated by basic medical and functional needs. The occupational therapist recognizes that **social and recreational activities** are also essential for a meaningful existence.

For all of us, a balanced life includes:
- Self care (activities of daily living)
- Work (the productive use of time)
- Recreation (relaxation, amusement, self-expression)

Each of these has physical, social and emotional elements and a balance between dependence, independence and inter-dependence.

Assessment will include review of previous occupation and interests, previous activity levels, the limitations imposed by the disease, mental concentration, emotional preoccupation and the important priorities for that person.

★ **Most patients usually want to go on being as independent and useful as possible.**

Rehabilitation to full previous normal living is always the goal, but may not always be possible. The occupational therapist will encourage independence in some areas, and appropriate dependence or inter-dependence in others. As the patient's condition deteriorates this balance shifts and activities may need to be re-graded. Continuous reassessment is more important than a single appraisal. (see *Rehabilitation*)

Occupational therapy may involve:
- Assessment (living skills, work, leisure)
- Home visits, environmental changes
- Provision of aids and adaptations
- Training in the use of equipment
- Work simplification
- Energy conservation, time management
- Group activities
- Group therapy (touch, role play, psychodrama)
- Social skills or assertiveness training
- Education in coping with change (patient and family)
- Relaxation and stress management
- Therapeutic activities (arts, crafts, poetry, music)
- Reminiscence therapy

Maintaining normal social activity and **conversation** is often the best form of occupational therapy. Reminiscence therapy has proved a very useful tool. (see *Spiritual Pain*)

When a normal lifestyle is no longer possible, learning new skills can be a way of reducing the frustration of losing previous abilities. Craft work (such as embroidery, leatherwork, knitting, weaving, sewing, pottery, basketry, or making soft toys) can be therapeutic for many patients. **Projects should be short-term**, easy to pick up and set down, and have a pleasing result. They can then be given as presents, or left behind, or even sold as a donation. They allow the patient to give rather than to keep receiving.

A **day hospice** brings opportunities for group activities and games. Group entertainments are often enjoyed, such as demonstrations of crafts or cooking, or musical or theatrical performances, or short trips. (see *Day Hospice*)

Attention to **personal appearance** (barber, beautician, manicurist) and **personal well-being** (relaxation techniques, meditation, massage, aromatherapy) can raise morale and restore a person's spirits.

Occupational therapy encourages patients to lift themselves out of the **passive sick role** (often associated with feelings of helplessness and loss of control) and to be more **independent, creative and productive**. It emphasizes "doing" rather than "being done to". This can restore a sense of purpose and accomplishment.

PAIN

(see Bone Pain, Central Pain, Liver Pain, Nerve Pain, Pain Pathways, Pain Threshold, Pelvic Pain)

Pain in cancer patients can be:

- Cancer-related   70%
- Treatment-related   15%
- Incidental   15%

★   **Many cancer patients assume they will get severe pain and are relieved to learn that 30% of cancer patients do not get pain.**

The best clinical classification of cancer pain is:

1. **Continuous cancer pains** (visceral or soft tissue) which usually respond well to opioid analgesics.

2. **Variable cancer pains** which tend to respond poorly to opioid analgesics.
   - Bone pain
   - Nerve pain
   - Pleuritic pain
   - Colic (see Intestinal Obstruction)

3. **Incidental pains** not caused by the cancer, which need specific treatments.
   - Tension headache
   - Anal fissure
   - Reflux esophagitis
   - Osteoarthritis
   - Angina
   - Renal colic
   - Treatment-related (scar pain, neuropathy)

★ **Cancer pain is relatively easy to control in about 85% of patients. About 15% of patients need specialist knowledge or techniques.**

★ **The aim of pain control is an alert, pain-free patient.**

Pain Control Involves Three Steps

I. Detailed assessment

II. Plan of management

III. Monitoring

I. **Pain assessment** — The clinician must decide what type of pain it is in order to institute the correct management. The purpose of assessment (usually history and physical examination suffices) is to consider the likely cause of each pain. (In one survey 34% of patients had more than 4 different pains.)

★ **The main purpose of the initial assessment is to assess the CAUSE and not the severity of the pain. Estimating severity of pain is only useful in monitoring response to treatment.**

The **body chart** is a useful tool in assessing a patient's pains. Since pain is a wholly subjective symptom, it can be difficult to convey information about it. Poor communication can cause poor pain control. A body chart makes the problem more visible and helps to improve communication. Ideally it is filled in by the patient with the doctor or nurse (or preferably both) present. It emphasizes that patients often have more than one pain, and it encourages analysis of the likely cause of each pain (visceral, bone, nerve, pleuritic, colic, incidental), which improves management.

The patient's initial description may be enough to suspect the type of pain:

"Aches all the time." - visceral

"Worse when I move" - bone

"Burning, stabbing" - nerve

"Worse when I breathe" - pleuritic

"Comes and goes" - colic

Some questions usually help to clarify the diagnosis:

• Where is it?

• What is it like?

• Does it spread?

- What makes it worse?
- What improves it?
- Does it come and go?
- Is it severe?

These questions need to be asked about **each** pain.

A detailed analgesic history is essential both to assess the cause (bone and nerve pains usually respond poorly to opioid analgesics) and to help with appropriate prescribing of analgesia later.

- Which drugs tried?
- Dose actually taken?
- Did it help? For how long?
- Interval between doses?
- Side-effects?
- Reason for stopping?

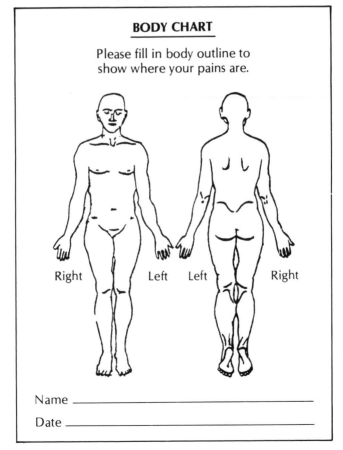

BODY CHART

Please fill in body outline to show where your pains are.

Right   Left   Left   Right

Name _____

Date _____

II.   **Management options:**
   1. Morphine (or other opioid)
   2. Co-analgesic drugs
   3. Radiotherapy (for bone pain)
   4. Nerve block
   5. Physical methods
   6. Psychological methods

   1. Visceral and soft tissue pains respond well to the correct dose of **morphine** (or other opioid).

★   **There is no known opioid drug superior to morphine.** (see Morphine)

   2. **Co-analgesic drugs** may be required when morphine is not effective or only partially effective:
   - NSAIDs for bone pain
   - Steroids for nerve compression pain
   - Tricyclics for nerve pain (burning)
   - Anti-convulsants for nerve pain (stabbing)
   - Anti-spasmodics for colic
   - Antibiotics for cellulitis

   3. **Palliative radiotherapy** is the treatment of choice for bone pain. (see Bone Pain)

   4. About 7% of patients with cancer pain benefit from a **nerve block**. (see Nerve Blocks)

   5. **Physical methods** of pain relief include:
   - Heating pad
   - Local injections (steroids, local anesthetic)
   - Skin traction (see Fractures)
   - TENS (see TENS)
   - Massage

   6. **Psychological methods** of pain relief are important, particularly for the few patients whose pain (most commonly nerve pain) can be reduced but not abolished. (see Nerve Pain, Pain Threshold)

III.   **Monitoring pain control** — The key to effective pain control is **constant reassessment (at least daily)** and modification of treatment until the patient is pain-free.

The best measurement of the severity of pain is the patient's verbal report. The difficulty is that often different professional carers need to assess pain control at different times, and are not present together with the patient to listen to his description of the pain.

There are several methods of recording the patient's own assessment:

1. Verbal description
2. Pain score
3. Visual analog scale

1. **Verbal descriptions** can be used (none, mild, moderate, severe, excruciating), and the patient is asked to supply or check off the appropriate word.

2. The patient can be asked to give a **pain score** from 0 to 10, and the number is recorded by carers on the patient's chart.

3. A **visual analog scale** can be used. The patient puts a mark on a horizontal line which reads "no pain at all" at one end, and "worst pain imaginable" at the other. Since nurses have the most contact with patients, it is a good idea for these assessments to be recorded by the nurses on the team.

The **Happy Face-Sad Face scale** (a variation of the visual analog scale) is a useful tool in assessing pain in younger children.

Indirect assessment of severity of pain is by:

- Observing behavior
- Observing mobility
- Asking about sleep
- Reviewing analgesic requirements

The patient with severe pain is less able to carry on with normal activities of daily living, less able to be independent, less able to concentrate, may have disturbed sleep due to pain, and needs escalating doses of analgesics.

Good communication among physicians, nurses and other members of the team is essential. One reason why pain control is often achieved more quickly in a hospice setting than in a hospital is because, **in a good hospice program, the doctor and nurse in charge discuss the treatment plan of each patient at least once a day.**

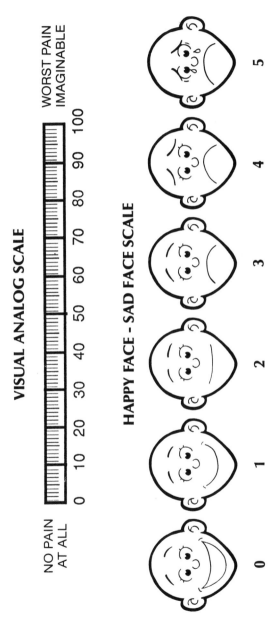

VISUAL ANALOG SCALE

NO PAIN
AT ALL

0 10 20 30 40 50 60 70 80 90 100

WORST PAIN
IMAGINABLE

HAPPY FACE - SAD FACE SCALE

0   1   2   3   4   5

PAIN PATHWAYS

Although we talk of a "pain pathway", it is more accurate to think in terms of a complex and constantly changing system. The neurological pathways involved send signals to the cortex where they may be interpreted as pain.

Pathway	Method of pain control
Cortex	General anesthetic
↑ Thalamus	Opioids
↑ Spino-thalamic tracts	Cordotomy
↑ Dorsal horn of spinal cord	Opioids
↑ Sensory (nerve) fiber	Local anesthetic
↑ Nerve endings	Prostaglandin inhibitor

Nerve endings are sensitive to prostaglandins (and other chemicals) released by tissue damage such as bone metastases. Most tissues of the body give rise to pain when appropriately stimulated. (The exceptions are liver, lung, spleen and some regions of the brain.)

Sensory nerves are not specific for pain. For example, visceral sensory nerves that signal bladder or rectum distention, with increased activity will signal pain.

Sensory nerves from the internal organs run with the sympathetic nerves, as follows:

T2 - T5	Lungs
T4 - T5	Esophagus
T6 - T8	Stomach, pancreas, liver
T9 - T10	Small bowel
T10	Ovaries, testes
T10 - L3	Colon
T11 - L1	Bladder
S2 - S5	Prostate

All sensory nerve fibers pass into the posterior nerve roots and then synapse (make contact) with cells in the dorsal horn of the spinal cord.

The **dorsal horn of the spinal cord** acts as a computer to collect and analyze sensory information. Cells in the dorsal horn send axons up the spino-thalamic tracts to the thalamus. The cells in the dorsal horn are connected by interneurons which regulate nerve activity.

Cells in the dorsal horn are strongly influenced by the activity in other dorsal horn cells in adjacent spinal segments (up or down). Thus pain in the hand due to median nerve compression can eventually spread up the arm. This is an example of **hyperalgesia**, when surrounding normal areas of the body can become sensitive or painful.

Chronic pain can produce permanent changes to the connections among the cells in the dorsal horn. Therefore, cutting a sensory nerve may not stop pain, because the (altered) pattern of nerve activity in the dorsal horn may continue to signal pain. For example, pain from an ischemic foot can continue even after the foot is amputated (phantom nerve pain).

There is considerable overlap. A single cell in the dorsal horn of the spinal cord may receive input from bladder, colon, skin and muscle. Input from skin and viscera can summate at the dorsal horn. Pain can thus be **referred** (for example, diaphragmatic irritation can cause pain in the shoulder).

Sensory nerves contain both touch fibers and pain fibers. **Increased input from touch fibers can inhibit pain transmission.** Touch fibers release encephalins in the dorsal horn, and if the touch stimulus is strong enough this can inhibit pain. (This effect is abolished by naloxone.) This is the basis of the "gate theory" of pain transmission, and the observation that rubbing the skin near a painful area can make it less painful. It also explains the effectiveness of TENS and high-frequency electro-acupuncture. It provides a theoretical model for future methods of analgesia.

Descending pathways descend from the midbrain to the cells of the dorsal horn of the spinal cord. They release encephalins. These descending pathways were discovered in 1969 by Reynolds (a psychologist working with rats). He found that minute quantities of morphine injected into a certain point of the midbrain of the rat could achieve whole-body analgesia, but the effect was lost by cutting descending pathways. These descending pathways inhibit pain transmission in the dorsal horn. They are activated by pain. Thus a severe pain in one part of the body can mask a less severe pain in another. Expectation of pain will activate these descending pathways in experimental animals. **This provides an anatomical basis for the well-recognized effects of psycho-social factors on pain perception. Explanation, reassurance and psychological support can all reduce pain.**

The **spino-thalamic tracts** convey fibers upwards from the cells of the dorsal horn of the spinal cord to the thalamus. They travel in the antero-lateral tracts of the spinal cord. A cordotomy (more correctly called an antero-lateral tractotomy) divides these fibers and renders parts of the body below the lesion analgesic. A bilateral cordotomy would render all parts of the body below the lesion analgesic. Some spino-thalamic fibers also pass to the midbrain (forming a feedback loop via the descending pathways) and to the hypothalamus (accounting for the autonomic response to severe pain of sweating and tachycardia).

The **thalamus** is an important part of the system of nerve pathways that can eventually signal pain. The cell fibers in the spino-thalamic tracts synapse with cells in the **lateral thalamus**. These cells are arranged somato-topically (each group of cells corresponds with an area of the body). However, some fibers pass to the **medial thalamus**, where each cell can receive input from a very large area of the body. The medial thalamus is concerned with the quality of pain. Electrical stimulation of the thalamus in conscious humans can cause burning pain in extensive areas of the body. Fibers from the thalamus pass to the cerebral cortex.

The **cerebral cortex** is the place where the pattern of nerve impulses is finally interpreted as pain. Hence the pathways are more correctly called nociceptive pathways (which may or may not cause the sensation of pain). The cerebral cortex also provides information about the location and intensity of pain.

The **encephalins** are small peptides (discovered in 1975) which act on opioid receptors (particularly in the midbrain and the dorsal horn of the spinal cord). There are five main receptors now recognized. The encephalins act as the chemical messengers of a primitive inhibitory signaling system in the CNS. Morphine (a plant extract) happens to bind to the same receptors and is therefore an analgesic.

PAIN THRESHOLD

Pain threshold is a concept that has arisen from experimental work on animals. Nerves usually have to be stimulated above a certain intensity or frequency to signal pain. It is everyone's experience that the severity of a pain depends on morale and behavior. Pain may not be felt in the heat of a battle, whereas pain seems worse if we are already frightened or anxious.

One physiological basis for a pain threshold is the endogenous opioid system (encephalins, endorphins and other molecules) which is activated by the descending pathways from the mid-brain. Pain activates the system. In experiments, rats can raise their pain threshold to an expected pain by behavioral conditioning. In humans, explanation and preparation for a painful procedure probably does the same thing. The endogenous opioid system is not active all the time. (Intravenous naloxone which inhibits the system does not cause pain in normal subjects.) (*see Pain Pathways*)

Pain threshold cannot be measured. It is best to assume that the complaint of pain means the person **is experiencing pain**. It is inaccurate and unhelpful to say that a person has a "low pain threshold". This is a value judgment which really means "This person complains a lot about pain."

Pain behavior differs from pain threshold. A person may exhibit pain behavior one moment and then (unaware of observers) may appear free of pain (as judged by activity levels, facial expressions, sleep, or behavior such as not needing analgesics). The question then is not "What is this patient's pain threshold?" but "What does this person gain by behaving as if he had severe pain?"

★   **The concept of pain threshold is clinically useful because it helps with pain control.**

The problem of pain control is seen as having two components:
- Reducing pain
- Raising the pain theshold

The pain threshold is raised by:
- Reducing physical discomfort (sore mouth, nausea, etc.)
- Ensuring adequate sleep
- Discussing worries and fears
- Resolving emotional problems
- Maintaining contact with family and friends
- Developing a feeling of security
- Relaxation
- Diversional activities

★   **"I could stand the pain so long as I knew that progress was being made."** (Norman Cousins, *Anatomy of an Illness*)

PANCOAST'S SYNDROME

(see Lung Cancer)

Pancoast's Syndrome involves:

- Apical lung cancer
- Rib erosion (2nd and 3rd ribs)
- Vertebral involvement (about 5% get cord compression)
- Brachial plexus (pain and weakness)
- Sympathetic nerve damage (ptosis)

C8, T1 nerve roots are affected, with wasting of muscles in the hand and forearm and nerve pain up the medial aspect of hand and arm. Sympathetic nerve damage causes ptosis (dropped eye-lid), a small pupil, and sometimes flushing and absent sweating on that side of the face (Horner's Syndrome).

Palliative radiotherapy (with the field usually including the vertebral bodies since it is known these are commonly involved) can abolish or reduce pain in 80% of patients. Average survival after treatment is 9 months, and some patients survive 2 years.

The most difficult symptom to treat is usually the nerve pain radiating into the arm, which can be severe. Once the nerves are destroyed by advancing tumor the pain may stop. *(see Nerve Pain)*

PARANOIA

Paranoia in terminal illness can be classified as:

- "Normal"
- Organic
- Depressive
- Excessive denial

Mild ("normal") paranoia is common in very ill patients, who are often understandably preoccupied with themselves. It is important to avoid behavior that can be misinterpreted, such as laughing in a group that excludes the patient.

If accompanied by disorientation and memory failure, paranoia suggests an **organic cause** such as drugs, infection or brain metastases.

Paranoia may be one feature of **depression**. (*see Depression*)

Paranoia is often a manifestation ("externalization") of **fear or denial**. ("I am getting weaker, you must be poisoning me with these drugs.") In this case a trusted carer needs to spend time with the patient. Discussion should focus on the patient's illness to reality-test ideas. ("If you stopped taking the drugs do you think you would feel strong again?")

PELVIC PAIN

Cancers of the cervix, uterus, bladder and rectum can cause recurrent disease in pelvic lymph nodes with:
- Pain
- Leg swelling (lymphedema)
- Urinary frequency
- Hydronephrosis

The best method of diagnosing recurrence is by CT scan. A pelvic mass may not be palpable. Recurrence after surgery can be treated and sometimes cured by radiotherapy.

Pelvic pain has several components:
- Visceral (supra-pubic and back pain)
- Pelvic floor (perineal pain)
- Posterior infiltration (sacral pain)
- Lumbo-sacral plexus infiltration (buttock and leg pain)

The continuous visceral component of pain usually responds well to morphine, but the nerve pain can be difficult to control.

A number of other options exist:
- Radiotherapy (for bone pain)
- High dose of steroids (reduces peri-neural edema)
- Epidural steroids (for nerve pain)
- Intrathecal neurolysis (for perineal pain)
- Sacral cryo-analgesia (for perineal pain)
- Epidural morphine
- Epidural bupivacaine

Careful selection of patients for these specialized procedures is essential. (*see Nerve Blocks, Nerve Pain, Spinal Opioids*)

PHENOTHIAZINES

Thiethylperazine and **prochlorperazine** are useful drugs in preventing and controlling nausea and vomiting. They are less sedating than chlorpromazine. The usual oral dose of thiethylperazine is 10mg 2 or 3 times a day. It is also available in suppository form (10mg every 12 hours). The usual oral dose of prochlorperazine is 5mg 3 times a day, or 25mg by suppository every 12 hours.

Chlorpromazine is too sedative for routine use as an anti-emetic; it is useful when an anti-emetic and anxiolytic action are needed together. It is useful as an adjunct to benzodiazepines for severe insomnia, with a 25mg to 50mg dose at 5:00 p.m., followed by temazepam 40mg to 60mg at bedtime.

Methotrimeprazine is best thought of as a double-strength chlorpromazine. It is a powerful anti-emetic and is particularly useful in a continuous subcutaneous infusion. Methotrimeprazine is also very useful in the management of terminal agitation. (see *Subcutaneous Infusions, Terminal Phase*)

Haloperidol is a useful drug in terminal care, as a non-sedating anti-emetic or anxiolytic. 1.5mg at bedtime is the usual dose in the prevention of nausea; 5mg 2 times a day is the usual starting dose in the drug management of anxiety. It can be used to calm a severely agitated patient, using 10mg subcutaneously per hour until the patient settles.

PHYSICAL THERAPY

The physical therapist can offer:
- Advice on exercise
- Advice on walking aids
- Passive exercises
- Advice on positioning and turning
- Teaching family members
- Chest physiotherapy
- Breathing exercises
- Relaxation
- Massage
- Edema control

Over 50% of terminally ill patients can benefit from physical therapy. It is almost always welcomed by the patient. The aim is to improve independence lost because of pain, immobility or loss of confidence. Achieving realistic short-term goals boosts morale. Many patients are surprised and pleased to have physical therapy and often say, "Nobody told me how much I should do." (see Rehabilitation)

Exercise programs encourage patients to take an active part in their own care. They should be taught an exercise regime, and encouraged to practice.

Walking re-education is often required for patients who have lost confidence. If a patient can straight leg raise in bed, it is usually realistic to try walking with a frame. For patients who have trouble lifting (due to back pain, for example) a wheeled frame can be used.

Passive exercises reduce stiffness and are usually welcomed by patients who are unable to move their limbs. Family members can be taught a program of exercises which helps them contribute to patient care. (Family members should also be taught how to lift, turn and position the patient.) (see Pressure Sores)

Chest physiotherapy using gentle techniques of percussion, vibration, coughing exercises or forced expiration can increase the volume of sputum expectorated from the main bronchi, and can improve lung function. These techniques can be very helpful but must be used carefully. Postural drainage is not indicated, and even the gentler approaches can cause bronchospasm or short-term hypoxia in very ill patients. (see Dyspnea)

Breathing exercises are useful in almost all cases of dyspnea, because episodes of panic and hyperventilation are common. (see Dyspnea)

Relaxation therapy is especially useful for patients with dyspnea, but most patients have episodes of anxiety and benefit from relaxation. (see Relaxation)

Massage is helpful to ease stiff muscles and to reduce a feeling of isolation. It can be taught to family carers. (see Touch)

Lymphedema can often be reduced by a determined program of compression therapy. (see Lymphedema)

PITUITARY ABLATION

Ablation of the pituitary gland can produce pain relief by an unknown mechanism. Pain relief can occur within hours. It can have a place for widespread cancer pains (soft tissue or bone) unresponsive to other treatments. **It is very rarely indicated.**

Results of the procedure are:

- Complete pain relief   40%
- Partial effect   30%
- No effect   30%

The pituitary injection of alcohol is a relatively simple procedure in expert hands. The transnasal transpenoidal route was described by Bonica in 1968. It requires a light general anesthesia and is performed under x-ray image intensifier. 2ml of alcohol is injected. A cisternal puncture is then performed to inject 40ml hydrocortisone to prevent damage to the optic nerve.

The procedure may have to be repeated.

Complications:

- 6% mortality
- Nasal hemorrhage or rhinorrhea
- Diabetes insipidus (give desmopressin)
- Cortisone replacement needed
- Thyroxine occasionally required

PLEURAL EFFUSION

A pleural effusion is a collection of fluid in the pleural cavity. The fluid may be transudate (as in heart failure) exudate, blood or chyle (lymphatic fluid leaking from the thoracic duct). It occurs most commonly with malignancies of bronchus, breast, lymphoma, ovary and mesothelioma.

Mechanism — In normal individuals there is 10ml to 20ml of pleural fluid acting as a lubricant between the parietal pleura (lining the chest wall) and the visceral pleura (covering the lungs). There is a daily flow of about 500ml of pleural fluid. Malignant effusions are mainly due to direct infiltration of the pleura causing capillary damage and leakage of protein, or reduced absorption of fluid due to damaged pulmonary lymphatics. Ascitic fluid can also spread into the pleural space via lymphatic connections crossing the diaphragm.

Prognosis — A pleural effusion does not necessarily imply a short prognosis. Median survivals of 6 to 16 months have been reported depending on the primary tumor (bronchus 6 months, breast 14 months, mesothelioma 16 months).

Assessment — A pleural effusion may be silent if the fluid accumulates slowly. The usual history is increasing dyspnea over a number of days, sometimes with a dry cough or pleuritic pains (which resolve as fluids separate the pleural surfaces). The typical signs are stony dullness and absent breath sounds. Chest x-ray shows a basal opacity.

Management options:

1. Leave untreated
2. Aspiration
3. Intra-cavity instillations
4. Talc pleurodesis or pleurectomy
5. Radiotherapy or chemotherapy

1. A pleural effusion should be **left untreated** in a patient with advanced metastatic disease (and a known diagnosis) if it is not causing breathlessness.

2. **Aspiration** of 500ml or more of fluid will often relieve dyspnea but the fluid tends to re-accumulate over 1 to 7 days. A simple aspiration under local anesthetic is a useful technique for a patient with advanced disease. It takes 20 to 30 minutes and can safely be performed in the home.

Technique:

- Stop or reverse any anti-coagulants!
- Use bupivacaine 0.25%, 5ml to 10ml.
- Use a small-bore needle or wide gauge IV catheter.
- Use a 3-way tap and large syringe.
- Pass on top of a rib (avoid neurovascular bundle).
- Do not remove more than 1 to 1.5 liters (pulmonary edema).
- Stop if there is pain, coughing, or dizziness (mediastinal shift).

The procedure is much easier if the needle is pre-attached to the 3-way tap by a long, flexible plastic tube. This allows the operator to move the 3-way tap without moving the needle in the chest wall.

Sudden removal of fluid can cause pulmonary edema in the rapidly expanded lung.

★   **Simple aspirations should be performed first in patients with advanced disease, before using instillations.**

Aspiration is quick and painless and may relieve dyspnea for several days or until the patient dies. **Simple procedures such as aspiration of fluid should be painless.** By using plenty of local anesthetic and waiting a few minutes for it to take effect, patients rarely experience discomfort. Some patients dread these simple procedures because they have needlessly experienced a lot of pain when these were previously performed.

3. Aspiration of fluid can be followed by the **instillation of either cytotoxics or sclerosants** in an attempt to stop the fluid re-accumulating. Intracavity cytotoxics have little effect on tumor cell counts and act as irritants to cause pleural inflammation. Sclerosant agents are inserted via an intercostal drain, which is clamped for 3 to 4 hours and the patient placed in various positions to promote a diffuse pleural response. A variety of agents have been used.

Agent	% Control of Effusion
Quinacrine	75
Doxorubicin	73
Tetracycline	71
Bleomycin	55
Thiotepa	27

Instillations can be painful and should only be considered for rapidly recurring effusions in a relatively fit patient. Instillations cause an intended pleurisy with pain and fever for 24 hours. A tetracycline instillation is very painful, and must therefore be mixed with lidocaine.

4. **Talc pleurodesis** has a 90% success rate and should be considered in patients with a prognosis of 2 to 3 months or more. Large effusions in malignant disease tend to recur rapidly. For patients in good general condition talc pleurodesis or **pleurectomy** can give a better quality of life than repeated aspirations. It requires general anesthetic and skilled operators. 10g of sterilized talc is insufflated. It is painful for 24 hours and opioid analgesics are required. Two chest drains have to remain in place for at least 4 days post-operatively to allow the pleural surfaces to remain in opposition.

5. **Chemotherapy** (for breast cancer, small (oat) cell cancer of the bronchus, or lymphoma) may effectively prevent recurrence of a pleural effusion.

PRESCRIBING

★   **Good prescribing is a skill.**

★   **The single most important step in prescribing is the routine use of a drug card.**

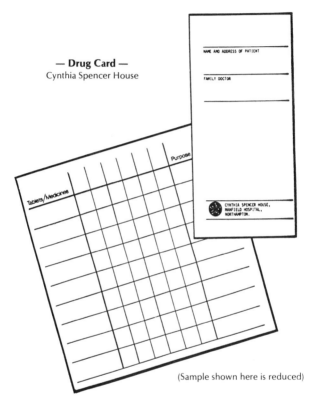

— **Drug Card** —
Cynthia Spencer House

(Sample shown here is reduced)

The **drug card** lists medications, and gives times each drug should be taken, together with the purpose of each. It should be filled in with the patient, and with his carers. It should be explained clearly and reviewed regularly with them. Any changes to the patient's medications should be noted clearly on the card. The drug card also improves communication about the patient's current medication among team members. Ask the patient to bring the card to all appointments.

It is important to ask about **drug preferences** when pre-scribing new medications. Many patients have already tried a variety of pills and potions, and have developed strong feelings about some of them.

Consider the **best route** for each drug — oral, sublingual, by suppository, continuous subcutaneous infusion, or IM injection. (IV drugs are rarely if ever necessary.)

Carers often like to know how much flexibility they can have. (For example, can they increase the analgesics?) They need to know which drugs are essential, and what to do if the patient is vomiting and unable to take them orally.

Review regularly. In good hospice practice the drug orders for the patient are reviewed every day by doctor and nurse together.

It is a good principle to make only **one drug change at a time**, so that if changes occur (for better or worse) it is possible to pinpoint which treatment has been responsible.

It is important to **stop unnecessary medications** whenever possible. For example, some patients have been on anti-hypertension medication for years, and this may become inappropriate. Similarly, patients are usually willing to stop unnecessary iron tablets because of their constipating effect.

★   **Stop drugs that have not helped.**

Most patients have several symptoms and **polypharmacy is unavoidable**.

A retrospective survey of 676 patients at St. Christopher's Hospice showed the following patterns of prescribing:

Drug	%
Phenothiazines	87
Morphine	80
Corticosteroids	57
Night sedation	54
Anti-emetics*	44
Daytime sedatives	35
NSAIDs	32
Anti-depressants	19
Anti-convulsants	8

*excluding phenothiazines

Always explain any drug changes. It is distressing to patients if medications change without explanation.

Be flexible. Treatments may need to be changed if priorities change.

Do not use prescribing as a barrier. When patients complain of anxieties it can be tempting to prescribe drugs when what is often needed is a sensitive discussion of their true situation.

Patients sometimes blame the drugs for the weakness or drowsiness of advanced disease. **Changing drugs can sometimes be the doctor's excuse to avoid discussing the difficult issues of dying.**

"In the practice of our art, it often matters little what medicine is given, but matters more that we give ourselves with our pills." (Alfred Worcester, *The Care of the Aged, the Dying and the Dead*, 1935)

PRESSURE SORES

Pressure sores (decubitus ulcers) affect 20% of terminally ill patients. They occur over bony prominences and weight-bearing areas, most commonly sacrum, hips, heels (but also elbows, spine, side of knee, ears and back of head).

There are two types:
- Superficial (capillary damage)
- Deep (large vessel damage)

Superficial sores begin with capillary damage. They can occur on normal skin if excess pressure is applied (within 30 minutes on a hard surface for an elderly patient or a diabetic). They are painful. They can become deep if neglected.

Deep sores (usually seen only in chronically bedridden patients) start with deep tissue damage. The overlying skin appears intact until it dies and breaks down to reveal a large necrotic cavity. They are full thickness from the beginning and can go down to bone. They are rare in terminally ill patients and will not be discussed further.

Pathophysiology — Pressures on the skin above 30mm Hg (capillary blood pressure) cause tissue damage. After 1 to 2 hours there is irreversible cell damage. Early redness (hyperemia) which still blanches on digital pressure (showing the capillaries are intact) will reverse after 4 hours of pressure relief. Non-blanching hyperemia takes 48 hours of pressure relief to reverse.

★ **Pressure damage occurs more rapidly if the skin is also subject to friction (skin damage) or lateral shearing forces (capillary damage) — both of which occur if patients are pulled instead of lifted. All carers should be taught the correct techniques of lifting and turning.**

★ **Prevention is better than cure (which is often impossible).**

Prevention:

The principles of prevention are relief of pressure and friction, which are aided by the following:

- Whirlpool baths (to relieve pressure)
- Spenco chair cushions
- Careful lifting and turning (to avoid friction or shear)
- Regular turning in bed (at least every 2 hours)
- Sheepskin mattress and chair covers
- Spenco (siliconized) mattress covers to reduce friction
- Ripple or water mattresses
- Heel and elbow protective siliconized pads

A simple baby sponge taped onto the sacrum (and changed regularly) can bring considerable relief when a bony sacral prominence makes sitting uncomfortable.

Avoid ring cushions which restrict blood flow and increase the risk of tissue damage.

Specialized Dressings:

★ **Specialized dressings promote healing only if pressure is relieved.**

The concept of moist wound healing was developed in the 1960s. The aim of these newer specialized (and expensive) dressings is to accelerate healing by promoting the ideal micro-environment in terms of temperature, moisture and oxygen supply, and by preventing adherence which damages new granulation tissue.

Stage of Damage	Dressing
1. Blanching erythema	Semi-permeable membrane
2. Red ulceration	Hydrocolloid dressing
3. Yellow exudate and cavitation	Absorbent dressing plus foam covering
4. Black necrotic tissue	Irrigate with streptokinase and treat as in #3

1. **Semi-permeable membranes** (Opsite, Bioclusive, Tegaderm) are useful for early pressure areas with little exudate, particularly on elbows, hips and insides of the knees. They can reduce pain. The membrane is waterproof and protects the skin if there is incontinence. It can be used successfully on the sacral area but it needs to be skillfully applied.

The area must be carefully cleaned to remove skin grease, avoiding broken skin and the anal margin. Two carers are needed: one to hold the skin tight and the other to apply the membrane. Several overlapping pieces may be needed to cover awkward areas. A piece of stomahesive plaster cut to a triangle can be used to fill the sacral cleft. If the membrane is applied unevenly it can cause friction and more damage.

Small amounts of exudate can be aspirated with a needle (the hole is sealed with another piece of membrane). Larger amounts of exudate prevent the membrane from adhering.

Unfortunately, a significant number of patients develop an allergic reaction to these membranes.

2. **Impermeable hydrocolloid dressings** (Duoderm, Comfeel) are occlusive, adhesive and waterproof. They have an inner layer that converts to gel when in contact with wound exudate. This provides a good environment for moist wound healing. The lack of oxygen transfer promotes formation of granulation tissue.

The indications for use are:
- Partial thickness skin loss
- No infection
- Little or moderate exudate

The dressing should overlap normal skin by 3cm to 4cm. It can be used alone as it is adhesive. It is changed when the liquid becomes visible as a yellow bubble (when the dressing begins to disintegrate). It can be left in place for 4 to 5 days, but may need changing more frequently. On changing the dressing, yellow gel may be found on the wound surface. This is normal (it is not pus) and should be washed off with normal saline.

The brands of dressings vary in pliability and absorbency.

3. **Alginate dressings** (FDA approval pending for Kaltostat, Kaltocarb) are particularly useful in promoting healing of deeper pressure sores. The dressings are highly absorbent and convert to a gel which promotes moist wound healing. It is important to pack loosely.

The material conforms to the cavity and is non-adherent and easily washed off with normal saline. It is also hemostatic and controls capillary bleeding. It can be used to hold fluid (such as metronidazole to control smell) in contact with the wound. It needs a secondary covering, preferably a foam dressing.

These dressings need to be changed daily.

Foam dressings (Lyofoam, Synthaderm) absorb excess exudate and maintain a warm, moist environment conducive to healing. Lyofoam-C is impregnated with activated carbon to reduce smell. The foam should overlap the wound by 3cm and is held down by hypoallergenic adhesive tape.

Absorbent powders (Debrisan beads, Duoderm granules) and pastes (Debrisan Wound Cleaning Paste) are occasionally useful if there is a large quantity of exudate. These can cause discomfort. If used excessively they dry out the wound and can be difficult to remove.

4. Black necrotic tissue delays healing and can become infected causing odor. **Enzymatic debridement with streptokinase** is better than using acidic desloughing agents which can damage granulation tissue. Streptokinase is expensive, but it is superior to chemical debriding agents, and is only occasionally needed. Streptokinase can be applied on an alginate dressing. A dry hard black area (on the heel, for example) can be softened and removed by applying a hydrocolloid dressing.

★   **It is important to understand that a pressure area will heal if it is kept clean and relieved of pressure.**

Healing can be enhanced by some of the **newer dressings** which promote moist wound healing — **but only if pressure-relieving techniques are adequate.**

Routine **irrigation** of pressure sores with warm saline is recommended to remove exudate. Antiseptics can delay healing. Infected or smelly exudate is best removed with 10% Betadine solution, diluted to 5% with normal saline to avoid damage to new tissue. (**Avoid** hypochlorites which damage granulation tissue.)

Avoid "remedies" like sugar, honey, oxygen, wine or egg white. There is no evidence that they help, and they distract from the essential treatment, which is pressure relief.

Pressure relieving aids (specialized cushions, mattresses or beds) are useful for both prevention and treatment. A large cell ripple mattress, properly inflated, will reduce interface pressures between skin and surface, as measured by pressure sensors. Sequentially inflated chamber mattresses can reduce pressure enough to heal pressure sores without turning the patient. However, the effect of surface pressure on capillary flow remains poorly understood. More study of preventive techniques is needed to develop optimum methods.

Physical methods of treatment are sometimes used (in addition to pressure relief) to promote granulation tissue and speed healing. They include ice therapy (to reduce the skin edema in early pressure areas with redness only), ultraviolet light, ultra-sound, ionized water vapor and pulsed high-frequency energy. (These methods should **not** be used to deslough or treat infected wounds.)

Avoid massage which can increase skin damage — any benefit it seems to have is due to associated pressure relief.

Surgical excision of black necrotic tissue may be necessary to reduce infection and smell. Pain in a deep pressure sore is unusual and suggests pus under a necrotic slough, which can be painlessly excised without local anesthetic to release the pus.

Drugs — There is some evidence that oral zinc (such as zinc gluconate tablets) improves skin healing. Zinc is an essential trace element, and it is low in 80% of patients with chronic disease.

In the treatment of pressure sores it is logical to give Vitamin C daily if nutrition has been poor for several months. Vitamin C is essential for the maintenance of healthy collagen and connective tissue in skin. White cell Vitamin C levels are low in 70% of patients with chronic disease.

Broad spectrum antibiotics with anti-staphlococcal action should be given if there is cellulitis.

Comfort care — Even with a short prognosis of a few weeks, wound healing may still be an important aim (to maintain positive attitudes for both patient and carers). During the last few days of life wound healing is secondary to comfort.

Simple and effective management of superficial pressure sores in the last few days of life can be achieved with one of the barrier creams, applied generously and covered with soft gauze. It is cooling and soothing, and reduces friction and lateral shearing forces on the skin. Combined with pressure-relieving techniques it can still produce gradual healing of the skin. Turning routines should be relaxed in the terminal phase if the patient is most comfortable on one side, or if turning causes discomfort.

Patients find washable Spenco (siliconized fiber) mattress covers very comforting, as these reduce pressure and lateral shearing forces.

QUALITY OF LIFE

"In the hospital they seemed to think that being termi-nally ill meant you have to crawl into a corner and die, but there is still a quality to my life." (Sandra C. - a patient)

A good quality of life can be said to exist when the **hopes of an individual are fulfilled by experience**. A useful question to ask an ill patient can be "What would you be doing today if you were well?" This can reveal a gap between "life as it is" and "life as I wish it was". (This applies to well people as well as sick people.)

Objective measurements such as physical independence indexes do not equate with quality of life. For example, a woman with advanced ALS in a hospice was just able to write but was unable to speak, had severe difficulty swallowing and was unable to move her body. Yet she would often write "I feel well today, I am happy." There was a good quality to her life as far as she was concerned. Quality of life assessed by a patient can and usually does change from day to day, and will depend on many factors including physical comfort.

A sense of well-being can give a good quality of life even if a person is able to do very little.

When a doctor advises against a treatment such as chemotherapy he may be assuming that the reduced quality of life due to side-effects outweighs any advantages in terms of prolonging life. If treatment will simply harm and has no chance of helping, then the doctor has a duty to resist treating (the principle of "do no harm!"). If there is even a small chance of prolonging life, however, a few patients will opt for aggressive treatment. They may opt for quantity rather than quality. **It is important to avoid making assumptions about the patient's wishes by asking the patient.**

Various methods of measuring quality of life have been devised, looking at physical, social and psychological well-being. These rating scales can help us to avoid making assumptions. In one study, for example, patients with limb sarcomas were treated conservatively (on the assumption that limb-sparing treatment would improve quality of life), but they had as many problems as those treated by amputation.

When thinking about the quality of life of ill people, it can be helpful to know about some common worries and concerns.

In one study, 250 patients with advanced cancer were asked **"What are your main concerns at present?"**

Responses were

Concern	How often mentioned (%)
Regaining health	45
Religion or philosophy of life issues	22
Concern for spouse	19
Concern for children	12
Confidence in doctor	8
Dissatisfied with care	6
Anxiety about treatment	5
Pain relief	5
Loss of independence	5
To get home again	4
To help others	4
Inability to function	3
Effects of treatment	3
Thoughts of dying	2
To die peacefully	2

The patients were also asked **"Are you making any plans for the future?"**, a question which correlated with whether life was felt to be worth living.

Responses were

Plans	How often mentioned (%)
Travel	15
Make the most of time left	8
To go home	7
To sort out affairs	7
To return to work	5

Quality of life cannot be assessed by observation because it is subjective. Needs and concerns are highly individualistic and can vary from day to day. There is some evidence that quality of life is mainly determined by the extent to which the person has come to terms with his situation.

This can be explored with such questions as:
- Do you feel life is worth living?
- Do you look forward to the future?
- Do you feel low in spirits?
- Do you feel afraid?
- Do your beliefs help you?
- Do you get support from your church?

Other important issues concern:
- **Symptoms, especially:**
  - Pain
  - Poor appetite
  - Nausea
  - Bowel function
  - Breathing
  - Drowsiness
  - Knowledge of disease or treatment
  - Support
- **Worries for partner or family:**
  - Opportunities to express love
  - Feeling needed
  - Able to share feelings with someone
  - Practical support
  - Contacts outside family

Patients tend to score their quality of life higher than observing doctors and nurses, perhaps because they have lower expectations. The **use of a questionnaire** on quality of life may itself improve quality of life by encouraging patients to communicate about their problems and thus to make adjustments.

"Quality of life" must not be confused with "meaning of life".

RADIOTHERAPY

Palliative radiotherapy is given to relieve symptoms. It is important to give the shortest treatment that is known to be effective (because many patients have a short prognosis). Half of all radiation therapy treatments have palliation as the primary goal.

Palliative radiotherapy can be useful in the following situations:

- Bone pain (*see Bone Pain*)
- Bone collapse (spinal cord compression)
- Fungation (cutaneous spread)
- Control of hemorrhage
- Relief of obstruction (SVC, airway, esophagus)
- Brain metastases
- To reduce tumor bulk (sometimes reduces pain)
- Joint pains in leukemia

★　　　**Palliative radiotherapy is the treatment of choice for bone pain.** (*see Bone Pain*)

★　　　**Symptoms respond best when treated early.**

Radiotherapy is unlikely to help with:

- Ascites
- Pleural effusion
- Abdominal carcinomatosis
- Nerve plexus pain

The difference between low-dose palliative and high-dose radical radiotherapy often needs explaining.

With **radical radiotherapy** the maximum tolerated dose is given to attempt **cure**. A common treatment plan utilizes a dose of 6,000 cGy over a 6 week period. Treatment planning identifies the volume to be irradiated, avoiding, as far as possible, sensitive tissues (skin, mucous membranes, spinal cord, small intestine, lung, kidney). The treatment is given in fractions to allow normal tissues to repair between doses. The dose goes to the limits of tissue tolerance and therefore side effects are more common. Further radiotherapy (even low dose palliative radiotherapy) to the same area is often not possible.

A common dose of **palliative radiotherapy** might be 2,000cGy over 4 days. This shortened course of treatment will usually induce enough tumor shrinkage to relieve symptoms. In long bones a **single dose** of 800cGy is as effective as multiple fractions. In some sites (head, neck, pelvis) the dose of radiation may need to approach curative doses to produce an effect (4,000cGy over 4 weeks). (see *Bone Pain*)

With palliative radiotherapy **side effects are uncommon**. Nausea and vomiting usually occur if the field includes the abdomen (particularly around L1), and sometimes also after irradiation of the mediastinum or pelvis. Hair loss only occurs if the head is irradiated. Nevertheless, radiotherapy should never be used as a placebo. Apart from wasting time, any form of deception erodes trust.

Skin care is important. The mega-voltage machines (commonly used for radical radiotherapy) have a skin-sparing effect (the 100% dose occurs below the skin surface) but the ortho-voltage machines (particularly useful for the treatment of bone metastases) cause a skin reaction. Usually there is minimal redness and soreness followed by pigmentation which fades after about 1 year. During treatment (and for 1 or 2 weeks afterwards), the patient is advised not to wash or wet-shave the area, to avoid lotions or make-up, and exposure to sunlight. Cotton clothing is recommended. Skin soreness is treated with topical hydrocortisone cream.

Skin reactions commence about 21 days after the first treatment and last 1 or 2 weeks after the last treatment (with longer treatments).

The skin-sparing effect of mega-voltage machines does not occur on the contra-lateral side (where the x-rays exit the body). Unexpected hair loss or skin redness can occur (for example, radiotherapy to the groin may cause soreness over the sacrum or buttocks).

REASSURANCE

We talk of "the doctor (or nurse) as a drug". Reassurance is an important part of controlling symptoms. It is based on a trusting relationship. (Trust mainly depends on whether the patient likes you, and that is significantly correlated to whether you spend some time talking with the patient about non-medical issues.) (see *Trust*)

A common fear is that any new symptom means that the cancer is spreading, or that the situation is worsening. It is very important to **explore fears behind symptoms**. An important question is, "Have you known anybody else with cancer?"

It is very important to **pin-point the worry before giving reassurance**. It is useless to reassure a patient that he won't get pain, when his real terror is of suffocating to death.

★ **Never just say "don't worry". This implies there is something to worry about, without giving the patient the chance to discuss it.**

Examination is usually an essential part of reassuring someone about a physical problem, to demonstrate that you are in full possession of the facts prior to starting to reassure. The final step in reassurance is **explanation**. Even when the situation is as bad as it can be, explanation still reduces uncertainty and thus raises morale. (*see Explanation*)

People sometimes feel embarrassed at having to complain about all their discomforts and physical problems. It is sometimes helpful to reframe this situation by explaining that telling you about symptoms is not "complaining", but is, in fact, helping you to do your job efficiently.

★ **False reassurance is a distancing tactic, and destroys trust. It is important to be honest. ("We can't completely cure that liver of yours, I'm afraid.") It is also important to be optimistic — which is where expertise in symptom control comes in. ("I'm sure we can help you.")**

REHABILITATION

★ **Controlling symptoms often enables rehabilitation.**

"I have learned never to underestimate the capacity of the human mind and body to regenerate, even when the prospects seem most wretched." (Norman Cousins, *Anatomy of an Illness*)

Rehabilitation demands a team approach to the problems of immobility and lack of confidence. It may require physical therapy, occupational therapy, and adaptations to the patient's home. Sometimes patients have lost confidence and independence because family members have been too kind.

A graded approach to rehabilitation from hospital to home includes:

- Self care (washing, feeding)
- Sitting out of bed
- Getting dressed
- Walking with support
- Walking with a cane or a frame
- Climbing steps
- Assessment of daily living activities
- Home assessment by an occupational therapist and a home care nurse
- A visit home
- A few days at home
- Home with day care support

This gradual approach allows the patient and family members to build up confidence. Achieving short-term goals without loss of security often boosts morale.

Opportunities for rehabilitation are too often lost because professionals lack imagination and initiative. Planning with patients and families can enable the patient to return home, sometimes for weeks and months.

Comments from a patient — Mr. C.B., paraplegic from an advanced cranio-spinal ependymoma (adapted by permission from a recorded conversation):

"When you start thinking about other things apart from the hospital, it starts to clear your mind and I think it really helps. That's another thing I'd say — if at all possible, argue to try and get out of the hospital, even if its only for a couple of hours. Go into your favorite McDonald's and have a Big Mac. Maybe not even eating it, but smelling it, and being in the same place you've been when you were well. Very, very important to me. That's where good family and friends come in handy.

There are a lot of things you can do, that you probably think you can't. And too, you may well struggle, but to have achieved it in the end is a very big plus, and very helpful. And you go home at night and think 'Geez, I got up that step, and got around that park, and went fishing today, and never thought I would do.' And its very important in my mind. Very important for me."

Comment from a family member — Mrs. M.H., 59, with colon cancer and brain metastases, was admitted to an in-patient hospice, immobile due to weakness in the left arm and leg. Intensive physiotherapy and rehabilitation enabled her to walk independently and to return home for a month (after a brief home visit with the occupational therapist and physiotherapist to give her husband confidence). She enjoyed her time at home, was able to go to her husband's retirement party, and continued to visit the day hospice twice a week. She was readmitted to the in-patient hospice (after a seizure) and despite being weaker she continued to enjoy walking exercises and graded limb exercises up to 3 weeks before she died. A year later her husband Fred wrote:

> *"We were married for 36 years, and yet it's those last few months I remember most vividly. We were so grateful for all that hard work — otherwise those precious moments of triumph would never have taken place."*

RELAXATION

Stress releases adrenaline causing sympathetic stimulation ("fight or flight") with tachycardia, increased respiration and mental arousal. Relaxation opposes the effects of anxiety. It increases parasympathetic activity with slowing of both pulse and respiration associated with mental calmness (and increased regularity and amplitude of alpha wave activity in the brain).

Relaxation therapy is of considerable benefit to many patients facing terminal illness. It can raise the pain threshold, reduce dyspnea, reduce fear and anxiety, and increase patients' abilities to cope by fostering a sense of mastery over their situations. Relaxation therapy can also be useful for family members and carers.

There are four essential elements:
- Quiet environment
- Constant stimulus (sound or touch)
- Passive attitude
- Decreased muscle tone

There are many approaches to relaxation therapy, including:
- Massage
- Progressive muscular relaxation
- Breathing exercises

- Biofeedback
- Meditation
- Hypnosis
- Spiritual healing
- Visualization

The best form of physical and mental relaxation is provided by **regular deep meditation**. However meditation demands a degree of concentration and can be difficult for some patients who are very tense and who need to focus on **physical relaxation**, initially with **massage, progressive muscular relaxation** (contracting then relaxing different muscle groups) and **breathing exercises** (encouraging full expiration, lowering of the shoulders and diaphragmatic breathing so a hand on the chest remains still). These are best taught on an individual basis, then practiced daily with the help of tape recordings.

Simple techniques that the patient can grasp easily are usually best. It is important in a panic situation that the patient feels some relief right away. It is useful to involve family carers, as they can confirm any instructions, and they will usually be the ones present to help the patient through a panic situation.

Biofeedback can be useful for people who find it difficult to relax, particularly as they start a program of relaxation. Measurements of pulse, galvanic skin resistance (sweat) and electromyography (muscle tension) can demonstrate control of autonomic responses and boost confidence in self-control.

Meditation is a method of focusing attention which reduces the body's state of arousal. The focus of attention may be a visual image, a repeated sound (mantra) or a physical repetition (breath pattern). Meditation is a simple technique, but it needs to be taught and practiced. Correct posture is important (sitting, not lying).

Hypnosis is a form of guided meditation during which suggestibility is increased. **"Glove and stocking anesthesia"** can be easily induced, which demonstrates the power of the mind over the body. The patient can then be taught a method of **self-hypnosis** (which is similar to meditation).

Spiritual healing, which includes emotional counseling, positive thinking and physical touch (often in a religious context), can result in deep relaxation.

Visualization (a technique developed from motivational psychology) means the regular practice of visualizing a desired outcome, such as shrinkage of cancer cells. Even if cancer is spreading, visualization can still be used to create positive mental attitudes, and to help the patient have a sense of control over a worsening situation. Visualization is best when combined with a program of relaxation, exercise and healthy diet. Drawings of imagined symbols can be useful to explore attitudes to disease, to overcome resentments and to identify new goals. (see *Visualization*)

Art therapy and **music therapy** can be important tools in achieving relaxation, and in exploring the patient's attitudes and fears. Relaxation is also an important component of some of the complementary therapies such as reflexology and aromatherapy.

★ **These techniques are properly used as adjuncts to competent pharmacological symptom control, not as attempted substitutes.**

RESEARCH & AUDIT

Research and audit are an essential part of caring. It is important to analyze the effectiveness of care, to ask hard questions, and to look for ways of improving standards.

"Gaining knowledge has risks . . . it is costly . . . it focuses blame; so ignorance always seems attractive." (Duncan Vere)

It is not enough to rely on our own clinical experience which is limited and biased by memory (we tend to remember successes more than failures), nor on anecdotal information, although these can serve as starting points for inquiry.

Clinical trials are justified in patients with advanced disease because they are needed to answer unresolved problems in controlling symptoms. There should be no ethical problems if trials are well designed and supervised so that all patients are given sound treatment, even though treatments differ. Patients with far-advanced disease are often particularly willing to assist with research, seeing it as a way of leaving behind a contribution of life and learning.

Prospective, randomized, double-blind, controlled clinical trials are time-consuming and difficult. In the hospice or palliative care setting, 50% to 90% of patients are unable to complete the studies. The few that have been performed have been helpful. As multi-center studies are undertaken, greater numbers of patients will enter clinical trials.

Because controlled trials are so difficult in hospice and palliative care, we often have to depend on reviewing our past experience (**retrospective surveys** of clinical practice) or on formulating new treatment plans (based upon new information from elsewhere) and monitoring the effect. (In other words, **organizing our experience**.) Careful documentation and computerization of significant clinical findings will enable retrospective surveys to discover significant correlations to increase our understanding, and to audit our practice.

Another method of research is the **careful analysis of symptoms and comparison with subsequent post-mortem findings**. Three such studies at St. Christopher's Hospice have looked at malignant intestinal obstruction and malignant dysphagia. In this way our understanding of the pathophysiology of symptoms is increased.

Many questions remain unanswered. Does hospice and palliative care improve quality of life and reduce suffering? Is in-patient care better than home care? Which parts of the morphine molecule cause the side-effects of constipation and drowsiness? Does counseling reduce distress? What factors, if any, predict which persons are likely to experience pathological grief reactions? What is the most effective way of teaching symptom control to doctors?

RESPITE CARE

Respite care is the planned short-term admission of a patient to a hospital, hospice, or nursing home, in order to provide temporary rest and relief for the family carers. In some areas, "respite volunteers" will move into the patient's home for a few days to replace or relieve the family carers. There are a few respite care holiday homes (usually in resort areas) which offer a short vacation to both the patient and the carers.

Carers may be elderly or in poor health, may be parents with young children, or may have other family and job responsibilities. Caring for a patient at home is hard work, and creates many stresses even for young, physically fit carers. Carers can become physically, mentally and emotionally exhausted. (see Burn Out, Home Care)

Intermittent **planned** short-term respite care gives the carers a change to rest, relax and recoup. Just knowing that respite care will be available when needed increases the carers' coping abilities. The goal of respite care is to support family carers **before** a crisis point is reached.

Admissions for short-term respite care can be stressful for the patient. In-patient staff must be aware of the special needs of terminally ill patients, and make special efforts to help the patient feel at home. If an in-patient hospice is available, it should be used for respite care. If not, the same hospital ward or nursing home should be used each time, so that the patient can build relationships with the professional staff.

RETROPERITONEAL METASTASES

Retroperitoneal lymphatic spread can occur with cancers of the pancreas, breast, cervix, endometrium, kidney, colon or prostate. Primary tumors can also arise in the retroperitoneal space (sarcomas, germ cell tumors, lymphomas).

The retroperitoneal space lies in the lumbar region between the peritoneum and posterior abdominal wall. It extends from the ribs to the pelvis, deep to the quadratus lumborum muscles. The space includes the kidneys, adrenal and para-aortic lymph nodes.

Retroperitoneal tumor masses can reach a large size before symptoms and signs develop:
- Backache
- Palpable abdominal mass
- Hydronephrosis
- Urinary frequency
- Venous thrombosis
- Lumbo-sacral plexus involvement (pain, impotence)
- Lymphedema (of legs, scrotum)

Procedures to decompress or bypass the ureters are only indicated where further investigations, or treatment of a primary tumor, are considered appropriate. (see *Ureteric Obstruction*)

SEIZURES

Seizures occur in only 1% of terminally ill patients.

Causes:

- Brain tumor
- Brain metastases
- Uremia (rare)
- Hypoglycemia (rare)
- Hyponatremia (very rare)

Seizures are rare with brain metastases. Routine prophylaxis with anti-convulsants is unnecessary, and need only be started after the first seizure.

Controlling seizures:

- Diazepam enema 10mg
- IV diazepam 10mg
- IM phenobarbital 200mg
- IM paraldehyde (5mg to 10mg) (or 10ml in 50ml saline rectally)

Of the above options the **diazepam enema** is the simplest treatment. The effect is often almost instantaneous. It can be repeated after 5 minutes if necessary, and it is safe to give 4 enemas over a period of 30 minutes. If convulsions recur later that day 4 more enemas can be given over a period of 30 minutes. (Diazepam enemas are not available commercially in the United States, but some enterprising pharmacists prepare them for use in hospice and palliative care.) IV diazepam 10mg can be used instead of the diazepam enema.

In the rare case where convulsions are not controlled by diazepam, IM phenobarbital 200mg can be given (although it is absorbed slowly). Alternatively, paraldehyde IM or rectally is virtually always effective.

A new method is to use water-soluble phenobarbital in a **separate** continuous subcutaneous infusion (400mg to 600mg per day). It cannot be mixed in the same infusion with other drugs.

Preventing seizures — If a patient requires regular anticonvulsant medication to prevent seizures, oral phenytoin 300mg at bedtime is usually the drug of first choice.

If seizures recur, ensure that plasma levels are in the therapeutic range (10mg/L to 20mg/L [40μmol/L to 80μmol/L]). If low, increase phenytoin gradually by 50mg per day, because small increases in dose can cause large increases in plasma levels (saturable metabolism). Levels above 25mg/L [100μmol/L] can cause drowsiness and ataxia. Avoid combinations of anti-convulsants whenever possible. Drug interactions occur.

If phenytoin is ineffective or not tolerated, change to valproic acid 200mg 3 times a day. If seizures recur, increase the dose to a maximum of 400mg 4 times a day. It can cause nausea and is best taken after food. Plasma levels do not accurately reflect activity with valproic acid, so routine monitoring of plasma levels is not helpful.

Carbamazepine and valproic acid both lower effective phenytoin levels. Phenytoin potentiates diazepam.

Focal seizures (twitching of the corner of the mouth, or in one finger, or in one arm or leg) are distressing because the patient is often still conscious. They can develop into a generalized seizure. Focal seizures are best controlled by diazepam (enema or IV). The best drug for prophylaxis is carbamazepine, starting with 100mg to 200mg 2 times a day, and increasing gradually up to 400mg 4 times a day if necessary. Drowsiness and dizziness can occur. Plasma levels should be monitored initially (optimum levels are 4mg/L to 12mg/L [17μmol/L to 50μmol/L]).

Valproic acid is effective in generalized and focal seizures. It is best reserved for cases where other drugs are ineffective or cannot be tolerated. Start with oral valproic acid 200mg 3 times a day (after food to avoid gastric irritation and nausea), increasing by steps to 300mg to 600mg 4 times a day if convulsions are not controlled. Plasma levels do not correlate with effect and are not helpful. Side effects include drowsiness, altered lung function, reduced platelets, increased appetite, edema and (rarely) jaundice.

If the patient cannot swallow prophylactic anti-convulsants because of dysphagia, vomiting or unconsciousness, give IM phenobarbital 100mg 2 times a day, or water-soluble phenobarbital 200mg per day in a **separate** continuous subcutaneous infusion.

Seizures are very frightening for the family (and for the patient with focal seizures) and explanation is essential.

Common worries include:
- Will they cause brain damage?
- Is the cancer spreading?
- Will they shorten the life span?
- Will the patient die during a seizure?

★ Seizures should be controlled even in an unconscious patient, for the sake of the family.

SEXUAL NEEDS

★ A patient's sexuality does not end with the diagnosis of terminal illness.

Patients are likely to discuss sexual concerns only if their professional carers routinely take a sexual history and are comfortable doing so. Many doctors and nurses assume that a patient's sex life is satisfactory if the patient does not specifically bring up the subject (an assumption not made about other aspects of health).

The sexual needs of patients with advanced illness are often neglected. Sex is associated with living, not dying, and a couple (and their doctors and nurses) may wrongly feel it is not a legitimate problem. Most couples, however, welcome an opportunity to discuss problems of physical intimacy. It may be important to discuss the couple's sex life before the illness occurred, to put their current needs into context.

Patients who are perhaps too ill to have sexual needs still have **sensual needs**, and in the loneliness of facing death may want nothing more than to be close to their spouse or lover, and to express their feelings in physical language, even if it is simply stroking each other's body. Discussing sexual needs is a form of permission-giving, and it can boost the morale of patients to realize they are still considered as sexual persons.

Questions such as "How has this illness affected your relationship?" or "Are you still able to kiss and cuddle?" open the way. It may sometimes be necessary to provide more specific language for a discussion, by asking "Do you have trouble getting an erection . . . reaching a climax . . . finding a comfortable position . . . etc?"

Specific problems that sometimes occur are:

- **Shame** of a disfigured body ("I don't feel nice enough to be touched.")
- Fear of **damage** ("We thought it might do some harm.")
- **Guilt** ("I didn't like to mention it when she was so ill.")
- Fear of **contagion** ("I thought I might catch the cancer.")

• **Misinterpretation** ("I thought he must have found someone else.")

★   **Sexual counseling is part of emotional rehabilitation.**

SKULL METASTASES

Skull metastases are most commonly seen in naso-pharyngeal tumors but can occur with any tumor that metastasizes to bone. Pain can precede neurological signs by several weeks, but they can present as painless cranial nerve palsies. Metastases in the base of the skull can be difficult to see on x-ray (CT scans are needed).

Metastases in the base of the skull are a particular feature of breast cancer. Isolated cranial nerve lesions can occur, commonly in the 6th nerve causing squint, or in the 12th nerve causing difficulty in moving the tongue (chewing, speaking). Radiotherapy to the base of the skull can some-times reverse the nerve damage. Steroids are usually given simultaneously.

Other recognized syndromes include:

Jugular foramen:
- Occipital pain (worse on head movement)
- Occipital tenderness
- Dysphagia, dysarthria (cranial nerves 9, 10)
- Weak shoulder (cranial nerve 11)
- Ptosis (sympathetic nerves nearby)

Sphenoid sinus:
- Bifrontal headache and nasal stuffiness
- Retro-orbital pain
- Diplopia (lateral rectus palsy)

Fractured odontoid:
- Severe pain on neck flexion
- Tingling and weakness in both arms
- Leg signs if spinal cord compression occurs

SMALL STOMACH SYNDROME

Small stomach syndrome consists of:

- Epigastric discomfort (dyspepsia) after food (gastric distention)
- Retrosternal discomfort (heartburn) after food (reflux)
- Nausea, hiccup
- Flatulence
- Early satiety

It is due to inability of the stomach to distend, usually because of:

- Gastric carcinoma
- Partial gastrectomy
- Hepatomegaly (possibly)

★   **The pain does not respond to opioid analgesics.**

Many patients with massive hepatomegaly have no gastric symptoms. Symptoms are **exacerbated** by anxiety (and air swallowing), irritant drugs (iron, NSAIDs, steroids), delayed gastric emptying (opioids, anti-cholinergics), or decreased tone in the lower esophageal sphincter (alcohol, diazepam, nitrites, verapamil, nifedipine). An esophageal tube for dysphagia causes reflux and gas.

Management options include:

- Explanation
- Review of drugs
- Small frequent meals
- Simethicone after meals
- Metoclopramide after meals
- H_2-receptor antagonist
- Remember anxiety (air swallowing)

Simethicone (silica activated dimethicone) is a defoaming agent available in a number of antacids (Mylanta, Riopan Plus, etc.). It clears gas bubbles by allowing bubbles to coalesce, and by facilitating eructation (belching) which reduces gastric distention.

Metoclopramide is a gastro-kinetic anti-emetic. (The usual dose is 10mg to 20mg after meals.) It increases gastric emptying by increasing the tone of the lower esophageal sphincter, decreasing the tone of the pylorus and increasing gastric and small bowel peristalsis.

Ranitidine 150mg 2 times a day should be added for severe or persistent symptoms.

SMELLS

Offensive smell is miserable and embarrassing for a patient. It is a constant reminder of disease and isolates the patient from the close contact of family and friends. It may be due to **fungation, fistula, stoma leakage, pressure sores** or **rectal discharge**.

Management options:
1. Change dressings frequently
2. Use charcoal pads
3. Treat infection
4. Use deodorant sprays
5. Use air cleaners/extractors

1. Regular **cleaning and changing of the dressings and soiled beddings** is essential. Use of scented soaps, talcum powder and colognes can help. (*see Fungating Tumors*)

2. **Charcoal pads** in a dressing absorb smells. Some dressings contain a layer of charcoal.

3. Most odors are due to **anaerobic infections**. Metronidazole 500mg 3 times a day or chloramphenicol 500mg 4 times a day are often extremely effective. Once smell is reduced it can be controlled by continuing the medication at lower doses.

4. Specialized **deodorant sprays** are available for use when colostomy bags are emptied or dressings are changed. Scented air fresheners should generally be avoided because they tend to mix with existing smells rather than removing them.

5. Electric **air cleaners** and **extractors** are helpful and can be left on provided the noise does not unduly disturb the patient.

SPINAL CORD COMPRESSION

Incidence — Spinal cord compression affects 5% of patients with advanced cancer.

★ **It is a medical emergency. Treatment within 24 to 48 hours can sometimes restore function.**

Presentation — Spinal cord compression usually occurs in advanced disease, but in 8% of patients it is the presenting feature.

Typical features and common sequence	% at diagnosis
• Back pain	95
• Weakness (both legs)	75
• "Funny feelings" (both legs)	50
• Urinary hesitancy or retention	50
• Loss of rectal sensation (late)	—

★ **Motor and sensory loss may be denied by a frightened patient. Examine carefully for a sensory level.**

Investigations — Plain x-ray may show bone destruction, loss of a pedicle or vertebral body collapse (sparing of the intervertebral discs is a classical sign of malignant damage).

Myelogram can give valuable information about site and extent of the compression.

CT scan can be useful to delineate soft tissue masses.

★ **It is essential that investigations do not delay treatment.**

Management options:
1. Immediate high dose steroids
2. Same-day radiotherapy
3. Surgical decompression

1. **Steroids** — Give an immediate dose of dexamethasone 30mg IV as soon as possible.

2. **Same-day radiotherapy** is most suitable for direct extradural compression of the cord by radio-sensitive tumor deposits (myeloma, lymphoma, leukemia). It cannot restore stability to an already collapsed vertebra.

The results of radiotherapy are better than surgery with less morbidity. If treatment is started within 48 hours of signs occurring there is a chance of complete recovery. Treatment is usually 3,000cGy over 10 to 14 days.

3. **Surgical decompression** usually should only be considered if:

- Diagnosis is in doubt (biopsy possible)
- Symptoms worsen during radiotherapy
- Patient has already had maximum radiotherapy
- Tumors are radiotherapy resistant

Results are disappointing in terms of mobility. 75% of patients present when already unable to walk, when the chances of restoring mobility are poor. Overall only 35% retain or return to the ability to walk.

Nevertheless treatment may still be worthwhile for the patient, even when prognosis is short, if it is possible to **rescue sphincter function**, and thus avoid the demoralizing symptoms of incontinence.

Prevention — Prophylactic radiotherapy should be considered if a patient has thoracic metastases with any degree of vertebral collapse, since this can prevent total vertebral collapse and spinal cord compression. A spinal support corset and advice on avoiding lifting or twisting can be important.

SPINAL OPIOIDS

Spinal is a collective term meaning **epidural** or **intrathecal**. Opioid receptors in the brain and spinal cord were identified in 1973. Wang reported the use of spinal morphine for analgesia in humans in 1979. By delivering morphine close to the receptors much lower doses are required.

The main indication is **severe pain** (visceral, soft tissue and bone pains respond best) **uncontrolled by oral or systemic opioids**. The spinal route, which is rarely needed, has the single advantage over recommended systemic routes (oral, subcutaneous, rectal, IM) of fewer side-effects such as constipation and drowsiness.

Spinal opioids occasionally cause dose-dependent nausea, itching and urinary retention, but the incidence of respiratory depression is very low, and tends to occur only in opioid-naive patients. Tolerance can develop if high doses are used in excess of the required analgesic dose.

The usual starting dose of epidural morphine is 50% of the systemic dose. For intrathecal morphine the starting dose is 5% to 10% of the systemic dose. For example, if the patient requires 10mg morphine by IM injection, an equi-analgesic dose by epidural injection would be 5mg, and an equi-analgesic dose of morphine intrathecally would be 0.5mg to 1mg. The effect lasts 8 to 12 hours.

If the patient is morphine-naive (i.e., has not been on regular doses of morphine) the recommended starting dose for epidural morphine is 2mg to 3mg every 12 hours. This would be an unusual situation because most patients will already have been on regular oral morphine well prior to considering the epidural route.

The **epidural route** is preferable to the intrathecal (no headaches, less risk of infection or neurological damage, safer if an inadvertent overdose is given), but pain can occasionally occur on injection, probably because the catheter tip is near a nerve root. This is sometimes overcome by slightly withdrawing the catheter. The position of the catheter tip is not critical because the analgesic effect is obtained by morphine suffusing into the CSF and is non-segmental.

The catheter is usually inserted at L1, and the free end tunneled under the skin. (A long IV catheter can be used to form the tunnel for the epidural catheter.) This ensures that any skin infection is trivial, and does not track down into the epidural space. The catheter entry point can be covered with a small piece of transparent membrane (Opsite). Vigilant nursing care is needed to observe for signs of infection.

Morphine for spinal injections (epidural or intrathecal) should be preservative-free and given through a filter attached to the free end of the catheter.

Various **advanced opioid delivery systems** are available. An indwelling subcutaneous access portal can be implanted. This allows injections through the skin into the portal and reduces the risk of infection. Implantable reservoirs have also been developed to give a continuous infusion of morphine. These systems are expensive. The reservoirs are large and although they can function for months, they tend to block or become infected and need replacing.

In summary, the use of spinal opioids is rarely indicated. The technique has few advantages over oral medication that is carefully titrated. It has the major disadvantage of requiring the patient to have a permanent in-dwelling catheter in his back.

Note — Intraventricular opioids have been used to control intractable head and neck pain. Under local anesthesia an intracranial reservoir can be stereotactically placed with the catheter tip in the frontal horn of one lateral ventricle. A usual dose range would be 0.25mg to 1mg of morphine by injection into the reservoir every 24 hours. The theory is to reach the cerebral opioid receptors with morphine.

However, since the CSF has a continuous circulation, drug flow would normally occur to the brain **within 30 minutes of a lumbar intrathecal injection**. The indications for intraventricular opioids are therefore very, very few indeed.

SPIRITUAL PAIN

"The spiritual aspects of an illness concern the human experiences of sickness (or 'dis-ease') and the search for meaning within it." (Peter Speck)

★   **Symptom control has to precede spiritual support. A person cannot think about the meaning of his life while he has pain or keeps being sick.**

Spiritual anguish is universal as people face death. Dying can involve extreme loneliness, sadness and fear (as well as physical distress).

Spiritual support occurs in the context of an equal human relationship which allows a person to work through his feelings of anger or hopelessness, and achieve a sense of integration and a sense of responsibility. In a secure environment, free of physical suffering, where a person feels accepted and not completely alone, it is possible to come to terms with death and view it not simply as a giving up out of weakness, but as a **letting go out of strength**.

Recognizing spiritual problems — It is easy to miss or to ignore spiritual pain. A common example is the patient who says "I seem to be wasting away ", or "I'm not eating enough." It is tempting for the doctor to respond by asking about diet or dysphagia, when it is fear of not existing that the patient is struggling to express.

There may be a sense of:
- Unfairness (Why me?)
- Unworthiness (I don't want to be a burden.)
- Hopelessness (What's the point?)
- Guilt (It's a punishment.)

- Isolation (No-one can really understand.)
- Vulnerability (I'm a coward.)
- Abandonment (God doesn't care.)
- Punishment (But I've led a good life.)
- Confusion (Why does God allow suffering?)
- Meaninglessness (My life's been wasted.)

All these things are made worse by physical suffering, social isolation, practical worries or unfinished emotional business.

Spiritual anguish can be considered in terms of:
- The past (painful memories, guilt)
- The present (isolation, anger)
- The future (fear, hopelessness)

Spiritual "work" can be considered in terms of:
- Releasing the past
- Balancing hope and fear
- Relinquishing responsibilities
- Preparing for death

Reminiscence as therapy — Remembering the past can bring new sense to the present. It can be very helpful at the right moment to say "Tell me your life story." One technique is to record and transcribe conversations about childhood and early life. Encouraging reminiscence has a number of benefits. It is usually enjoyed. It provides companionship and helps to overcome the problem of boredom. It improves self-esteem and helps a person to feel recognized as an individual. It helps in distinguishing the causes of emotional reactions (some of which are related to past events more than present ones). It can increase confidence as a person is reminded that he overcame past difficulties. It helps to integrate the patient's present experience of illness into the context of his whole life. Finally, the healing of painful memories can occur in the context of a sensitive relationship of mutual trust. Acceptance from another can increase self-acceptance.

★   **A useful way of encouraging reminiscence is by using the patient's family photograph album.**

Integration can be both internal (through dreams or sorting memories) and external (being or becoming a useful part of something bigger than oneself). Integration is never complete. The main thing is to make some progress and not approach death by disintegrating. Almost everyone facing death searches for some way of making sense of his situation. This has been called "autobiographical reconstruction". One young man with a bone sarcoma which started in his left arm believed it had been partly caused by his mother's desertion of the family when he was 13, leaving him to "mother" to his younger brother and sister and straining "my left side, which is the feminine side of the body". Listening patiently to these personal searchings (and putting aside our own scientific notions) is part of spiritual support.

Companionship is an essential part of spiritual support. Spiritual support can only occur through a meaningful human relationship. This is not necessarily time-consuming. The key qualities of openness, sensitivity, and a willingness to be yourself and to listen can be conveyed within minutes.

Establishing a relationship with someone who is very ill can be difficult, but there is more to spiritual support than talking. Just sitting with someone for a while conveys a powerful message. Regular prayer and/or meditation greatly increase our capacity to listen. They also put us more in touch with the metaphysical, unknowable part of life that is an important concern for many people who are facing death. (see Listening)

★ **A good companion talks of life as well as death. Above all, a good companion knows how to listen.**

Professionals working with dying persons sometimes talk of the importance of "coming to terms with our own mortality", but our own honest fear of dying can be an essential element in this relationship of spiritual support. We must never minimize the dread that some people have of death. Compassion means "suffering with".

Spiritual support is a two-way process. Patients and families facing death very often provide spiritual support for the professional carers around them. When this occurs we should say so. It boosts morale. One of the rewards for professional carers is seeing the difference that true acceptance and companionship can make to a person approaching death.

Anger — We should expect to encounter anger, which occurs when a person is threatened, frustrated, helpless or rejected. Anger is a common reaction to advanced disease, both for patients and family members. Anger is also a common response to grief. Many people find anger less uncomfortable than sadness. The professional management of anger (in self and others) is important, because anger can be either creative or destructive. Anger is close to love. (The opposite of love is not anger, but indifference or calculated hatred.) Suppressed anger distorts relationships and can cause depression. Anger can be a positive force for change — it can be used creatively to improve communications.

Anger is commonly projected or displaced (onto situations, doctors, nurses, family members, God). The person may not be fully aware of the true source of the anger. Anger can be associated with bodily arousal (the adrenalin response of fight or flight), and this has to be allowed to subside before feelings can be discussed.

Acknowledge anger. It can help to say "All this would make me feel very angry." Once anger is acknowledged and expressed it will subside. Analyze the problems and frustrations, not the anger itself (ask "What?" and "When?" **not** "Why?"). The source of anger may be linked to earlier life experiences (childhood rejection by parents, for example).

Fear almost always relates to the **imagined future** rather than the reality of the present. It can be helpful to reality-test fear by asking "What is the worst thing that could happen?" Even if the person says "I might die" it is still possible to reduce fears by discussion. Is it fear of the process of dying or what happens afterwards? Is it fear of being alone or being buried alive? Professionals often believe that discussing fears will make them worse, whereas sharing thoughts and feelings always reduces anxiety. Fear may be disguised as denial, insomnia, nightmares or attention-seeking behavior.

When patients mention **dreams or nightmares** it is important to ask for details, not to analyze, but as a way of encouraging patients to discuss the feelings they had when dreaming. It sometimes becomes possible to talk of fear in terms of the dream, even if the patient cannot express his fears about the disease. Reviewing and verbalizing a dream can be an extremely helpful step in the process of adjusting to change.

> Mr. E.J., age 50, with advanced bowel cancer, was living alone at home, at 152 Sudborough Road. On one visit to the hospice out-patient clinic (as he became much weaker) he said, "I have some important questions to ask you this time." He wanted to discuss in detail what would happen if he could no longer manage at home. This was a noticeable change to his previous attitude of beating the cancer

and getting on with a vigorous life-style. During the discussion he said, "Something strange happened the other day."

Encouraged to continue, he described falling asleep one afternoon, and waking in the early evening. He said, "For the next two hours I knew only two things for certain. I was not E.J. and I did not live at 152 Sudborough Road. It was frightening. Gradually it began to come back." He went on to say, "I've told all sorts of people about my dream, and no-one can explain it." After a pause he added with a sigh, "I'm just not myself at the moment."

The important realization that he was no longer his old self helped him to begin to make important and realistic plans for his future.

The changing nature of hope — In advanced disease hope of cure becomes inappropriate. This does not mean that patients should not go on hoping for a cure. It means it should not be their main hope. Becoming obsessed with hope for cure in the face of advancing disease is inappropriate and becomes disheartening.

Realistic and appropriate hopes may be:
- To walk again
- To get home for a time
- To feel better tomorrow
- To be remembered
- For the family to cope
- For stronger trust in God
- For a future beyond physical existence

It is often helplessness that makes people feel hopeless. If people are given back some control of their situation, they can often cope again and feel more hopeful. The sick person needs realistic short-term goals and projects (a weekend trip, a family anniversary, knitting for an expected grandchild). Leaving behind skills is a very therapeutic way of remaining hopeful. It helps with the difficult business of role adjustment. Even someone who is weak and ill can give instructions and enjoy seeing someone else's achievements.

Patients have the greatest confidence in professionals who allow for hope and who join in the hoping. **This does not mean we should tell lies.** When we realistically face up to the issues of the moment, provide what support we can, and restore control to the patient as far as possible, then there is nothing wrong with adding our hope to theirs — indeed it is always helpful and encouraging.

A sense of completion is very important. It is easier to leave a life that is tidied up. This includes making a will, handing over responsibilities and tackling any unfinished emotional business. It is a time to take stock and look back on what has been achieved and left behind. It is often a great relief to the patient when someone finally has the courage to ask if he has made a will. Making a will usually brings relief and reduces anxiety. It is a practical way of remaining in control of the situation. A will can be made whether one is well or ill, and many patients welcome a discussion of their future.

The concept of responsibility — Victor Frankl, a psychiatrist who survived the extreme suffering of a Nazi concentration camp, wrote a book called *Man's Search for Meaning*. He quoted Friedrich Nietzsche: "He who has a **why** to live for can bear almost any **how**." Frankl wrote **"We had to teach the despairing men that it did not really matter what we expected from life, but rather what life expected from us . . ."**

A dying patient is not responsible for his illness, but he is responsible for his reaction to his illness. Suffering itself has no meaning or value, but opportunities for good can arise out of any situation, even a situation of suffering. This concept is easier to accept when you are well than when you are ill, but it is still helpful. It emphasizes that a person copes best who remains realistic and yet hopeful in every situation. Respect for this responsibility can restore a person's self-esteem and sense of control.

Religious support — One purpose of religion is to make sense of life — to put meaning into a person's situation.

We may not understand or accept the religious beliefs of our patients, but we can **respect** them. It is not necessary to know the details and customs of every religion. It is necessary to take an interest, and to learn about their special observances. It is one more facet of good care to know about religious needs, which may be much more important to a person than medical or nursing needs.

Ask about prayer, rituals, festivals, diet, fasting, and the need for quiet. Learn about any special religious requirements the patient or family will have around the time of death.

It can be helpful to distinguish between spiritual and religious support. When a person has the comfort of a religious faith, we must help to ensure he has all possible support from that religion, whatever it is. Formal religious support is intended to provide complete spiritual support, and for many it does. But religious practice can sometimes fail to meet a person's deepest spiritual needs. Religious rituals and sacraments are very important, but devoid of genuine pastoral concern they can become another barrier for an anxious minister, priest or rabbi to hide behind.

STEROIDS

In a study of 373 hospice patients 50% received steroids and 40% derived some benefit from them.

A dose of dexamethasone 4mg per day is very useful in most patients to improve appetite and give a feeling of well-being (but with no effect on physical weakness). It is important to time this intervention carefully to avoid side effects, particularly facial disfigurement.

A trial of high dose steroids has a place in the management of many different symptoms in terminal care, such as:

- Superior vena cava obstruction
- Dysphagia from esophageal cancer
- Vomiting resistant to anti-emetics
- Vomiting from pyloric stenosis
- Dyspnea from lymphangitis carcinomatosa
- Edema from lymphatic obstruction

A trial of high dose steroids should last 7 to 10 days to see if symptoms are going to resolve. The aims of the treatment should be carefully explained to patient and family, emphasizing that any improvement in symptoms is likely to be of a temporary nature.

If the trial of high dose steroids is successful the dose should be reduced very gradually (2mg per week) to try to maintain the symptom control, but minimize the long term side effects. If the trial of steroids is not effective the steroids should be stopped (or continued as a low dose for non-specific effect, such as improved appetite).

Dexamethasone is the steroid of choice in terminal care.

Dexamethasone 4mg per day is the usual dose for anorexia, or to improve the patient's feeling of well-being.

Dexamethasone 8mg per day is the usual dose for symptoms of compression (superior vena cava obstruction, lymphedema, dysphagia).

Dexamethasone 16mg per day is the usual dose for raised intracranial pressure.

If the patient can swallow only liquids, **soluble predniso-lone** should be used (30mg prednisolone is equivalent to 4mg dexamethasone).

If the patient has been on steroids for more than one month, and is to be weaned off steroids, transfer the patient to prednisolone so that the dose can be reduced more gradually.

The particular problems in the use of high dose steroids include:

- Oral thrush
- Gastric irritation
- Facial swelling
- Striae and easy bruising
- Edema (sodium retention)
- Weakness (potassium depletion, proximal myopathy)
- Diabetes
- Insomnia or excitation (psychosis is **very** rare)

About 5% of patients have to stop steroids because of side effects, particularly facial disfigurement (swelling, hair growth, acne). The speed at which facial swelling develops is very variable. The timing of a trial of high dose steroids is important. High doses for too long can cause considerable disfigurement (including skin striae, bruising and abdominal distention).

Oral thrush can develop rapidly and can be particularly severe if the patient is on steroids. Consider prophylactic anti-fungal treatment.

About 5% of patients develop **dyspepsia**. Ranitidine 150mg 2 times a day should then be added, and should be started with steroids if there is a history of peptic ulceration.

Agitation and restlessness can occur (but psychosis is rare). Some patients notice that steroids taken late in the day cause **insomnia**. Agitation may be controlled by halo-peridol 3mg to 5mg 2 times a day. If not, the steroids need to be reduced or stopped.

In a known **diabetic** steroids will increase insulin requirements. A trial of high dose steroids is still possible, provided glucose levels are closely monitored.

Proximal myopathy can occur after several weeks on high dose steroids, particularly affecting the quadriceps (difficulty climbing stairs).

Hyperphagia (a distressing increase in appetite, sometimes with a craving for food day and night) occurs in about 3% of patients.

Other rarer side-effects include myoclonic jerks, cataracts, arthralgias (on increasing or decreasing the dose) and re-activation of tuberculosis.

SUBCUTANEOUS INFUSIONS

The portable syringe pump was invented by Wright in 1979 to deliver desferrioxamine to patients with thalassemia. In the same year Russell suggested its use for infusions in terminal malignant disease.

The continuous **subcutaneous** infusion of drugs by a small portable pump (sometimes called a "syringe driver") is a major advance in terminal care, particularly for symptom control in the home. It has a number of advantages over intravenous therapy. It is safer (much less risk of infection and no risk of air embolus). The patient can remain fully ambulant. Tolerance does not develop to subcutaneous morphine as it does occasionally to IV morphine. (see Morphine)

The main **indications** for continuous subcutaneous infusions are vomiting, dysphagia, severe weakness or unconsciousness. They can be particularly useful for patients at home, either to control nausea and vomiting, or during the last days of life if the patient is no longer managing oral medication.

A continuous subcutaneous infusion of drugs is particularly useful in the management of malignant intestinal obstruction. (see Intestinal Obstruction)

★ **Continuous subcutaneous infusions are rarely needed for pain control alone.**

★ **Each drug in an infusion must be individually titrated to the patient's needs. Do not use "fixed cocktails" of drugs.**

The following drugs can be used in continuous subcutaneous infusions and mixed together in any combination:

Drug	Usual Starting Dose per 24 hours
Morphine	½ the 24 hour oral dose
Cyclizine	100mg to 150mg
Haloperidol	5mg to 10mg
Methotrimeprazine	50mg to 100mg
Scopolamine	0.8mg

Do not use chlorpromazine, prochlorperazine or thiethylperazine in continuous subcutaneous infusions, because these cause skin irritation. Cyclizine above a concentration of 10mg/ml may precipitate with morphine or hydromorphone.

When a patient needs regular injections of antiemetics, it is usual to start a continuous subcutaneous infusion with cyclizine 100mg to 150mg per day. Haloperidol 5mg to 10mg per day can be added if necessary. In nausea resistant to these drugs, methotrimeprazine 50mg to 100mg per day is usually adequate, although very sedating. (If the patient is warned of this, he or she will usually prefer sedation to nausea.) Very often, once nausea is controlled, the dose can gradually be reduced over a period of days without the nausea returning.

The following drugs can also be used in continuous subcutaneous infusions, but experience with them is more limited:

Drug	Usual Starting Dose per 24 hours
Hydromorphone	½ the 24 hour oral dose
Metoclopramide	30mg to 60mg
Dexamethasone	2mg to 12mg
Atropine	1.2mg
Midazolam	10mg to 30mg
Phenobarbital (water-soluble)	200mg
Hyaluronidase	1ml

Midazolam, a short-acting water-soluble benzodiazepine, can be useful for terminal agitation.

Phenobarbital must be in water-soluble form, and **cannot be mixed with other drugs**. A second (separate) continuous subcutaneous infusion can be started when phenobarbital is used to control seizures.

Hyaluronidase can reduce any swelling at the infusion site, but is **contraindicated** if there is a history of asthma or allergy.

★　　　**The only contraindication to continuous subcutaneous infusions is severe thrombocytopenia.**

When the subcutaneous route is chosen, the pump must be small, portable and battery-operated. The use of larger and more complicated pumps merely adds to expense, and reduces mobility in the conscious patient. In the United States, several companies sell small, portable, battery-operated pumps suitable for hospice and palliative care use. For example, Baxter/Auto Syringe Division (Hooksett, New Hampshire) makes the Model AS30C Infusion Pump (Weight: 9.7 ounces — Size: 4.0 x 4.4 x 1.5 inches), and Medfusion (Duluth, Georgia) makes the Infumed Model 200 and 300 pumps. Infusaid (Norwood, Massachusetts) sells the British-made Graseby Syringe Driver, Models MS26 and MS16A.

Explanation — The patient and family must be prepared before a continuous subcutaneous infusion is set up. Most patients willingly accept it, and quickly adapt to it, provided the pump is small, easy to use, and unobtrusive. (One patient attended a very elegant formal reception with the pump hidden in her evening bag.) Some people dislike the thought of being "hooked to a machine", and explanation about the size and portability of the pump is important. Most patients soon forget it is there. Patients can still take showers and baths, but should avoid dropping the pump in the bathwater.

Technique — A small (25g) butterfly with a long (100cm) cannula attached is inserted **subcutaneously** in the abdomen, chest, thigh or upper arm, and is covered with a small piece of transparent membrane (Opsite) which holds it firmly and allows the site to be inspected for swelling or redness. This site normally has to be changed every 2 or 3 days.

SUPERIOR VENA CAVA (SVC) OBSTRUCTION

This is one of the few emergencies in terminal care. It is due to pressure from involved nodes in the superior mediastinum (usually the right paratracheal chain) and is seen most commonly in carcinomas of the bronchus (especially on the right) and breast, and in lymphoma.

The SVC drains blood from the head and upper body.

The full neck veins can be mis-diagnosed as heart failure (but are non-pulsatile).

The important early features are:
- Headaches (worse on bending)
- Blackouts
- Pink eyes
- Infra-orbital swellings (especially in the morning)
- Cyanosis and edema of the arms
- Thickening of neck ("tight collar")
- Dilated veins (arms, neck, upper chest)

The enlarged nodes may also compress other structures in the superior mediastinum, including:
- Trachea (stridor, dyspnea)
- Esophagus (dysphagia)
- Recurrent laryngeal nerve (hoarseness)

Urgent radiotherapy is the treatment of choice, together with high dose steroids (dexamethasone 8mg per day). Chemotherapy (in lymphoma or small (oat) cell carcinoma of the bronchus) is occasionally indicated.

SUPPORT

Coping with advancing disease produces moments of crisis from time to time for both patient and family. Independence and coping are normally encouraged, but at times of crisis patients and family members regress, and additional support is required. Professional carers have to be sensitive to the balance required.

The principles of giving support are:
1. Emphasize **warm nurturing care** (using first names, touch, eye contact, and showing a concern for the other's comfort).

2. Arrange **practical help** with day-to-day routines (releasing the person's energy for "worry work").

3. **Interpret** new information. (Stress reduces concentration, causing "cognitive erosion".)

4. **Rehearse problems** such as anticipated medical procedures. (Surprise increases stress. Give "anticipatory guidance" by explaining what will happen and how the person may feel.)

5. Be **optimistic**. (Optimism reduces stress.)

6. Tolerate **abnormal behavior** (irritation, anger).

7. **Mediate between family members.** (Stress can cause destructive fighting, and the needs of individuals may have to be explained to each other. Foster mutual support.)

8. **Encourage rest.** (Mental stress causes exhaustion.)

Coping with advancing disease also causes stress to the carer. The unsupported, fatigued carer is at a disadvantage in coping with a crisis. The support of a multidisciplinary team, the reassurance of a well-managed and adequately staffed organization, and a suitable personal balance between work and recreation can help to minimize stress and avoid "burn out". (see *Burn Out, Crisis Theory, Respite Care*)

SURGERY

Palliative surgery can occasionally have a place even in patients with far-advanced disease. The aim is always to achieve **optimum quality of remaining life**.

Surgical procedures are occasionally indicated as follows:

- **Ascites**

    Paracentesis

    Peritoneovenous shunt

- **Bronchial obstruction**

    Laser therapy via bronchoscope

- **Colonic obstruction**

    Palliative resection of tumor

    Palliative bypass (entero-colostomy)

- **Dysphagia**
    Esophageal tube
    Esophageal laser therapy
    Anastomosis of stomach to cervical esophagus
    Intraluminal radiotherapy

- **Feeding enterostomies**
    Pharyngostomy
    Gastrostomy
    Jejunostomy

- **Laryngeal obstruction**
    Tracheostomy

- **Liver metastases**
    Hepatic segmentectomy

- **Malignant ulceration and fungation**
    Partial resection (and sometimes skin graft)
    Debridement with cryotherapy

- **Pancreatic cancer**
    Gastro-jejunostomy (for gastric outlet obstruction)
    Bile drainage procedures
    Biliary stent insertion
    External drainage of bile

- **Pathological fractures**
    Internal fixation
    Total hip replacement

- **Pleural effusion**
    Pleural aspiration
    Closed tube thoracostomy and pleural sclerosis

- **Rectal tumors**
    Palliative colostomy with mucous fistula
    Palliative colostomy with closure of distal limb
       (Hartmann's procedure)

- **Small intestine obstruction**
    Enteroenterostomy (bypass)
    Resection or anastomosis

- **Urethral obstruction**
  Supra-pubic catheter

- **Urinary obstruction**
  Ureteric stents
  Nephrostomy
  Ureterostomy
  Ileal conduit

SWEATING

About 5% of cancer patients have tumor-induced fever and sweating. Tumor proteins may act as endogenous pyrogens on hypothalamic temperature regulators. Sweating is under cholinergic control. It is made worse by anxiety or infection.

Heavy sweats, especially night sweats, can occur in a variety of cancers, but are especially common in:

- Lymphomas
- Mesothelioma
- Small (oat) cell carcinoma of the bronchus

Management options:

1. General measures
2. NSAIDs
3. Acetaminophen
4. Antibiotics
5. Anxiolytics
6. Aluminum chloride anti-perspirant
7. Plasma exchange (in lymphoma)

1. **General measures** include frequent baths or sponge baths, air conditioning or an electric fan to improve skin cooling especially in hot weather, regular changes of bedding to reduce smell, and adequate replacement of salt and fluids.

2. **NSAIDs** block prostaglandin synthesis which is the final pathway in fever production. Aspirin, ibuprofen, indomethacin or naproxen can all be effective.

3. **Acetaminophen** is anti-pyretic and useful for patients who cannot tolerate NSAIDs.

4. Sweating may be due to an infection (infected pressure sores or a urinary tract infection, for example). If the patient is on steroids there may be no fever. Blood cultures may be indicated. A **broad-spectrum antibiotic** (chloramphenicol 500mg 4 times a day) may be indicated for a suspected silent infection.

5. Anxiety can cause sweating. Propanolol 20mg to 40mg 4 times a day reduces the somatic effects of anxiety (sweating, tremor, palpitations). **Anxiolytics** such as chlorpromazine 10mg to 25mg 3 times a day may be helpful, the anti-cholinergic action possibly also reducing sweating.

6. 20% **aluminum chloride solution** is a potent anti-perspirant useful for localized sweating in the arm-pits.

7. **Plasma exchange** has been effective in patients with lymphomas.

TALKING ABOUT DYING

All professionals and volunteers who work closely with dying patients are aware of the positive benefits of honest and open discussion. Elizabeth Kübler-Ross in *On Death and Dying* wrote about her in-depth interviews with many dying patients. She observed that the majority wished to share their concerns. Some who were depressed or morbidly uncommunicative reacted with relief and (paradoxically) more hope.

Those who doubt the truth of this need to experience for themselves, through role play, the powerful feelings of misery and tension a person experiences if he, and his family, remain unable to discuss the one thing uppermost in their thoughts.

Doctors often fear talking directly about dying in case it increases the patient's fears. In fact, the opposite is almost always the case. Sharing and discussing feelings and worries almost always helps to reduce fear and to raise the patient's morale.

Common fears include:
- Severe pain
- Choking or suffocating
- Making a mess
- Being helpless
- Dying alone
- Being buried alive

Many patients find it reassuring to discuss (often just once) the process of dying. Fears are often reduced simply by sharing them. Death itself is very rarely painful or unpleasant if symptoms are carefully monitored. Many hospice in-patients who have never seen a death find it very reassuring to witness the peaceful death of another patient.

It is helpful to be aware that, as people become weaker and weaker, their own attitudes to dying can change. **"Death is almost always preceded by a perfect willingness to die."** (Alfred Worcester)

If a person has never dared to consider what dying involves, it can be helpful to encourage some thinking about it. (For example, one patient found it reassuring to realize that birth and death were related and possibly similar experiences.)

★ **Talking about dying does not lessen the sadness of dying, but it can lessen the fear.**

Timing is important. Patients, like everyone else, have times when they want to be cheerful and times when they want to discuss what burdens them. We need to perceive their cues. At times a dying patient may prefer not to talk too openly about death and we must also be sensitive to this. (see Coping with Dying)

★ **It is almost always possible to be both honest and optimistic.**

> Mrs. M.M., age 27, with carcinoma of the ovary, had a sudden hemorrhage and was dying of acute renal failure. She had always denied her disease. She wanted a normal life and had continued working up to the week before she died. She had enjoyed a very active social life for the 3 years of her illness, partly in compensation for years of being repressed by over-protective parents. Talking with her doctor two days before she died, she began to sob and said defiantly "I am still going on holiday at the end of the month!" Then she asked "Do you think I will?" The doctor, who had had several conversations with her over a period of months and knew she coped by denial, felt to say "No", even at this stage, seemed unkind. To say "Yes" would be lying. After a pause, the doctor said "Looking back on these past months, you have done more living than most people pack into a lifetime." She stopped crying and smiled, and began to talk of some of the good times she and her husband had recently enjoyed.

When discussing dying, and sharing the sadness, it can be helpful to lighten the conversation at times. It can be helpful to ask a question such as "If you woke up tomorrow and found you were well again, what would you go and do?" This can give the person a rest from his emotions and restores balance to the conversation.

TALKING ABOUT PROGNOSIS

Patients sometimes ask the question "How long have I got?" A great deal of anxiety and fear surrounds the issue of prognosis. Sometimes the patient mistakenly believes that death is going to occur within a few days, or at any moment. An honest discussion can then greatly reduce anxiety.

If an explanation is wanted (and it is not always wanted) a useful initial sentence can be "We know you have a serious illness which will shorten your life, and I don't think you have years ahead of you any more." This can lead into a discussion of "months rather than years", or even "weeks rather than months".

★   **Never limit prognosis to a specific figure.** ("You have 6 months.")

This prediction almost always turns out to be unhelpful because it increases fear and is seldom accurate. (Several studies have shown that professional predictions of prognosis are usually wrong.) Overall survival statistics for a particular disease are seldom helpful to an individual patient.

A patient may hint verbally or non-verbally that he is plucking up courage to ask about the frightening subject of prognosis. It can then be a relief when the doctor or nurse takes the initiative and says something like "Most people who are ill like this worry about how long they might have — does that worry you?" The patient then usually gives a clear message about how much he or she wants to know at this stage. Sometimes a patient's attitude can be difficult to judge, and a question like "How long are you hoping (or planning) to live anyway?" — possibly asked in a lighthearted moment — can throw a lot of light on feelings and fears. (see *Talking with Patients*)

Provided the person breaking the news is hopeful and supportive, it is usually possible to be honest without destroying the patient's coping mechanisms. Adjusting to the idea of having a short time to live rarely happens overnight. The person may need to "try out" various emotions and attitudes. The same information is often requested several times in different ways. (see *Breaking Bad News, Coping with Dying*)

Most patients want to live as long as possible, but a few patients are greatly relieved to know that their time is short, and even take comfort from this news.

There is some evidence that people can postpone their death until after an important occasion (such as a religious holiday, a birthday, or a wedding). This suggests that family and social events may have an effect on quantity as well as quality of remaining life.

TALKING WITH CHILDREN

Talking with children can demand different techniques than talking with adults. There is growing evidence that the involvement of children around the time of death greatly reduces later psychological problems. Children must not be excluded from family discussions. The family myth that "children should be protected from distress" must be gently challenged. (see *Family Meetings, Grief, Talking with Families*)

Some techniques to encourage children to talk openly include:

1. **Chat freely.** Be prepared to give a monologue, and tell stories until they pick up on something. Don't start by asking questions.

2. **Make mistakes or silly remarks**, and allow them to correct you.

3. **Use drawings or dolls.** Children express thoughts and feelings through play.

4. Work through, and **do not displace**, the parents.

5. Avoid asking "How do you feel when . . . ?" Instead ask "What happens when . . . ?"

6. Children need even more **affirmation** than adults. The whole conversation needs to be affirming. ("You seem good at . . . ")

7. When explaining avoid concepts. Children find concepts very difficult to understand and they distance the child from the discussion. Children communicate through play. Use analogies. ("It's a bit like . . . ") **Be simple and direct.**

8. **Children have strong feelings.** They can usually only take them in small doses. They feel sad one moment and laugh the next. You have to work with small doses of sadness. If an issue is rejected because it is painful, change the subject but return to the painful issue because it is the important one. Children understand the idea of unwrapping a parcel.

9. **Children are self-centered.** Their world revolves around them. Fantasies (especially magic thinking) are common. ("I made Mommy sick because I was naughty.") You may need to spend time carefully explaining the true situation in an age-appropriate way. (see Children)

TALKING WITH FAMILIES

Most families welcome the opportunity to meet a professional (usually doctor, nurse, social worker or chaplain, or ideally two or more together) to discuss the illness, ask questions and express feelings. (see Family Meetings)

Some families have communication problems. The aim of intervention is to help the family develop its level of openness in the face of stress. (see Communication Problems)

A great deal can be achieved in a single family meeting. The first few minutes are particularly important. Make initial contact, especially eye contact, with every person present. If one person feels left out or resentful it can prevent the whole family from communicating. Every individual present has an equal right to speak and be heard. Include children and talk to each one briefly (which demonstrates that they are involved).

Set clear boundaries for the first meeting. ("We have an hour now. At the end we can decide whether we need to meet again.") Towards the end find an opportunity to say "We have five minutes left now so I think we should . . . "

Avoid premature interpretations of a family's behavior (which can rightly cause anger). Affirm their strengths. ("You have cared for him so well.") They will volunteer their weaknesses.

★ **You can challenge a family to change only when they feel their behavior has been understood, accepted and affirmed as their very best effort to cope with the crisis.**

Allow the family to choose the first subject and to discuss what is important to them ("content"). This gives you the time to observe the "process" (who is dominant, who interrupts, who looks to whom for confirmation of what is being said, who is quiet, who agrees with whom). "Process" happens in any meeting. All behavior communicates something. Always observe "process" as well as listening to "content".

Early in the discussion, focus on the principal aim of the meeting. This can be an opportunity for you to emphasize that the **family is a system**. ("This problem must be affecting you all. It often helps for everyone to talk together when there are worries.")

You should view the family as a **resource group**. Examining a problem together makes it more manageable. ("Has this happened before? What else have you tried to do about it?") The more the problem is re-enacted the better. Taking responsibility for the problem empowers a family to do something about it. The attitude that "Someone should do something about all this." leaves the family powerless. Help the family to think of helpful things they can do to improve the situation. They then begin to feel better and communicate more openly.

Once the family feels you are on their side and that you like them, they will allow you to **challenge assumptions**. ("Why do you think his weakness is due to the medicine?") Challenging assumptions does not involve disagreeing or imposing your opinions. It involves asking questions, often that nobody has dared to ask before. Change is painful and resisted. Families can only proceed at their own pace. By a process of affirming and then challenging ("the stroke before the kick") it is possible to move a family towards looking at painful issues together.

A fixed idea in a family is usually a **group defense**. ("In this family we don't want sad talk.") This need not be directly challenged. It is overcome by discussing practical issues and allowing the feelings to emerge. ("She's stuck in her room all day long. Anybody would be sad.")

Misunderstandings and upsets in a family are usually due to untested assumptions about each other. It is helpful to allow the family to listen to each other's distress. ("How have things changed for each of you? Betty, will you start?") Focus on the practical issues and the feelings will emerge.

Criticisms within a family ("the blame game") happen during a crisis as a way of coping, and of avoiding discussion of painful topics. If a family focuses on the negative side of behavior it causes escalating tension. You should remember that all behavior (even unhelpful behavior) is usually adopted for good reasons. The counselor can reinterpret ("re-frame") behavior as positive. ("So when you shout at your Mom it stops her worrying about your Dad?")

Be open and factual. Present information in a straight-forward way. **Avoid euphemisms** such as "passing away", which reduce openness and imply that you are unable to speak directly about death (and therefore the family should not either). It is important, however, to use the family's word for a particular concept before introducing new words. ("I knew I had a tumor but now you've said its cancer.")

★ **The family's understanding and attitudes need to be understood so that the therapist can relate to their belief system.**

★ **By being open and factual the counselor provides a model for the family to copy.**

The counselor must establish at least one open relationship with the family members. **Open discussion** with an individual should best occur in the context of a family meeting. It demonstrates the safety of openness to the rest of the family. A discussion that occurs in isolation from the rest of the family can reduce communication within the family.

A common problem is **collusion** between family members to help avoid painful topics, leaving you unable to hold an open discussion. Identify the family member who seems most uncomfortable with the discussion, and gently explore that person's experience of death, so that he can express his feelings. ("Have you known anyone else with cancer?") You can also increase openness by offering reading materials or videos of other families in open discussion, or by getting two or more families together to discuss some of the issues. These methods can have a powerful effect in normalizing the family's experience.

Respect the hope for life. It can be a great insult to discuss death with a family without discussing life. No one can think about death all of the time. The professional may be eager to assist a family with the issue of dying, but the family may have other important life issues to focus on, and we need to respect a family's timing, and their need for balance.

Remain calm. The family is already stressed and will not be helped by further upset. You may feel powerful emotions but these need to be understood and controlled, otherwise you can collude with their responses (by avoiding certain topics or overreacting to particular issues). You may decide to express your own emotions, and even cry, if you feel this will encourage openness.

Allow crying but don't let it block communication. Have tissues ready, but as they are handed to the person it is helpful to say "What made you cry just then?" or "Do you mind talking to me while you're crying?" or "Does anyone else feel like crying?" or "Have you cried together before?" The moment of heightened emotion often comes when an essential topic is touched upon (or thought of) and discussing crying often opens up communication and brings great relief.

A family meeting should end with affirmation. Families who have had difficulty communicating and coming closer together can sometimes be greatly strengthened by a simple suggestion such as moving closer to each other in the room, or holding hands together for a few moments, or an exercise where they say the words "I love you " to each other. You need to demonstrate ("Come together and hold hands, like this, let me do it too, that's it.") rather than give instructions.

You should end with affirming words. ("This is a family that is good at . . . " or "You have had the courage to face up to the worst and this can make you stronger together.") (*see Communication Problems*)

TALKING WITH PATIENTS

★   **"Medical care flows through relationships. The spoken word is the most important tool in medicine."** (Eric Cassell)

★   **"The doctors' misconception is in thinking their usefulness is in medications."** (Norman Cousins, *Anatomy of an Illness*)

Symptom control demands that we come alongside the patient to meet his needs. Sometimes professionals say "How do I talk to dying patients?" which makes the incorrect assumption that dying persons are different from other persons.

It is usually more important to listen than to talk. (*see Listening*)

Getting close to a dying person reminds us that we too will die some day, which can raise uncomfortable questions about our beliefs and the direction of our own life. Patients are often far more realistic than we are. They are hoping for kindness, not miracles.

A commonly expressed fear is "What if the patient asks me a question I can't answer?" This is one worry that prevents many professionals from approaching too closely. The answer is that we needn't always give answers, and there may not be any.

When asked a difficult question the important principle is to ask it back (**reflective listening**). The most feared questions are "Is it cancer?" and "How long have I got?" It is surprising how often patients will answer these questions for themselves.

It is essential (especially initially) to reflect the question back:

- "Is that what you've been thinking?"
- "What do you feel about that?"
- "What have you been told already?"
- "How long are you hoping for?"
- "Why have you asked me that just now?"

It is never necessary to answer questions "blind". Feelings are more important to patients than facts, and this approach helps meet the patients' primary need to express feelings. When facts are clearly being requested, it is usually more comfortable and straightforward to discuss facts after the patient's feelings are known.

One of the biggest mistakes in talking to patients is making assumptions about what they mean, how they feel and what they need. This can be avoided by **asking questions**. Combined with listening skills, questions are the key to identifying real needs.

★ **Open questions open up communication.**

Open questions starting with "Why . . . ?", "When . . . ?", "What . . . ?", "How . . . ?" invite more than "Yes" or "No" answers. They encourage patients to express feelings.

For example:

- "What do you understand about your illness?"
- "What is the hardest part of this illness for you?"
- "How do you feel about changing the treatment?"

- "Why do you think you feel frightened?"
- "How do you see the future?"
- "How is this illness affecting your children?"

The immediate response may be "I don't know." but allowing time often leads on to other responses.

Closed questions starting with "Do you . . . ?", "Have you . . . ?", "Will you . . . ?" can be answered with a "Yes" or "No". They are useful occasionally to pinpoint particular areas.

For example:
- "Have you known anyone else with cancer?"
- "Are you still able to cuddle together?"
- "Is there anything else on your mind?"
- "Have you seen anyone die?"
- "Are you an active member of a church?"

Leading questions should be avoided. They close conversation down. ("You seem fine today — are you?" "You don't need anything, do you?")

★ **There is more to conversation than waiting to talk. The words we use should be influenced by what has just been said. It is helpful to use the same words and phrases as the patient to improve communication and build empathy and trust.**

Transactional analysis can be a helpful way of looking at professional-patient relationships. All of us (even young children) can fluctuate between three ego states:
- "Parent" (protective)
- "Adult" (capable, logical)
- "Child" (in need of support)

An interaction between patient and carer may be adult-adult (logical discussion) or parent-child (reassuring, supporting, protecting). All human beings (patients included!) need adult-adult interactions at some times, and parent-child interactions at others.

It is helpful if professional carers can be aware of the patient's need to be a "child" at times and to regress and receive encouragement, warmth and physical touch. Patients often have good reason to be irritable and miserable and carers need to make allowances for such behavior. At other times patients need to be "adult" and assume responsibilities again.

Professional carers also have needs and feelings. In a therapeutic relationship it can be all right to become a "child" occasionally. ("I feel tired today.") This can bring balance and normality to what is, or should be, an adult-adult exchange most of the time.

Somtimes it is necessary to change the interaction from parent-child to adult-adult. For example, a patient who is inappropriately dependent for his degree of physical disability might be asked "What are your thoughts about getting home again?" This may re-focus the conversation on adult responsibilities. (Professional carers who are comfortable with traditional parent-child medical interactions may on occasion feel threatened by a patient who demands an adult-adult relationship.)

All patients, even children, have responsibilities. They are responsible, not for the disease, but for their own responses to having an illness.

First words are remembered best. First impressions are often difficult to reverse. If time is limited, first words are even more important. Compare "Hello Mrs. Jones, I'm Doctor Smith. I've come to spend a few minutes to talk with you about your illness " (while preferably sitting down on a nearby chair) to "Hello, I can only spare a few minutes to talk about your illness." Since first words and first impressions are so important, some preparation is essential before meeting new patients.

Good manners (proper introductions, use of correct names, courtesy, respect for social expectations, etc.) are essential.

Non-medical talk is important. To talk to someone about illness and dying without talking about life and living is a great affront. It has been shown that to discuss non-medical matters, even briefly, increases the chances of the patient liking you, which in turn increases the likelihood that the patient will trust you. Skillful "talkers" find a point of contact with each patient early in the conversation and build on it in subsequent conversations.

Be aware of the **juxtaposition of words**, which can convey information (just as avoiding a subject can convey information). Introducing a new topic of conversation may simply be due to bad listening, but it can convey an unintended message. For example, if a patient mentions weight loss and the doctor then asks a question about the family, the patient may assume (rightly or wrongly) that the doctor has gone from thinking about weight loss to thinking in terms of a poor prognosis and how it will affect the relatives.

Be aware of the **power of words**. In an emotionally charged situation, such as a first visit to see a hospice or palliative care doctor, words can take on an extraordinary power. ("He said he'd see me soon, I must be getting worse.") Words can be "mis-taken" by patient or family to mean impending doom. Use words carefully and sparingly. Use kind, positive words rather than harsh or negative words whenever possible. ("Your strength is not so good today ", not "You are getting weaker.") Choosing to use technical words carries a message. It is a way of signaling emotional distance.

Be encouraging. To encourage means "to fill with courage" and it is one hallmark of leadership. Emphasize and affirm a person's strength when possible. ("Look how strong you have been up to now.") A person's role may finally be restricted to being a patient. ("You are a good patient — we enjoy looking after you.") Telling of other patients' successes and triumphs, small as well as large, can be encouraging and can reduce the sense of isolation.

Words can reframe a situation. Words not only describe reality but can also change a person's perception of reality. ("I hadn't seen it that way before.") Words can re-label a situation to give it positive connotations. This can increase a person's confidence and ability to cope.

<u>Negative</u>	<u>Positive Reframing</u>
"I've been ill for so long."	"You're through the worst."
"We can't cope any longer."	"How have you managed to cope so well?"
"I'm terminal."	"You're living with an incurable illness."
"I hate complaining."	"We need to know everything so we can help."
"He's giving up."	"He's letting go."

"There is nothing good or bad, but thinking makes it so."
(William Shakespeare)

Use silence. As we talk to someone and tell him things, he is also telling himself things, if we allow time and space for this to happen. Learn to recognize the signs that a patient is dealing with important material (loss of facial expression, absence of blinking, immobility). New information may need to be integrated with current beliefs and memories if it is to bring about useful changes. "New" information may not come directly from another person but may be re-awakened from memory.

> *Miss J.W., a woman with advanced cancer, met a hospice nurse for the first time. She talked at some length about her feelings and her fears. The nurse said very little, but reflected back some of her comments and encouraged her to talk. A week later she surprised the nurse by saying "I've been thinking about what you said and I've decided to accept my illness."*

Avoid giving advice when discussing feelings or reactions. Listen instead. The answers lie within the person. Advice is only helpful when discussing facts. (*see Advice, Explanation, Reassurance*)

Respect secrets. It is important to balance the need for emotional openness with the need for personal uniqueness. Patients are vulnerable and often confide their deepest secrets to their carers. These secrets must be respected because secrets can give a person strength. People who have survived prolonged torture often speak of focusing their thoughts on some secret information that only they knew about.

(Occasionally a patient may confide a harmful secret. The question then arises whether the carer should keep this secret, or share it with other members of the team. The key issue is whether keeping the secret is likely to result in harm to other indivduals. The principle of confidentiality is extremely important but cannot support keeping secrets which are harmful.)

Change insight into empathy. Sharing insights can be threatening. It is often better to use insights to increase empathy and build trust. For example, if you notice that a patient's pain seems worse whenever his family visit, avoid pointing that out directly. It can be useful to make a comment such as "It is difficult to cope with pain especially when you have a lot of other pressures on you." Such an observation can encourage the patient to discuss his real problems.

An **honest reappraisal of the situation** can sometimes bring great relief.

Mrs. D.D., a woman of 60 with a brain tumor, had struggled for several weeks to get walking again, but her legs gradually became weaker. She and her husband became increasingly frustrated and depressed, having decided to try for her mobility above all else. One day the doctor explained to them "Times change, and times have changed for you; your legs simply don't have the strength left now for you to walk any more." Initial sadness was soon replaced by relief that the unsuccessful battle to walk was over. They started to have more realistic aims. She enjoyed going out for "walks" with her husband pushing her wheelchair.

Avoid colluding with unrealistic statements or aims.

Miss G.E., a woman of 62 with far advanced abdominal cancer said to a doctor "Well, I'm glad I'm getting better." The doctor made a point of going back to the woman, sitting down and saying "I'm glad you are feeling better and the pain and sickness are gone, but we cannot make this tumor go away." The woman smiled and accepted this statement. By avoiding collusion the doctor was able to continue visiting the woman every day, without feeling awkward or embarrassed, right up to the day she died, 10 days later.

Honest description of our own feelings can sometimes provide a breakthrough in communications.

Mr. R.H., a man of 58 with recurrent cancer of the larynx, seemed withdrawn and negative at every visit to the out-patient clinic of the hospice. On the fifth visit the doctor said "You always make me feel helpless and hopeless!" The man smiled and from that time communication was improved. The patient had finally succeeded in communicating the way he felt.

Anecdotes (true stories) can sometimes be a helpful way of gently and indirectly conveying an idea. Therapeutic suggestions can be passed on by means of an amusing story (perhaps with no obvious relevance at the time). This leaves the patient with new information or new possibilities, and allows time for change to be self-initiated. Anecdotes are usually memorable and non-threatening. They can be used to encourage or motivate a person. People often have in their own history the forgotten resources to overcome a problem. Anecdotes can stimulate memories and associations and can bring change in awareness or attitudes over a period of time.

> Mr. R.C., a younger patient struggling to walk again with the help of a walking frame, was amused to hear about the efforts of the doctor's one year old daughter, who was just learning to walk. The doctor mentioned this in conversation without thinking of the implications. From then on, the patient asked about the little girl and seemed keen to talk about her. Learning to walk had somehow been reframed by the anecdote as something normal, healthy, entertaining and fun.

Wrong or hurtful words are those spoken without kindness. **It is usually the lack of kindness and not the words themselves that cause pain.** Our words flow from our attitudes. Our attitude to the incurably ill often reveals our appraisal of our own self-worth.

Humor is important. It can be strengthening and unifying. Humor enables us to rise above a situation. It can be a way of mutually regressing to childhood, if only for a few moments, to allow a rest from powerful emotions. Humor also involves reflecting on experience. It helps to put things in perspective. It can be a way of allowing discussion of a painful or difficult problem. Humor can sometimes be used alternately with sadness, so the sadness is dealt with in small doses. (This technique can be especially useful when discussing sad things with children.) Laughter can allow us to ventilate and release intense feelings. (Many jokes are about otherwise taboo subjects.) There is truth in the saying "laughter is the best medicine". Laughter can be therapeutic and can raise the pain threshold. Laughter, like play, brings a sense of shared experience and can convey friendliness and raise morale. Patients who are very ill continue to enjoy amusing events or stories and appreciate being told "You haven't lost your sense of humor." Sometimes as professionals we "cry with those who cry" but forget to "laugh with those who laugh".

Important — Do not hide behind an insincere, hearty joviality. This is one way of avoiding the real issues and distancing ourselves from emotional pain. ("Come along now, it can't be that bad, give me a smile!") Similiarly some patients display a persistent joviality to mask their anguish and carers must not be pulled into behaving the same way, which keeps all conversation superficial.

Who should talk to the patient? A sick person can relate in depth to only one or two carers. Repetitive questioning by members of different professional disciplines is tiring. This is one reason why good communication within the team is essential.

The **context of talking**. Most patients cope because of the support of family and friends. Words can be especially therapeutic in the context of a family group. Often the best way of supporting a patient is to support the family. (*see Family Meetings, Talking with Families*)

TASTE CHANGES

About 20% of terminally ill patients complain of taste changes. Commonly there is an aversion to meat (which tends to taste metallic), or sweet food becomes more difficult to taste. Zinc deficiency has been implicated as a cause. Cytotoxic drugs (especially cytarabine) can affect taste. Aberrations in taste are not necessarily permanent and even after many weeks taste can return to normal.

Management options:
- Exclude gingivitis and oral thrush
- Adapt diet

A bad taste in the mouth may be due to gingivitis and slight bleeding. Examine for thrush. (*see Candidiasis, Mouth Care*)

Extra seasoning (herbs and spices) can help. Try adding salt if food is too sweet, or sugar if too bitter. It can help to change the temperature at which food is normally eaten.

Learned aversion may occur to food eaten around the time of chemotherapy. Avoid favorite foods at treatment times.

TEAMWORK

★ **"No one can carry out hospice care in isolation. Each one of us, in whatever discipline, has to learn to work as a team, to appreciate and draw on the expertise of other members and make a commitment towards them as well as those we serve."** (Cicely Saunders)

★ **"The team is a flexible blend of skills to meet the ever changing needs of patient and family."** (Elisabeth Earnshaw-Smith)

A team approach can and should be applied whenever a person is facing a fatal illness. It need not be confined to hospice care.

In *Motivation and Personality* (1954), Abraham Maslow described a "hierarchy of needs". If we are released from basic needs like food, warmth, shelter and physical comfort we can address higher needs like social relationships, security, self-esteem and a sense of meaning. The holistic approach to care addresses all these issues simultaneously. This demands teamwork.

For a team to function properly, good communication is essential. Uncoordinated care and conflicting advice destroy trust. Communication is hard work. It requires a structure, such as weekly team meetings plus daily updates.

Good teamwork involves respect for other professionals (and volunteers) and a realistic view of our own skills.

A good team requires good leadership. A team leader has three overlapping areas of concern which must be kept in balance: **achieving the task, building the team, and developing individuals**. The leader should convey enthusiasm about the task, brief the team together about policy and plans, and delegate tasks and develop individual skills.

There will always be tensions in a team of people committed to a task. These can be overcome by goodwill and regular discussion. **"If a group fails in its task it is most probably because its members have been more concerned with establishing their own status . . . "** (Nicolo Machiavelli)

Good terminal care is inevitably multi-disciplinary. Communication is essential to coordinate efficient care. Regular reassessment avoids the danger of the team members assuming that "someone else must be doing it".

The nature of the help that is offered can depend upon searching out private facts, opinions or emotions. If these are shared in the context of a team it must be with respect for individual privacy, and with the purpose of enhancing quality of life.

Talking about patients is an essential aspect of caring for patients. The way professionals discuss patients (and each other) affects standards of care.

Gossip (speculative discussion of an absent person) is one of the major forms of communication between people. Gossip can provide information, which helps a group to function, and can be supportive to the person discussed.

However, gossip is wrong if it is:

- A breach of confidence
- False (or based on hearsay)
- Irrelevant
- Demeaning
- Judgmental

Gossip can be harmful to patient care. For example, a derogatory comment about a patient by a senior member of staff can affect the attitudes of all the team. Gossip tends to talk of all persons, however gifted or unusual, in the same terms. It is a way of distancing ourselves from the distress of the real situation. Gossip is attractive because it provides a sense of superiority over others, but it encourages hypocrisy (moralizing about others without having to moralize about ourselves).

TELLING THE TRUTH

★ **"How much to tell lies somewhere between too little and too much."** (Tom West)

In the past many doctors held the view that patients with serious diseases should not be told. Apparently doctors felt that knowledge of the true diagnosis would cause demoralization and despair. However, the idea that avoidance is somehow protective is a false assumption. **Avoidance does not help patients adjust to their situation.**

The principle of "primum non nocere" (first do no harm) is sometimes used to defend the stance of deception. The patient will of course be distressed by the doctor's words when bad news is broken, but to argue that a discussion (skillfully conducted) should therefore be avoided is analogous to saying that a surgeon should not cut his patient as it would cause avoidable suffering.

Against the anguish of finding out must be set the benefits of knowing. Several studies have shown that the great majority of cancer patients want to be told the truth.

Patients tend not to press for information and yet they need information for many different reasons:

- Relief of uncertainty
- Discussion of future needs
- Planning for the future (legal, financial)
- Attending to unfinished emotional business
- Avoiding deceit
- Maintaining open communications
- Preparation for death

Giving a patient the opportunity to ask in detail about the diagnosis also avoids the all-too-common devastating situation when a patient discovers the true diagnosis by accident, perhaps by overhearing a conversation.

A better question than "Can the patient stand being told?" is "Can the patient stand **not** being told?" However, the decision to be honest brings with it a duty to explain and support.

It is tempting to tell too little, perhaps to avoid upsetting and disappointing the patient, but it can destroy trust, and can cause anger and resentment later on. Telling too much can cause anxiety and fear. (*see Breaking Bad News*)

★   **"Truth, like medicine, can be intelligently used, respecting its potential to help and to hurt."** (Avery Weisman)

TENESMUS

Tenesmus is a very unpleasant recurrent sensation of wanting to move the bowels. It is usually due to pressure on stretch receptors in the levator ani muscles from a pelvic tumor. The same sensation can occur after an abdominal-perineal resection of the rectum (when it is known as the "phantom rectum syndrome"). Low doses of morphine and/or chlorpromazine sometimes reduce this sensation.

★   **Always exclude impacted feces.**

Radiotherapy can be useful when a large cauliflower lesion is filling the rectum. It is **contraindicated** if there is vaginal involvement because of the risk of a rectovaginal fistula.

High dose steroids (dexamethasone 8mg per day) can help by reducing peri-tumor edema.

A bi-lateral lumbar sympathetic nerve block is some-times successful in reducing or abolishing tenesmus.

★ **Tenesmus due to large inoperable rectal tumors can be reduced by trans-anal resection or laser therapy.** (see *Lasers*)

TENS

TENS means transcutaneous electrical nerve stimulation.

TENS was developed as a result of the **gate theory** of pain (stimulating skin mechano-receptors produces pre-synaptic spinal inhibition of pain transmission). High fre-quency TENS (80Hz to 200Hz) is thought to work this way, but conventional low frequency TENS (2Hz to 6Hz) is thought to release endogenous opioids in the spinal cord and midbrain (like acupuncture).

There has been little research into the use of TENS in cancer pain, but individual reports suggest it can be helpful. In one descriptive study 34 out of 49 cancer patients had improved pain control, and some were able to reduce pain medication.

It is reasonable to try TENS on any patient who is open to the idea. Many cancer patients have musculo-skeletal pains (cervical spondylosis, for example, is a common condition) for which TENS can be helpful.

TENS is rarely helpful in nerve pain and tends to exacer-bate it.

Summary of optimum conditions for TENS:
- Compliant patient
- Competent patient or carer
- Self-adhering 2.5mm electrodes
- Use of good contact medium
- Frequency of 4Hz
- Intensity set to cause distinct pulsation (not pain)
- Electrodes applied to acupuncture points
- 15 to 20 minute treatment (usually daily)

The TENS machine should be small, portable, and have a frequency range of 0Hz to 200Hz, and a minimum of two channels. The patient should rent the machine for a trial, before considering purchase.

Electrode location needs to be precise, and is most effective when anatomical acupuncture points are used. Small electrodes are more effective.

Duration of treatment — Low frequency TENS should be used for only 15 to 20 minutes to prevent habituation (the nervous system tunes out a repetitive signal). The effect can last for hours or days. If low frequency TENS is ineffective, a trial of high frequency TENS is worthwhile, but the effect is usually short-lived (from a few minutes to 2 hours). A newer TENS device stimulates multiple points in random fashion (to avoid habituation) and may prove more effective.

Contraindications:
- Cardiac pacemaker
- Inflamed or infected skin

TERMINAL PHASE

Most patients become unconscious only for the last few hours of life, although sometimes (especially with primary brain tumors) the period of unconsciousness can last for several days.

Important Issues in the Terminal Phase

I. Drugs

II. Care of the weak or semi-conscious patient

III. Management of terminal agitation

IV. Support of the family

I.   **Drugs** — The commonly used drugs in the terminal phase are:
- Morphine
- Chlorpromazine or methotrimeprazine
- Scopolamine
- Diazepam

A continuous subcutaneous infusion of drugs can be useful during the terminal phase, particularly at home. (see *Subcutaneous Infusions*)

If a patient has needed regular oral morphine he will continue to need it to remain pain-free and peaceful. The equivalent IM dosage is half the oral dose (for example, a patient who was well-controlled on oral morphine 30mg every 4 hours will need IM morphine 15mg every 4 hours). The dose is increased if the patient seems restless due to increased pain. Occasionally two indomethacin 50mg suppositories are helpful if a patient with bone metastases gets pain on being turned.

Sedatives are quite often needed for agitation. Chlorpromazine 25mg to 50mg every 4 hours is usually adequate. Methotrimeprazine can be thought of as double-strength chlorpromazine and can be used in a continuous subcutaneous infusion 50mg to 100mg per 24 hours.

Scopolamine is a very useful drug for the terminal phase, being anti-cholinergic, drying up secretions, and reducing or abolishing respiratory bubbling ("the death rattle"). The usual dose is 0.4mg IM every 4 hours, or in a continuous subcutaneous infusion 0.8mg to 2.4mg per 24 hours. It is also very sedating.

Diazepam enema 10mg is useful for terminal twitching or focal seizures which can be very distressing for relatives. Diazepam 10mg IM or IV is an alternative to the diazepam enema.

★ **Warfarin should be stopped or reversed before the terminal phase. Otherwise terminal gastrointestinal bleeding can occur, and as sphincters relax in the hours before death altered blood comes out of the mouth, which is very distressing to relatives.** (see Bleeding)

II. **Care of the weak or semi-conscious** — Retention of urine is common, especially if anti-cholinergic drugs are used. Examine regularly for bladder fullness (especially if the patient becomes restless) and insert an indwelling catheter if necessary. Turn the patient every 2 hours (unless turning causes the patient distress). Mouth care is needed every hour. Use "artifical tears" eye drops every 2 hours if eyes are getting dry or inflamed.

All procedures should be explained to the family, who may find staying with the patient easier if they are allowed to help.

III. **Terminal agitation** — Most patients dying of cancer enter a phase of unconsciousness before death but a few patients (about 1% to 2%) close to death become **restless and agitated.** (It is obviously important to exclude discomfort from a full bladder.) They are usually mildly confused, but may be physically strong enough to be sitting up or even walking around. Their skin is often mottled due to poor peripheral circulation. They become increasingly distressed and dyspneic, and after several hours finally die.

It is difficult to understand why terminal agitation sometimes occurs. It may be due to hypoxia. (Some psychosocial professionals have noticed a correlation with denial and unfinished emotional business.) The patient becomes too mentally anguished for counseling help and needs urgent sedation. Without adequate sedation these patients have a most unpleasant and distressing death.

Powerful sedatives are needed for terminal agitation, and a combination of drugs should be given by IM injections or continuous subcutaneous infusion:

Drug	IM Dose mg per 4 hours	Continuous Subcutaneous Dose mg per 24 hours
Morphine	½ 4-hourly oral dose	½ 24-hourly oral dose
Chlorpromazine	25mg to 75mg	—
Methotrimeprazine	25mg to 75mg	75mg to 150mg
Scopolamine	0.4mg	1.2mg to 2.4mg
Diazepam	10mg (IM or rectal)	—
Midazolam	—	20mg to 80mg

The dose of morphine should be roughly equi-analgesic to previous doses. If the patient has not previously needed opioid drugs, start with 5mg morphine IM every 4 hours, or 30mg morphine in a continuous subcutaneous infusion every 24 hours. (If the agitation appears to be due to pain, higher doses of morphine may be needed.)

It can be worrying for both doctors and nurses to sedate someone just before he dies. ("Did the injection I gave kill him?") It is important to emphasize to carers that the above combination of drugs does not cause death (and indeed is occasionally used for severe insomnia quite safely). If the patient is sedated but does not die, the drugs can be reduced or stopped for a time, and the patient observed.

The level of sedation may be an important issue for the family and explanation is important. If the patient's level of consciousness is allowed to lighten it is important to observe carefully, and not to allow him to become agitated and distressed.

★   **This agitation is a terminal event, occurring only in the very last hours of life. It is NOT to be confused with the anguish and distress of many patients who are not yet dying and who need company and counseling and NOT sedation.**

IV.   **Support of the family** — Family members may find it difficult to concentrate properly or think clearly. They can need a surprising amount of guidance. ("You can sit down and hold his hand, like this.") They will tend to take on the role that is expected of them, but may need guidance about what is appropriate. They benefit from comfort and touch (people under stress regress). They may not remember details of any information given them at this time. (see *Support*)

If other deaths have not been seen there may be misconceptions about what death will be like. As death approaches simple explanations are greatly appreciated.

Some common questions, asked or unasked, are:

- Should we stay?
- Will it be long?
- Is he suffering?
- Can he hear us?
- What will happen?
- Why has the breathing changed?
- Why has the skin color changed?
- Why is he still getting injections?

Dying patients can sometimes still hear from time to time even when they are semi-conscious. It can be helpful for the family to know this. Very lightly touching the eyelashes of the patient to see if the eye-lid flickers can be a helpful guide to the level of consciousness.

Grief from previous deaths may be reawakened and it is a time when sympathetic listening is important. A common feeling is guilt at wishing the person would die, to end his suffering.

Keeping a vigil can become exhausting. It can be helpful to suggest a schedule of visitors, so that some keep watch while others rest. It is often difficult to judge how long a semi-conscious patient may live. The volume of the pulse is a guide — a full volume usually suggests that there are several more hours. The degree of difficulty in breathing, and the skin color (mottling or blueness suggesting shutdown of the peripheral circulation) are other guides.

Family members may be very distressed at the physical appearance of the body, and may feel unable to stay. They need permission not to be there.

After death allow time for the family to do what is important for them. Gently encourage them to see the body and say good-bye. Prayers at the time of death can be very comforting if appropriate for the family. Family members who have been very involved may want to help with laying out the body, and should be allowed to do so. The amount of time a person needs to spend with the body after death varies. Some people need to spend many hours in order to say good-bye. Others do not. Be flexible.

★ **It is rarely helpful to transfer a dying patient from home to a hospital or in-patient hospice simply to die.** (see Home Care)

THIRST

Patients who are ill and dehydrated complain of a dry mouth (and need regular mouth care) but rarely complain of thirst.

Thirst and polyuria suggest:

- Hypercalcemia
- Diabetes mellitus (steroid-induced)
- Diabetes insipidus

The combination of thirst with nausea or drowsiness is very suggestive of **hypercalcemia**.

High dose steroids can precipitate **diabetes mellitus**.

Diabetes insipidus occurs rarely due to primary brain tumor or hypothalamic secondaries (most commonly from bronchus and breast). The onset of thirst can be sudden, and a fluid balance chart shows an output of 3 to 6 liters per day (10 to 20 liters per day in very severe cases). There is nocturia. Urine osmolality is low (50 to 100 mosmol/L) and plasma osmolality is normal or slightly high (normal range 285 to 295 mosmol/kg), whereas in compulsive water drinking plasma is diluted and therefore low. It is treated with intra-nasal desmopressin, which acts for about 12 hours. The dose is adjusted to between 10 micrograms to 20 micrograms 1 or 2 times a day, to allow one diuresis a day to prevent water intoxication. (Often a single dose at bedtime is adequate to prevent nocturnal polyuria and sleep disturbance.) Desmopressin can also be given by IM injection (1 microgram to 4 micrograms per day). The patient should produce a daytime urine output of at least 500ml to avoid water intoxication.

In **total dysphagia** patients complaining of thirst usually need IV fluids, but tap water enemas via a Foley catheter can be a useful substitute in home care.

Thirst can be reduced or abolished by morphine. (*see Dehydration, Diabetes, Hypercalcemia*)

TOUCH

Touch can have powerful therapeutic effects and can enhance psychological and physical comfort. Several studies have demonstrated the power of even minimal touch to affect feelings.

Touch, used appropriately, can:
- Convey empathy
- Facilitate conversation
- Encourage the expression of feelings
- Improve trust

The interpretation of touch varies. In some situations or cultures touch may appear flirtatious, condescending or even threatening. It is less likely to be misunderstood if it occurs in the context of a structured interaction.

Individuals vary in the amount of touch they normally give and receive, but in times of stress the need for reassuring contact is increased (a regression to infantile needs). The elderly and seriously ill are particularly responsive to expressive touch.

Massage can be very useful, not only to ease stiff muscles and improve circulation, but to reduce tension and a feeling of isolation or anxiety. (If necessary, massage may be recommended on the pretext of rehydrating dry skin with cream.)

TRACHEOSTOMY CARE

★   **A tracheostomy should be performed only on a relatively fit patient who is experiencing tracheal obstruction. A tracheostomy should NOT be performed on a weak or dying patient when tracheal obstruction occurs as a terminal event. This simply prolongs the process of dying.**

A tracheostomy is a stoma into the trachea (so the patient breathes through the neck). It is necessary when tumors of the pharynx or larynx cause airway obstruction (with stridor, intercostal recession, and eventually cyanosis).

For **the first 2 or 3 weeks**, after a tracheostomy is fashioned, there is a risk that the pre-tracheal tissues will close over the stoma if the tube is removed. When changing the outer tube for cleaning, which needs to be done every few days, it must therefore be done quickly, with two nurses present. A spare tube plus introducer and pair of tracheal dilators are kept by the bed in case the tube falls out and needs urgent replacement. The tube is taped around the neck to prevent it being dislodged by coughing.

After the first few weeks the patient usually manages the routine care of the tracheostomy, which involves:

- Cleaning inner tube
- Changing outer tube
- Suction
- Skin care around stoma
- Humidification

The **inner tube** usually needs cleaning 2 or 3 times a day with a tracheostomy brush, depending on the amount of secretions. A **speaking tube**, with a valve, can be used as an inner tube. It blocks exhaled air which is therefore redirected through the damaged larynx, allowing speech. The voice is usually quiet and husky and the patient may need a call-bell. The speaking tube should be removed at night.

The **outer tube** usually needs changing every week. The new tube is inserted with an introducer with a rounded end. Permanent tracheostomy tubes are made of silver.

Suction is usually only required for the first few weeks, until the patient learns how to cough up secretions. If the patient has a lot of secretions (for example, due to a respiratory infection) he needs a portable suction machine at home plus some sterile soft catheters. Most patients become skilled at doing their own suction.

Skin care usually simply involves the use of Vaseline around the stoma to prevent the skin from drying out. If dry crusts develop they can be softened by breathing humidified air. A piece of foam can be worn over the tracheostomy to prevent sputum exploding out when coughing.

Note on laryngectomy patients — Following laryngectomy a wide stoma is fashioned and these patients only require a tube for the first few weeks, post-operatively. With no larynx they have to learn artificial speech (either esophageal or using a vibrator placed on the jaw to amplify lip speech).

TRUST

Trust depends in part on **reputation** and **competence**, and in part on **liking**.

★ **Meeting a patient for the first time is a critical moment in establishing trust.**

First impressions are particulary important. The studies by ethologists on imprinting (recognition and attraction) in newborn birds and animals may also be relevant to new encounters between humans.

A trusting relationship does three things:
- Reduces fears and improves morale
- Improves compliance
- Saves time

Trust is the first step to reassurance. A person will not share deep-seated fears with an uncaring stranger. (*see Reassurance*)

A person is more likely to take the advice of someone he trusts. (*see Advice*)

Trust saves time because it reduces the need for detailed discussion or justification of every step in treatment or management, although open communication among patient, family and carers is always important.

Good leadership should maintain trust, reduce uncertainty and be optimistic in some way. Optimism is supportive (pessimism is not) and being supportive boosts trust. Honesty and openness also boost trust. It is always possible to be both honest and optimistic. (*see Talking with Patients*)

303

URETERIC OBSTRUCTION

Obstruction of the ureters occurs most commonly in carcinomas of cervix, prostate, rectum, bladder and ovary, or in retroperitoneal lymphomas or sarcoma.

Obstruction for more than a few days causes irreversible renal damage.

In patients **with limited disease** the cytoscopic insertion of a self-retaining **ureteric stent** is a useful procedure.

In patients with **extensive malignant disease**, urinary diversion procedures (nephrostomy, ureterostomy, ileal conduit) have a high mortality and morbidity. They may prevent uremia only to prolong suffering from the original disease.

URINARY CATHETERS

Urinary incontinence is one of the most dreaded symptoms of advanced illness, and can too often become the primary reason for in-patient admission even if the patient prefers to remain at home. A permanent in-dwelling urinary catheter is often the best solution, and a relief to the patient (and to family carers). A catheter is usually better than pads or pants which can be smelly, uncomfortable, and embarrassing, and which predispose to pressure sores.

A covered leg-bag should be used if the patient is still getting dressed.

A catheter can be a worrying prospect. Explanation and discussion are essential and go a long way towards preventing discomfort and fear. ("How does it work?" "How long will I need it?" "How will I empty the bag?") One patient suffered unnecessary incontinence for a period of time because she assumed "catheter" meant something that would have to be inserted each time she wished to urinate.

Technique of catheterization:
- Explain to patient
- Consider oral lorazepam 1mg if patient is anxious
- Give analgesia if pain is likely
- Observe sterile technique

- Apply lidocaine jelly
- Use silicone catheter if long-term
- Use small diameter (12Fr to 16Fr catheter)
- Use 5cc balloon

Normal care involves encouraging fluids, preventing traction on the catheter, and avoiding needless changes of catheter. (If problems occur, consult a specialist continence advisor.)

Large balloons (20cc to 30cc) are useful in chronically catheterized patients with lax pelvic muscles, but in most patients they can cause bladder irritation and leaking. Leakage is more likely (surprisingly) with wide diameter catheters or large balloons. A leaking catheter should usually be left in place (unless due to be changed anyway), because changing the catheter rarely helps (unless the catheter is too wide or has a large balloon).

Leakage may be due to fecal impaction.

Bladder spasms cause pain and leaking and can be reduced with terfenadine or imipramine.

Debris can be cleared with daily saline washouts. Use sodium citrate washouts if there are blood clots. Antiseptic washouts are unnecessary, often quite painful, and can cause a chemical cystitis. Debris is lessened by acidification (try oral Vitamin C 1g per day).

A blocked catheter must be promptly replaced.

Rejection of the catheter may be due to:

- Lax pelvic muscles (use a 30cc balloon)
- Bladder spasms (use terfenadine or imipramine)

If a catheter is pulled out by a confused patient consider incontinence appliances instead.

If a urinary catheter cannot be used (due to a stricture, for example) consider a supra-pubic catheter.

URINARY FREQUENCY

Urinary frequency can cause exhaustion, insomnia and (if patient is unable to reach a toilet) incontinence.

The common causes are:

- Urinary infection
- Fecal impaction
- Diuretics

- Atrophic vaginitis
- Bladder spasms
- Diabetes insipidus

Always analyze a specimen of urine to exclude infection, and examine rectally to exclude fecal impaction.

Stop unnecessary diuretics.

Atrophic vaginitis can cause urinary frequency in the elderly. (*see Urinary Incontinence*)

Urgency and supra-pubic pain suggests bladder spasms which occur due to radiation cystitis or tumors of the bladder or prostate. (*see Bladder Spasms*)

Large volumes of urine (polyuria) can be due to diabetes mellitus, hypercalcemia or diabetes insipidus. Diabetes insipidus is treated with desmopressin. Even in patients with a normal urine volume, desmopressin can be useful to reduce night-time frequency which disturbs sleep. (*see Thirst*)

Burning and stinging discomfort (dysuria) does not usually respond to morphine but may be reduced with one of the following:

- Potassium citrate 10ml 4 times a day
- Sodium bicarbonate 2g to 4g per day
- Phenazopyridine 200mg 4 times a day

URINARY INCONTINENCE

Urinary incontinence occurs in about 20% of hospice patients. Many patients require urinary catheterization during the terminal 48 hours.

Before catheterization, consider treatable causes:

1. Infection
2. Impacted feces
3. Drugs (diuretics, sedatives, alcohol)
4. Atrophic vaginitis
5. Fistula (continuous dribble)
6. Difficulty in reaching toilet or commode
7. Attention-seeking behavior

1. A **low-grade urinary infection** can cause incontinence in elderly patients with no other symptoms.

2. **Impacted feces** commonly cause urinary symptoms.

3. **Diuretics** (including alcohol) late in the day, or excessive **sedation**, may cause incontinence at night.

4. **Atrophic vaginitis** causes urgency, dysuria and sometimes incontinence, and can be treated with oral ethinyl estradiol 0.02mg once a day, which is more convenient and more effective than topical preparations. There is no need to stop treatment to allow a withdrawal bleed in terminally ill patients. Estrogens are contraindicated in pre-terminal carcinomas of the breast, uterus and cervix.

5. A **vesico-vaginal fistula** causes a continuous dribbling of urine. Tampons are usually ineffective (except for very small fistulas). A urinary diversion procedure (ileal conduit, uretero-sigmoidoscopy) should be considered if the patient has a reasonable prognosis.

6. Patients with urinary frequency must be situated near a toilet or commode. Immobility, drowsiness, confusion or embarrassment may all make it difficult to reach a toilet or commode in time. A patient with dysphasia or speech deficits will not be able to ask for assistance.

7. Feelings of **fear and isolation** can sometimes drive a patient (particularly in certain in-patient settings) to deliberate incontinence in order to be noticed. Attention-seeking patients need sympathetic attention.

Management options:
- Incontinence appliances
- Shields, undergarments and bedding
- Desmopressin
- Catheter

A **urinary condom** drains into a catheter bag. Worn at night it can greatly improve life for some male patients, who can sleep without the disturbance of urinary frequency. Worn day and night it can cause skin soreness and can leak. **Urinals** for women are useful for urge incontinence when it may not be possible to get to the toilet or commode.

Shields and undergarments are helpful for patients with intermittent or minimal incontinence, particularly when they are active. Disposable absorbent underpads and micropore drawsheets are helpful and convenient.

Desmopressin can sometimes be useful for nocturnal incontinence. (see Urinary Frequency, Thirst)

For the majority of patients with persistent incontinence a **permanent in-dwelling catheter** is the best solution. (see Urinary Catheters)

URINARY RETENTION

Sudden retention is painful but gradual retention is not, and may present as overflow incontinence. Palpate to identify a full bladder. Perform a rectal examination to exclude **impacted feces**.

Poor urine output may be due to **dehydration** (dark urine, dry tongue, stiff skin, tachycardia) when the bladder is not palpable.

Anti-cholinergic drugs (phenothiazines, tricyclics, antihistamines) can cause urinary hesitancy and can precipitate urinary retention. Urinary hesitancy together with weak legs and back pain suggest **malignant spinal cord compression**. This is a medical emergency. (see *Spinal Cord Compression*)

Benign prostatic hypertrophy causes hesitancy. It may be easier to void sitting down (or sometimes in a hot bath) while applying pressure to the bladder. In patients too ill to consider trans-urethral resection, phenoxybenzamine 10mg 2 times a day can help. It reduces urethral tone (but can also cause tachycardia and postural hypotension).

In patients with prostate cancer urinary hesitancy should be treated with trans-urethral resection.

Retention of urine normally requires a urinary catheter. With tumor of the bladder neck or a urethral stricture it may not be possible to pass a catheter, and a supra-pubic catheter may be necessary. The bladder should be palpable before inserting a supra-pubic catheter. Oral imipramine 25mg reduces bladder spasms after the procedure.

VISITORS

It is often visitors who improve a patient's quality of remaining life more than anyone or anything else. One aspect of caring for patients is caring for family members and friends by acknowledging their contribution and showing concern for their feelings.

★ **"We must ensure that those who visit are not neglected but receive appropriate support for themselves. This might be . . . transport, meals or interpretation of the illness and patients' behavior, and providing the necessary space for the visitors to share what they are feeling and experiencing."** (Peter Speck, *Being There*)

308

Some common worries of those visiting the sick include:

- What will I see in the hospital or hospice?
- What will I say?
- How can I help?
- What should I take?
- Will I catch anything?
- How long should I stay?
- How often should I go?
- What if other visitors arrive?
- What if I get upset?
- What if I feel embarrassed?
- What if I say the wrong thing?

The **ideal visitor** makes the patient feel more loved, more supported and more in touch with the outside world. He listens, helps with practical things (without making a fuss), and understands that illness can make you tired and irritable.

Too many visitors is a common problem, particularly for the terminally ill. (Do not make assumptions about how many visitors a patient wants. Discuss it.) It is often a dilemma for patients, wanting the support and yet finding constant visitors exhausting. Families can delegate one person to organize a schedule of visitors. The patient can then feel supported without being overwhelmed. Professional carers can assist patient and family by constructing boundaries. It is easier to say "The doctor and nurse have said visitors must only stay five minutes now ", rather than "You're tiring her out with all this visiting."

Relations with professional staff can become tense if communication among staff and visitors is neglected. Visitors are often frightened of procedures or equipment and often feel very inadequate, or "in the way". Family visitors may also feel guilty. ("We wanted to cope at home but we couldn't.") They may feel resentful if their own expertise and hard work in nursing the patient at home is simply ignored or not acknowledged.

Children should be encouraged to visit the sick and the dying. However, children have short concentration spans, so provision needs to be made for them to play for some of the time, if they visit for more than a few minutes.

Long-term visitors to a nursing home, hospital or hospice can become part of the establishment. Visiting becomes a major part of their life. If the patient dies they may need to continue the relationship with the caring team for a time. Many hospices make provision for this. (*see Grief*)

VISUALIZATION

Visualization (or guided imagery) is the regular practice of creating mental images of a desired outcome, for example, shrinkage of cancer cells.

Visualization is a technique developed from motivational psychology. It is used to help patients participate in maintaining their own health. It is most effective when it is repeated 2 to 3 times a day, combined with relaxation therapy and a program of exercise and healthy diet.

The aim is to **visualize the desired outcome**, not what is happening at the time. Therefore, even if the cancer is spreading, visualization can still be used to create positive attitudes.

Visual imagery is best used as part of an active program to improve physical, mental and emotional health. If stress can suppress the immune system (and there is some evidence that it can), these techniques are a logical adjunct for patients who want to fight their disease.

Active participation in treatment and mobilization of inner resources increases a person's **sense of control** and reduces the sense of helplessness that can cause depression. Many practitioners are convinced that these methods prolong survival and improve quality of life.

Effective visual imagery should symbolize:
- Cancer cells as weak and confused
- Treatment as powerful
- Normal cells as strong
- White blood cells as numerous
- White blood cells as vigorous and aggressive
- Dead cancer cells flushed away
- The body free of cancer cells

Patients' drawings of visual symbols can sometimes reveal unhelpful attitudes to the disease (for example, if cancer cells are drawn as large and powerful, or white cells as small and weak, or radiotherapy as dangerous instead of helpful). Discussing the drawings with the patient can be a useful way of changing negative attitudes to disease.

Mental imagery can be used to:

- Boost confidence in medical treatment
- Reduce pain
- Achieve goals
- Explore feelings and attitudes
- Overcome resentments

WEAKNESS

Management options:

- Consider causes
- Consider trial of antibiotics (rarely indicated)
- Consider trial of steroids
- Physical therapy
- Discuss adjustment in lifestyle

Possible causes — Almost all patients with advanced cancer complain of generalized weakness. Sudden onset suggests a neurological deficit. Sudden generalized weakness may be due to adrenal failure or septicemia and a trial of steroids and antibiotics may occasionally be indicated. The fever of bacteremia may be masked if the patient is already on steroids.

Exclude hypokalemia (due to diuretics or steroids — or rarely ectopic ACTH from a small (oat) cell carcinoma of the bronchus which can be helped by metyrapone 500mg every 4 hours) as a cause of weakness. Stop any unnecessary hypotensive drugs.

★ **There is no drug that restores strength. Blood transfusions do not help.**

Discussion — The complaint of "I feel so weak " may really mean "I feel so dependent " or "I feel bored " or "Am I dying?" It is helpful to explain that although strength is going to be limited, it fluctuates, and a resting day reserves some energy for the next day. Steroids (dexamethasone 4mg per day) do not improve strength, but can induce a feeling of well-being.

Physical therapy — Exercise seems the natural antidote to weakness and 50% of hospice patients can benefit from physical therapy. Weakness is sometimes due to prolonged bed rest. Mobility and independence can often be improved once symptoms are controlled and the patient regains confidence. Even small improvements boost morale. The physical therapist, working as a team with an occupational therapist and a recreation therapist, can also give invaluable advice about aids and adaptations to make the most of remaining strength and can teach the family how to lift and move the patient. The family home may need such minor modifications as non-slip mats, handrails, raised toilet seat or commode, walking frame, etc. (see *Occupational Therapy, Physical Therapy, Rehabilitation*)

WEIGHT LOSS

Weight loss occurs in almost all patients with advanced cancer. At any stage in the disease weight loss suggests a worsened prognosis. Gross wasting (cachexia) occurs in about 20% of patients.

Management options:

- Treat anorexia
- Nutritional supplementation
- Explanation about diet
- Readjust dentures
- Consider clothing alterations
- Counsel about body image, pressure areas

Discussion — Both the patient and family may feel guilty about poor food intake. It needs explaining that weight loss is not simply due to poor diet. Intensive intravenous feeding often fails to promote weight gain and does not increase survival.

Nevertheless it is worthwhile trying to improve dietary intake for psychological reasons and also in the hope that weight loss may be slowed down. Aim to improve appetite and add oral supplements to attain a positive energy and protein balance. The average sedentary individual needs 1,500 calories per day. There is no evidence that supplementary feeding "feeds the tumor" or increases tumor growth. (see *Anorexia, Diet, Nutrition*)

In advanced disease weight loss is inevitable and weight no longer has diagnostic usefulness, so **avoid routine weighing** which can be demoralizing.

The **previous body image** is lost and some patients find it frightening to feel they no longer recognize their own bodies. Old photographs are sometimes helpful to "explain" to new carers how the person thinks of himself. New clothes that fit are a boost to morale and recent photographs of the patient with his family can emphasize that there is still a place and a role for this "new person". (*see Body Image*)

Weight loss usually slows as the disease progresses and it can be helpful to explain this.

Loose dentures are a common problem. Dental relining is simple, restores chewing and improves facial appearances. Eyeglasses tend to get too loose, and need to be tightened to be worn comfortably.

NOTES

NOTES

NOTES

COMMON CANCERS
Summary Information

*These summaries provide
brief background information only,
and are not intended as
definitive statements.*

CANCER STATISTICS

In 1989, about 1,510,000 people in the U.S.A. will be diagnosed as having cancer. There will be an estimated 502,000 deaths from cancer in the U.S.A. in 1989.

The table below shows expected deaths from each site or type of cancer, and may help to give perspective to the incidence of some of the cancers you may encounter. (This data is taken from the American Cancer Society's *Cancer Facts & Figures - 1989*.)

Lung	142,000
Colon & Rectum	61,000
Breast	43,000
Prostate	28,500
Pancreas	25,000
Leukemia	18,000
Non-Hodgkin's Lymphomas	17,300
Stomach	13,900
Ovary	12,000
Liver	11,400
Brain/Central Nervous System	11,400
Bladder	10,200
Kidney	10,000
Esophagus	9,400
Oropharynx	8,650
Multiple Myeloma	8,600
Cervix	6,000
Melanoma	6,000
Endometrium	4,000
Larynx	3,700
Connective Tissue	3,000
Hodgkin's Disease	1,500
Thyroid	1,025
Testis	350
Other and unspecified sites	46,075

BLADDER CANCER

Background information — 90% of bladder cancers are transitional cell carcinomas. 10% are squamous cell carcinomas. (Bilharzia infestation is a common cause worldwide of squamous carcinoma of the bladder.) 20% are multiple carcinomas, arising most commonly on the posterior wall in the region of the ureteric orifices.

Bladder cancer is usually seen in patients over the age of 50. It has been associated with certain occupations (notably in the chemical, rubber and cable industries) because of exposure to urothelial carcinogens (especially napthylamine and benzidine). Between 30% to 40% of cases of bladder cancer have been attributed to smoking.

The typical presentation is painless hematuria in an elderly male, but dysuria and supra-pubic pain can also occur. Tumors tend to be multicentric and often start as superficial papillomas. The speed of progression is very varied. Some tumors remain confined to the bladder mucosa for years, while others spread to lymph nodes within months. Tumors that infiltrate the muscle wall of the bladder usually spread to lymph nodes (obturator, iliac, para-aortic) and eventually to blood (with metastases to lung, liver and bone). Peritoneal spread (and ascites) can occur in advanced cases.

Assessment involves cystoscopy and examination under anesthetic to judge the degree of local spread. CT scan is useful to assess spread outside the bladder and plan radiotherapy.

Stage	Spread	Treatment	Approximate % 5-year survival
1	Mucosal	Diathermy, plus intravesical chemotherapy	90
2	Superficial muscle	Partial cystectomy or radical radiotherapy	50
3	Deep muscle	Total cystectomy and ileal conduit, or radical radiotherapy	20
4	Pelvic spread	Palliative radiotherapy (chemotherapy)	—

Note that histology as well as stage of spread affects prognosis. High grade (poorly differentiated) tumors are more likely to become invasive.

Treatment — Superficial papillomas are treated by endoscopic resection.

Intravesical chemotherapy is given after resection of the tumor if it is large, multiple, high grade or recurs within three months, or if random bladder biopsies show carcinoma-in-situ (or if the patient is a smoker). A variety of agents, including thiotepa, doxorubicin and mitomycin, are known to reduce the rate of recurrence.

Stage 2 tumors can be treated by partial cystectomy if the lesion is small and in a mobile part of the bladder, and where a bladder capacity of at least 300ml can be retained. Radiotherapy can be external or by interstitial radium implants.

Stage 3 tumors (with invasion of the muscle wall) are usually treated by radiotherapy (6,000cGy over 6 weeks using megavoltage equipment and a 3 field technique) with salvage cystectomy for the failures.

Recurrent disease occurs in 50% of patients eventually, and in 30% of patients within three months. Treatment is with diathermy resection, intravesical chemotherapy or laser resection. Repeated recurrence may be an indication for total cystectomy. Following cystectomy the patient has an ileal conduit (a segment of ileum which is resected then isolated, still attached to its own blood supply, and brought out as an abdominal stoma, and the ureters are implanted into it). Alternatively the ureters can be implanted into the sigmoid colon. Overall survival is around 60%, but once the disease has invaded the muscle wall, only 30% survive 5 years.

Advanced tumors (Stage 4) with fixation to pelvic structures, rectum or vagina, have a poor prognosis whatever the treatment. They are usually treated with palliative radiotherapy — usually 3,500cGy over 10 days. This will control the hematuria in 50% of patients, and can be repeated if necessary if hematuria recurs. In patients who already have severely reduced bladder capacity, radiotherapy can worsen urinary frequency.

Problems in advanced disease:

1. Pain
2. Frequency and dysuria
3. Bladder spasms

4. Bladder hemorrhage
5. Ureteric obstruction
6. Radiation bowel damage
7. Leg lymphedema
8. Bone pain due to metastases

1. **Pain can be of several types:**
- Continuous visceral pain
- Bladder spasms
- Nerve infiltration pain
- Dysuria
- Bone pain
- Ache in heavy lymphedematous leg

Nerve infiltration pain is difficult to treat and may require a number of approaches. (*see Nerve Pain, Pelvic Pain*)

2. **Frequency and dysuria** are common complications of treatment. Urinary frequency can be very distressing, particularly for the 6 to 8 weeks following radiotherapy (proctitis and tenesmus can also occur). It can be particularly severe in a patient who already has a reduced bladder capacity. It is important to exclude infection. Dysuria may be reduced by potassium citrate 10ml 4 times a day, sodium bicarbonate 2g to 4g per day, or phenazopyridine 200mg 4 times a day. An in-dwelling urinary catheter usually causes unacceptable discomfort. High dose steroids have little effect.

3. **Bladder spasms** cause episodic supra-pubic pain and urinary urgency. Morphine is not usually helpful. Oxybutynin is a powerful anti-spasmodic with local anesthetic properties, and 5mg to 10mg 3 times a day can be very effective in reducing bladder spasms. Anti-cholinergic side effects (particularly a dry mouth) can be severe. (*see Bladder Spasms*)

4. Massive recurrent **bladder hemorrhage** can occur as a late complication of radiotherapy (10%) or due to tumor recurrence. Treatment is difficult.

Options include:
- Bladder instillation with alum
- Cystoscopic diathermy (or laser)
- Hydrostatic bladder distention

- Urinary diversion
- Cystectomy
- Arterial embolization of the bladder

Irrigation with **1% alum solution** is usually the best option, and does not require a preliminary washout or anesthesia. Continuous irrigation via a 2-way catheter is necessary and the bleeding usually stops in 1 to 4 days. Alum works by precipitating protein on the mucosal surface and causing constriction of the mucosal capillaries. It is painless and non-toxic and can effectively control bleeding.

Diathermy (via cystoscope) can control small bleeding points (but may sometimes worsen bleeding). Simple removal of clots is sometimes enough to stop the bleeding. **Laser** therapy may be useful. (see Lasers)

Bladder distention uses a large balloon catheter to distend the bladder to above diastolic blood pressure for several hours under epidural anesthesia. It is a good treatment for post-irradiation hemorrhage and is usually successful. There is a small risk of perforation.

Cystectomy is a final option but should only be considered if the patient has a good prognosis.

5. **Ureteric obstruction** usually suggests a poor prognosis, and is correctly left untreated in the advanced stages of disease. In a relatively fit patient a ureteric stent may be considered. (see Ureteric Obstruction)

6. **Radiation damage** can cause hematuria due to telangiectasis, a contracted bladder, fibrosis of the terminal ileum (sometimes causing intestinal obstruction) and damage to the sigmoid colon (with stricture formation of telangiectasia and bleeding).

7. **Lymphedema** can occur in one or both legs due to damage to pelvic lymphatics. Compression therapy may be beneficial. (see Lymphedema)

8. **Bone metastases** can occur and may require treatment with radiotherapy or other measures. Metastases can also occur to liver and lung but these are late features of the disease and rarely cause significant symptoms. (see Bone Pain)

BRAIN CANCER

Background information — Primary malignant tumors of the brain do not arise from neurons (which cannot divide) but from supporting glial cells (gliomas).

In children, primary brain tumors are the second most common malignancies. The commonest brain tumors in children and young adults are medulloblastomas, craniopharyngiomas and ependymomas. Brain stem tumors (which are rare) are mainly encountered in children.

Medulloblastomas usually occur in the posterior fossa and present with cerebellar features or raised intracranial pressure. Craniopharyngiomas are slow-growing and often calcified, and can cause pituitary or hypothalamic damage. Ependymomas are derived from cells lining the CNS cavities, and the tumor spreads by direction invasion and also via CSF.

In adults, the majority of gliomas are astrocytomas. (5% are oligodendromas, which are slow growing.)

The peak age for astrocytomas is 50 to 60. They tend to be diffuse and infiltrating (and can occasionally cross the midline). Primary brain malignancies do not metastasize to the rest of the body (except when a ventriculo-peritoneal shunt has been inserted, and distant metastases, particularly to bone, can occur). 95% occur in the cerebral hemispheres or basal ganglia. 20% are low grade (Grades 1 and 2), and 80% are high grade (Grades 3 and 4). Very aggressive high grade astrocytomas are called glioblastomas.

Astrocytomas are **graded** on both histological and cytological changes. Grades 1 and 2 are relatively benign (and are associated with a long preoperative history). 30% of patients will survive for 5 years. Grades 3 and 4 have a poor prognosis. Only 10% survive longer than a year, and most patients die within 6 to 12 months of diagnosis.

Malignant brain tumors present with:

- Seizures
- Raised intracranial pressure (headache, vomiting)
- Focal brain damage (arm, leg, speech, vision, continence)
- Impaired higher functions (intellect, behavior, emotions)

Even large tumors may cause minimal symptoms. The interval between first symptoms and diagnosis is usually 3 to 9 months (although it can sometimes be several years if seizures are the first symptom).

Mode of presentation is noteworthy because in the terminal phase the same problems tend to recur. The high grade tumors tend to cause neurological damage. This correlates with poor survival. If signs of damage can be reversed with high dose dexamethasone then neuron damage is not yet permanent, and treatment with radiotherapy may still be appropriate. Severe disabilities (due to irreversible brain damage) are usually taken to be a contraindication to treatment.

Diagnosis is by CT scan, but CT scan cannot accurately predict the grade of tumor. Biopsy is important whenever possible, because low grade tumors can occasionally mimic a brain infarct on a CT scan, and high grade tumors can cavitate and mimic an abscess. Patients who present with seizures or raised intracranial pressure usually have a better response to treatment than patients with prominent focal signs.

Treatment — Surgery in adults with malignant brain tumors is always palliative.

Options include:

- Burr-hole biopsy
- External decompression and biopsy
- Subtotal resection
- Total resection

Burr-hole biopsy is all that can be offered for deep-seated tumors or tumors involving the dominant parietal lobe (controlling speech). With very deep tumors (thalamus, brain stem) even a biopsy may risk brain damage.

Surgical resection can prolong survival by several months for high grade tumors, and delays a recurrence of symptoms. Few surviving patients have their condition worsened by surgery.

A **shunt** (usually ventriculo-peritoneal) can be used to decompress the lateral ventricles if a deep midline (non-resectable) tumor causes obstructive hydrocephalus.

Radiotherapy prolongs survival in virtually all patients, particularly those with Grade 1 and 2 tumors. Low grade tumors have a better prognosis (particularly with no focal neurological signs), and around 30% of patients survive 5 years, and 20% survive 10 years. These patients tend to be given radiotherapy treatment over a longer period (for example, 6,000cGy over 16 weeks) to prevent the late side-effects of brain irradiation (dementia).

In patients with high grade tumors (Grades 3 and 4) the prognosis (even after treatment) is poor. Only 10% survive 1 year. Most of this group are given 3,000cGy in 8 fractions.

Radiotherapy treatment requires generous margins (because the tumors infiltrate diffusely) but "whole brain" radiotherapy treatments are rarely needed.

Advanced disability is usually taken as a contraindication to treatment, but reversible causes of neurological damage must be excluded, such as:

- Blocked shunt
- Inadvertent stopping of dexamethasone
- Post-ictal paralysis
- Hematoma from burr-hole biopsy
- Internal hydrocephalus due to a reversible "kink" in 4th ventricle

Chemotherapy is presently of little value (most cytotoxic drugs do not cross the blood-brain barrier) but can produce a response in a minority of patients.

Problems of advanced disease — As the tumor re-grows it tends to cause the same problems that the patient experienced at presentation. Further attempts at surgical debulking are occasionally possible (if the tumor is in the non-dominant parietal or temporal lobe).

Particular problems include:

- Hemiparesis
- Speech difficulties
- Hemianopsia
- Urinary incontinence
- Seizures (may be focal)
- Impaired intellect
- Personality changes
- Confusion
- Headaches (rarely)

The general pattern is usually one of a **gradual decrease in function**, a blunting of emotions and increasing dependency. The principle is to anticipate needs, and to order aids and appliances so they are available when needed. Teamwork among professionals and family carers is essential. A home assessment by an occupational therapist can be invaluable in enabling some or all of the care to take place at home. A physiotherapist should teach family carers how to lift, move and transfer the patient. The strain on carers can be considerable, and brief in-patient respite admissions can be helpful.

A **speech therapist** can provide helpful advice about maintaining optimum communication. Lip and tongue apraxia causes slow, deliberate speech. Understanding may be intact (newspaper, magazines and TV may still be enjoyed) even when speech is dysphasic (expressive dysphasia). In receptive dysphasia (sometimes associated with hemianopsia and loss of position sense) simple conversation may still be understood, though levels of understanding and speech ability often fluctuate. The carers need to know about the patient's background, occupation, interests and hobbies in order to maintain the best possible contact.

Hemianopsia (loss of peripheral vision on one side) can be frightening. The patient can be reassured he will not go blind (a common fear). Carers need to remember from which side to approach the patient.

Urinary incontinence (which may be due to frontal lobe damage) is usually best managed by an indwelling catheter. (see *Urinary Incontinence*)

Focal **seizures** (when the patient remains conscious) are more distressing than generalized seizures. Common (unwarranted) fears are that seizures increase brain damage, or the patient may die from a seizure. (see *Seizures*)

Confusion is common as the disease progresses. It is minimized by maintaining a familiar environment. Agitated confusion may be due to pain (impacted feces, pressure areas, urinary retention, headaches, dyspepsia). Having excluded causes of agitation, haloperidol (usual starting dose 5mg 2 times a day) can be a useful drug. (see *Confusion*)

Headaches are surprisingly rare with advanced gliomas and usually respond to acetaminophen 1g every 4 hours. Severe headaches can be reduced by carefully titrated doses of morphine. The patient is usually taking (or has taken) steroids, and increasing the dose may be indicated.

BREAST CANCER

Background information — One in 12 women develop breast cancer. The risk is increased 3 times if there is a family history in first-degree relatives.

The great majority of breast cancers are poorly differentiated adenocarcinomas (from glandular epithelium lining the ducts). The wide variety of histological appearances (polygonal, scirrhous, comedo, mucinous or colloid) have little bearing on prognosis.

The important exceptions are:

- Medullary - slow growing (80% of patients survive 5 years)
- Inflammatory - rapid and aggressive
- Lobular - non-invasive (in situ disease)

Prognosis is better if the tumor is well-differentiated or estrogen-receptor positive.

Most present as a lump in the breast, but occasionally as pain, discharge or bleeding from the nipple, inversion of the nipple or a lump in the axilla. **Screening** of the female population (using mammography and aspiration of cysts) has reduced the death rate from breast cancer in some countries. It is expensive.

Diagnosis is based on percutaneous or excision biopsy. Before mastectomy is contemplated investigations should be performed to ensure no patient with obvious metastases is subjected to unnecessary mastectomy.

Treatment of the breast cancer depends upon the stage of disease.

Stage	Spread	Treatment	Approximate % 5-year survival
1	Breast	Surgery and radiotherapy	80
2	Axillary nodes	Surgery and radiotherapy	40
3	Locally advanced	Radiotherapy	15
4	Metastases	Hormones or chemotherapy	10

For many years the mainstay of treatment was Halsted's radical mastectomy, (a disfiguring operation with a high incidence of post-operative lymphedema of the arm). This reduced the incidence of local recurrence to 40%, but had no effect on distant metastases and no effect on long-term survival. (70% of patients have recurrent disease after 20 years.) Less mutilating operations are now performed to control local disease, since survival does not depend solely on the extent of the surgery.

These procedures all have similar survival statistics and include:

- Extended simple mastectomy (axillary nodes excised)
- Simple mastectomy (with radiotherapy to nodes)
- Lumpectomy (with radiotherapy to nodes)

Other forms of conservative treatment are under investigation (for example, lumpectomy followed by short-term iridium-192 implants).

Post-mastectomy patients should be promptly fitted with a suitable prosthesis by a well-trained professional aware of the physical and psychological consequences of such surgery. The option of breast reconstruction surgery should be offered as appropriate.

If **axillary nodes are involved (Stage 2)**, many surgeons advise post-operative radiotherapy which in one study reduced local recurrence from 30% to 10%.

Surgery and radiotherapy combined can damage axillary lymphatics and will cause some degree of edema of the arm in 30% of patients. Fibrosis of the chest wall and radiation pneumonitis can also occur.

Adjuvant chemotherapy or hormone therapy is frequently given if the axillary nodes are involved, because the majority of these patients will develop recurrence at distant sites and therefore must have had micro-metastases at the time of presentation. Adjuvant polychemotherapy (given for 4 to 6 months) to women under 50 with early (node-negative) disease reduces the 5-year mortality. Adjuvant tamoxifen can reduce 5-year mortality in women of 50 or over.

Locally advanced disease (Stage 3) can be treated with radiotherapy. Good control of fungating disease can be obtained over three or four weeks. Even in the presence of metastatic disease, the quality of life can be much improved by keeping the local disease under control.

After apparently successful surgery for breast cancer, 60% of patients will develop **metastases (Stage 4)** within 5 years, although 3% of patients present with metastases over 10 years later. Once there are metastases, only 10% of patients will survive 5 years. Median survival after recurrence has doubled in recent years to about 3 years, due to better hormone therapy, chemotherapy, and better supportive care.

45% of patients respond to hormone therapy:

- Oophorectomy (if pre-menopausal)
- Tamoxifen
- Aminoglutethimide
- Progestogens

It usually takes about 6 weeks for a response to occur to hormone therapy (chest wall disease, and metastases in lung, bone and liver can all regress). Median survival is 3 years after a response. (A response means lesions regress or the disease becomes static. In 10% of patients lesions disappear and median survival is then over 5 years after the response.)

Hormone therapy is more likely to be effective if:

- There is a lengthy disease-free interval
- The patient is over 60
- There has been previous response to hormones
- Tumor is receptor-positive
- There is non-visceral spread

Hormone therapy is more effective for local disease than for visceral metastases. Many patients who have a response to tamoxifen go on to have a further response to second-line treatment with aminoglutethimide or progestogens. Hormone receptor assay can be a useful predictor of response. 75% of tumors with both estrogen and progesterone receptors will respond to treatment (while only 10% of receptor-negative tumors respond). On occasion, irregular vaginal bleeding may occur.

Tamoxifen 20mg per day is the agent of first choice for most post-menopausal women. (Oophorectomy is preferred for pre-menopausal women.) Side effects are few, but nausea and fluid retention occasionally occur. A "flare" reaction (bone pain and hypercalcemia) can occur during the first 4 weeks of treatment, requiring analgesics and/or steroids. Treatment should be continued because the reaction indicates a good chance of a response. Tamoxifen is an anti-estrogen. It binds to estrogen receptors on the cells, preventing estrogen from promoting growth.

Aminoglutethimide 250mg 4 times a day is the agent of first choice for bone disease secondary to breast cancer in post-menopausal women. It causes a "medical adrenalectomy" inhibiting estrogen production in the adrenals. Steroid replacement with hydrocortisone 200 mg 2 times a day is necessary. 25% of patients develop a rash about the 10th day, but the drug should not be stopped since this reaction is almost always self-limiting. About 10% of patients get some nausea or dizziness.

Medroxyprogesterone acetate 500 mg 2 times a day, or megestrol acetate 80 mg 2 times a day can both be effective hormone treatments. Weight gain can be a problem (and occasionally hypertension and glycosuria can occur).

60% of breast tumors respond to **chemotherapy**, but the duration of response (around 9 to 12 months) is shorter than for hormone therapy.

Chemotherapy tends to be given after failure of hormone therapy, or as a first treatment in patients with rapidly progressive or life-threatening disease (for example, lymphangitis carcinomatosa). Several studies have shown that it is not detrimental to patients' survival to reserve chemotherapy until hormone therapy has failed. When both treatments are given together the response rate is higher, but survival is not improved.

As with hormone therapy, the highest response is seen in disease of the chest wall and regional lymph nodes. Good response can occur in bone and lung metastases. The response rate for liver disease is low, although occasional good results are seen. Chemotherapy is generally ineffective for brain metastases.

The decision to treat with chemotherapy can be difficult. If hormone receptor assays show the tumor to be receptor-negative a response to hormone therapy will be seen in only 10% of patients. Even elderly women can occasionally tolerate chemotherapy well, and can have prolonged remissions.

Problems of advanced disease:

- Chest wall fungation (see *Fungating Tumors*)
- Lymph node enlargement (see *Lymph Node Metastases*)
- Bone metastases (see *Bone Pain, Fractures*)
- Hepatomegaly (see *Liver Pain*)
- Lung infiltration (see *Lung Metastases*)
- Pleural effusion (see *Pleural Effusion*)
- Brain metastases (see *Brain Metastases*)
- Lymphedema of the arm (see *Lymphedema*)
- Ascites (see *Ascites*)
- Hypercalcemia (see *Hypercalcemia*)
- Cranial nerve palsies (see *Skull Metastases*)

CERVICAL CANCER

Background information — The disease seems to correlate with sexual intercourse, and the peak age of onset is falling, possibly due to changes in social and sexual habits. Recent interest has focused on herpes genitalis virus type 2 (HSV-2) which is found in the epithelial cells of most patients with cervical cancer but in only 2% of normal epithelial cells. 95% of cervical cancers are squamous, 5% are adenocarcinomas (which tend to spread into the uterus).

The classic presentation is post-coital bleeding. There is often vaginal discharge. Pain or urinary symptoms suggest an advanced lesion.

Efficient screening should be able to greatly reduce the incidence of the disease. Cervical (Papanicolaou) smears can detect pre-cancerous dysplasia. Colposcopy allows local treatment (laser or cryosurgery) and follow-up. If dysplasia is left untreated for several years 30% to 40% progress to invasive cancer.

Accurate evaluation involves examination under anesthetic (to allow deep palpation), curettage, intravenous urograms, chest x-rays, and assessment of pelvic nodes (by lymphangiogram or CT scan). Lymph nodes may be routinely treated (by surgery or radiotherapy) even in the absence of firm evidence of involvement.

Stage	Spread	Treatment	Approximate % 5-year survival
1	Cervix	Surgery or radiotherapy	90
2	Beyond cervix, but not to pelvic wall	Radiotherapy	50
3	To pelvic wall, lower 1/3 of vagina, hydronephrosis	Radiotherapy	30
4	To bladder, rectum, or distant sites	Chemotherapy	—

Note that in this disease 5 year survival almost always means cure, because recurrence is very rare after 5 years.

The disease spreads locally to the vagina, laterally to the pelvic side-walls and in lymphatics to para-cervical, pelvic (obturator, iliac and lateral sacral) and para-aortic nodes. Blood-borne metastases (lung, liver, bone) occur late (but can be an earlier feature of the more aggressive form of disease seen in younger women).

Treatment depends upon staging. Radiotherapy is the treatment of choice for Stages 1, 2 or 3 in most centers, although for Stage 1 disease surgery is equally effective. A radical (Wertheim's) hysterectomy includes pelvic lymphadenectomy (20% have involved nodes). Surgery has a number of advantages (the extent of spread is defined, ovaries can be conserved, and there are fewer late complications) although there is a risk of damage to the ureters. Surgery is the treatment of choice for adenocarcinomas.

Radiotherapy can cure patients, including those with advanced disease (50% of Stage 2 and 30% of Stage 3 patients can be cured). Both internal radiotherapy (to treat the cervix) and external beam radiotherapy (to treat pelvic nodes) are used. External radiotherapy can control pain, hemorrhage and discharge.

Early complications of radiotherapy include:

- Infertility (menstrual periods stop)
- Diarrhea (towards the end of treatment)
- Vaginal stenosis

Vaginal stenosis is preventable by regular intercourse or the use of dilators. Hormone replacement therapy is required for younger patients. Sexual counseling (particularly concerning feelings of guilt or fear of damage) is important before and after treatment.

Recurrent disease in pelvic lymph nodes typically causes:

- Leg pain (nerve infiltration)
- Leg swelling (lymphedema)
- Urinary frequency
- Hydronephrosis

The best method of diagnosing recurrence is a CT scan. A pelvic mass may not be palpable.

Recurrence after surgery can be treated and sometimes cured by radiotherapy. Recurrence after radiotherapy (with no evidence of distant metastases) can sometimes be treated with pelvic exenteration (removal of pelvic contents including bladder and rectum) but this procedure has a high mortality and leaves the patient with both colostomy and ileostomy.

Chemotherapy is very disappointing. Treatment with single agents such as methotrexate can sometimes produce a temporary response and may occasionally reduce pain in advanced disease.

Problems in advanced disease:

- Diagnosis (radiation damage or recurrence?)
- Pain
- Discharge
- Ureteric obstruction
- Leg lymphedema
- Fistula
- Hypercalcemia
- Psychological problems

Distinguishing between recurrent tumor or radiotherapy damage can be difficult.

Late complications of radiotherapy include:

- Ulcerated anterior rectum (pseudo-carcinoma)
- Rectovaginal fistula
- Vesicovaginal fistula
- Small bowel stenosis and obstruction

These complications can require colostomy, ureteric transplant or small bowel resection and anastomosis (and in some patients all three operations become necessary). When these problems first arise recurrent cancer is usually blamed. As time passes and the patient's condition remains stable, the true cause of the damage becomes apparent. Even CT scan and guided biopsy of suspicious areas is often unhelpful because radiotherapy distorts normal tissue architecture, and because the malignant area may be missed.

Pelvic pain has several components:

- Uterine (supra-pubic and back pain)
- Pelvic floor (perineal pain)
- Posterior infiltration (sacral pain)
- Lumbo-sacral plexus infiltration (buttock and leg pain)

The continuous visceral component of pain usually responds well to morphine, but the nerve pain can be difficult to control. (*see Nerve Pain, Pelvic Pain*)

Vaginal discharge can be profuse, foul-smelling and sometimes bloodstained. The best management is regular irrigation and douching and regular change of absorbent pads. Oral metronidazole 250mg 3 times a day can reduce smell.

Even unilateral **ureteric obstruction** is a bad prognostic sign, and suggests a prognosis of only 1 to 2 years. In a patient with advanced disease it is important not to exchange a peaceful death from uremia for prolonged suffering from pain and discharge. (*see Ureteric Obstruction*)

Surgical diversionary procedures are justified if:

- Prognosis seems reasonable (3 months or more of active life)
- Further treatment is possible
- Benign radiation stricture cannot be excluded

Unilateral **lymphedema** is a common feature of recurrent carcinoma of the cervix. As the disease progresses it can become bilateral. It is due to damaged pelvic lymphatics. If the patient has already received radical radiotherapy further radiotherapy is not possible. If the patient presented with advanced disease, radiotherapy may shrink the tumor enough to improve lymphatic circulation, but it is rarely completely effective.

The leg can be reduced in size by a program of exercise, massage and compression therapy. This is always worthwhile. Even if the reduction in size is not marked, it usually improves morale considerably to receive treatment. Avoid diuretics. If the leg is also painful (often due to nerve pain radiating into the leg) pain control takes priority over compression therapy. The patient may need considerable psychological support to adjust to the disability and disfigurement. (*see Lymphedema*)

Rectovaginal and vesicovaginal fistulas can occur, with feces and/or urine passing out of the vagina. Urinary diversion and/or colostomy is justified in patients with a reasonable prognosis to manage this distressing symptom. It can be due to radiation damage and not recurrent disease. Where bypass is not possible, the problems include mess, guilt, smell and social isolation. Regular gentle irrigation and douching help to clean the area and reduce the volume of discharge. Absorbent dressings should be changed frequently. An indwelling catheter may reduce the urinary leak. Careful explanation helps to reduce guilt and misery. Oral metronidazole 250mg 3 times a day, deodorant dressings and air purifiers help reduce smell. (*see Fistulas, Smells*)

Hypercalcemia in gynecological malignancy (where bone metastases are rare) was first reported in 1956. It is associated with squamous carcinomas and can occur in about 5% of patients with advanced carcinoma of the cervix. (*see Hypercalcemia*)

Patients with cancer of the cervix may have psychological problems adjusting to the disease because it is:

- Linked with sexual intercourse
- Preventable by screening

Guilt, anger and communication problems are common reactions in all patients, but in this situation they may relate especially to these particular issues.

COLON CANCER

Background information — No definite cause of colon cancer is known. It is rare in developing countries, and low fiber diet has been suggested as a possible cause (because of longer fecal transit time allowing more contact with possible toxins in feces).

Three conditions predispose to colon cancer:

- Familial polyposis
- Longstanding ulcerative colitis
- Villous adenomas

(These persons should be regularly screened by colonoscopy.)

Large bowel tumors are usually adenocarcinomas. The rectum (50%), sigmoid colon (20%) and ascending colon (15%) are the most common sites.

The classic **presentation** is altered bowel habits with blood and mucous in the stools. Fewer than 10% of patients have a palpable abdominal mass. Lesions in the right side of the colon rarely obstruct and tend to present with anemia and weight loss. Lesions in the left side can obstruct (causing colicky pains) or perforate. (Rectal tumors cause tenesmus.)

Investigations include sigmoidoscopy (75% of tumors can be located) and barium enema. 10% of cancers can be missed on barium enema, so if symptoms persist a colonoscopy is indicated.

Prognosis relates to the Dukes classification (1932) of degree of infiltration through the bowel wall:

Stage	Spread	Approximate % 5-year survival
A	Limited to mucosa	90
B	Penetrating mucosa	60
C	Spread to lymph nodes	25
D	Metastases	—

Treatment — Surgery is the mainstay of treatment. The segment of bowel containing the tumor is resected (together with lymph nodes draining it) and the bowel is sutured together (restoring normal bowel function). Colon cancer can involve adjacent bowel, stomach or abdominal wall without distant spread to lymph nodes (still Stage B, therefore), and cure may still be possible by multiple organ resection. There is no evidence to support the use of adjuvant chemotherapy.

Obstruction or perforation may be managed by a **defunctioning colostomy** to improve the patient's condition prior to attempting removal of the tumor. The colostomy can be reversed later. (*see Colostomy Care*)

Early treatment of recurrence may improve prognosis. If disease is localized with no evidence of metastases a second-look laparotomy with a view to resection should be considered. If recurrent disease is extensive and inoperable local radiotherapy can sometimes reduce symptoms.

Colorectal cancer spreads directly into surrounding structures, and metastases occur to lymph nodes (mesenteric then retroperitoneal), and via the blood to liver (and less commonly to bone, lung and brain).

Even in patients with liver or peritoneal metastases surgical removal of the tumor may offer the best means of palliation. Some surgeons recommend radical bowel resection if the patient has only a solitary hepatic metastasis which is simultaneously resected. (*see Liver Metastases*)

In advanced metastatic disease systemic fluorouracil can produce a response (for example, the resolution of ascites) in about 20% of patients, but survival is not improved. If multiple metastases are confined to the liver, intrahepatic chemotherapy (using an implantable infusion pump) has so far shown results little better than the 20% response rate shown for IV chemotherapy.

Problems in advanced disease:

- Pain

- Ascites (*see Ascites*)

- Intestinal obstruction (*see Intestinal Obstruction*)

- Problems with colostomy (*see Colostomy Care*)

Pain is visceral and usually responds completely to a correctly titrated dose of morphine. (*see Liver Metastases, Liver Pain, Morphine, Rectal Cancer*)

ENDOMETRIAL CANCER

Background information — The majority of endometrial tumors are well-differentiated adenocarcinomas. It is most common in women aged 50 to 70. Late menopause is a known risk factor. Hormone therapy with estrogens (without progesterones) can cause endometrial hyperplasia which may predispose to cancer.

Post-menopausal bleeding is the classic presentation, but 20% of endometrial cancers occur in pre-menopausal women and present as inter-menstrual bleeding. Pain or discharge suggests advanced disease. Diagnosis is made by curettage.

Prognosis is usually good since the tumor is slow-growing and presents early. The 5 year survival after treatment is 75% (or 60% following treatment with radiotherapy alone). The rarer tumors (adenosquamous or sarcomas) have a poorer prognosis and only 20% of patients survive 5 years.

Treatment is by total abdominal hysterectomy and bilateral salpingo-oophorectomy. Post-operative radiotherapy (usually 5,000cGy over 5 weeks) can be given for poorly differentiated tumors, or if there is invasion of the myometrium (when the risk of node metastases is around 30%).

Vaginal recurrence, usually seen in previously un-irradiated patients, responds to local radiotherapy using intra-vaginal cesium, or iridium wires. Medroxyprogesterone acetate 100mg 3 times a day produces a response in at least 30% of patients with recurrent disease, and prolongs survival, but causes fluid retention and weight gain. Pulmonary metastases are particularly likely to respond. Combined chemotherapy can produce a response in patients who fail to respond to progestogens.

Problems in advanced disease — In advanced disease the tumor invades the muscle layers and spreads to lymph nodes (pelvic, para-aortic and sometimes inguinal and supraclavicular nodes). Vaginal satellite nodules (not part of direct extension) can occur. Local spread can occur to other pelvic structures (broad ligament, ovaries) and to the peritoneum (causing ascites). Bloodborne metastases tend to occur late (mainly in bone and lung).

The main problems are:

- Pain
- Discharge, smell (see *Smells*)
- Bleeding (see *Bleeding*)
- Lymphedema (see *Lymphedema*)
- Ascites (see *Ascites*)

Pain usually responds well to a correctly titrated dose of morphine. (see *Morphine*)

Pelvic disease may involve the lumbo-sacral plexus. (see *Nerve Pain*)

Profuse foul-smelling vaginal discharge can occur. Prophylactic long-term broad spectrum antibiotics may be required, including metronidazole 250mg 3 times a day to reduce smell. (see *Smells*)

ESOPHAGEAL CANCER

Background information — 90% of esophageal cancers are squamous (usually well-differentiated). 10% are adenocarcinomas involving the lower esophagus near the stomach. Risk of esophageal cancer increases 200 times after a caustic soda burn. Smoking and alcohol increase risk. Most patients present late, when the tumor is already advanced. Prognosis is very poor: few patients survive more than 6 months from the time of diagnosis.

Dysphagia and weight loss are the typical features at presentation. Some patients complain of heartburn and acid reflux (due to loss of an effective lower esophageal sphincter). Sometimes food accumulates above the block causing irritation, reflux and regurgitation of blood-stained material. Constant pain is a sinister symptom and usually indicates advanced local spread. Examination is usually normal unless metastases are already present (hepatomegaly, supraclavicular nodes).

Diagnosis depends upon barium swallow, esophagoscopy and biopsy. If surgery is considered, CT scan is important to exclude mediastinal node involvement.

Treatment — The results of treatment (surgery or radiotherapy) are poor. Only 5% survive 5 years.

Surgery is usually reserved for a relatively fit patient with no evidence of metastases. There are two principal operations. Lower-third tumors are resected and the stomach is mobilized (via laparotomy) and pulled up through the diaphragm (gastric mobilization and pull-through). For middle-third tumors esophagectomy is performed, and a segment of colon is transposed to make a pseudoesophagus (colonic interposition). These operations have a 10% mortality, but can result in good palliation (90% have normal swallowing) and occasionally in cure. 30% of patients need repeated dilations of the surgical anastomosis to maintain swallowing.

Palliative surgery is occasionally performed to bypass (rather than remove) the tumors. The stomach is brought up and anastomosed to the esophagus above the tumor. (This procedure can be combined with radiotherapy.)

Radical radiotherapy (with hope of cure in 5% to 10% of patients) is reserved for squamous carcinomas (adenocarcinomas are relatively radio-resistant) and will improve swallowing, but causes initial radiation esophagitis for 2 to 3 weeks. Normally 5,000cGy to 6,000cGy are given over 5 to 6 weeks. It is technically difficult because the long length of esophagus must be treated (5cm above and below the lesion because submucous spread is common) and the spinal cord or lung can be damaged.

Radiotherapy often causes retro-sternal pain on swallowing due to inflammation, which can be soothed with oral administration of local anesthetic-alkali-aspirin mixtures. The pain may be due to esophageal spasm which can respond to nifedipine 10mg 4 times a day. Radiation pneumonitis can cause dyspnea and cough. About 50% of patients will need repeated dilations of a stricture, which can develop 6 to 8 months after radiotherapy.

Palliative radiotherapy using lower doses (3,000cGy over 2 weeks) can relieve dysphagia. Squamous carcinomas respond better than adenocarcinomas which are more resistant to radiotherapy. If the patient requires a tube and radiotherapy, it may be advisable to insert the tube first.

There is no effective chemotherapy for this tumor.

Endoscopic intubation is an effective way of improving swallowing and is possible in 90% of patients. Results are good. 30% have normal swallowing. 60% can manage semi-solids. Tube insertion is usually best performed under general anesthesia and x-ray control, although it can be performed under sedation. Previous radiotherapy does not preclude tube insertion. The tumor must first be dilated. This can cause a fatal perforation and mediastinitis (there is about a 10% mortality with this procedure). Occasionally a small laparotomy is required to suture the distal end of the tube in place. Intubation of tumors in the lower third of the esophagus (or for recurrent tumors at an anastomosis) can be difficult because the tumor may not hold the tube in place.

Following tube insertion, the patient is advised to:

- Chew well
- Avoid large boluses of meat
- Have frequent fizzy drinks with meals

Problems with tubes include:

- Migration upwards (pain)
- Migration downwards (blocking)
- Reflux and heartburn
- Blocking with food (rare)
- Erosion and perforation (very rare)
- Celestin tube disintegration (after 6 to 9 months)

If the tube slips it may need to be repositioned or replaced. If it slips up, there is discomfort on swallowing and aspiration can occur. (When the tube remains in place the patient is unaware of its presence.) If the distal end impacts on the stomach wall it will block. Tumor overgrowth can be treated with laser or by inserting a larger tube.

Perforation following the dilation of strictures (postoperative or radiation fibrosis) can be successfully managed by the insertion of a tube. A tracheo-esophageal fistula can sometimes be sealed by an Atkinson tube.

Problems in advanced disease:

- Dysphagia
- Local spread
- Fistula
- Metastases

In **dysphagia** management options include dilation, tubes, laser therapy and high dose steroids. Liquidize foods. Give soluble drugs or use a continuous subcutaneous infusion. If a tube is present it may have become blocked (by food or tumor encroachment) or displaced. High dose steroids (dexamethasone 8mg to 12mg per day) can reduce peri-tumor edema and can improve swallowing dramatically for several weeks. (see *Dysphagia, Steroids*)

Laser therapy is now increasingly available at major medical centers and offers good palliation for dysphagia. It is complementary to tube insertion, which still has advantages in certain situations (for example, laser therapy is **ineffective** for extrinsic compressing tumors). (see *Lasers*)

Local spread of the tumor can cause:

- Vertebral pain
- Pleuritic pain (pleural involvement)
- Hoarseness (recurrent laryngeal nerve)
- Hiccup (diaphragm)
- Arrythmias (pericardium)
- Tracheo-esophageal fistula
- Mediastinitis
- Metastases
- Massive hemorrhage (aorta)

Changes in the pattern of pain may be due to vertebral or pleural involvement. Pericardial involvement usually causes atrial fibrillation.

A fistula in the trachea causes coughing a few seconds after a drink. Occasionally a patient may complain of episodes of coughing but not relate it to drinking. A patient with a fistula will cough up orange sputum after a drink of orange juice. Use of semisolid foods (jello, custards, liquidized food) can reduce the problem of coughing. It may help if the patient sits in a particular position when eating, (for example, at an angle of 45 degrees).

Mediastinitis is usually a terminal event but a small leak may settle with broad-spectrum antibiotics.

Metastases (a late feature of the disease) can occur to:

- Liver
- Lymph nodes (supraclavicular, neck)
- Lung
- Bone
- Skin (nodules)
- Brain (rare)

HEAD & NECK CANCERS

Background information — Head and neck cancers are usually squamous cancers. They are related to smoking. They are three times more common in men. The overall cure rate is about 40%.

The main sites are:

- Larynx
- Pharynx
- Oral cavity
- Salivary glands
- Nasal sinuses
- Orbit

Cancer of the larynx classically presents with hoarseness of the voice. Radiation therapy cures at least 75% of patients where the vocal cord remains mobile. Where the cord is fixed the 5-year survival falls to 25%. 60% of tumors occur on the vocal cords. About 35% occur above the cords and these tend to present late with dysphagia. About 5% occur below the cords: these also tend to present late and may cause stridor.

The pharynx is divided into three parts, the nasopharynx, oropharynx and laryngopharynx. **Cancer of the nasopharynx**, particularly common in the Mongolian Chinese, tends to present late with nodal disease in the neck. Unilateral nasal obstruction and secretory otitis media are common presenting features. Invasion of the base of the skull can involve cranial nerves 3, 4 and 6 (double vision or opthalmoplegia). Lateral extension can involve cranial nerves 9, 10, 11 and 12 (dysphagia, dysarthria). Bony invasion of the nasal sinuses or the orbit can cause pain.

Cancer of the oropharynx (including the soft palate, tonsils and posterior third of the tongue) tends to present with pain, dysphagia or cervical nodes.

Cancer of the laryngopharynx tends to present with dysphagia or (sometimes) stridor.

Cancers of the oral cavity usually present as non-healing ulcers on the lip, tongue, cheek or floor of the mouth. Cervical lymph nodes may be enlarged.

Cancers of the salivary glands occur most commonly in the parotid gland. The tumor usually presents as a painful lump or a facial palsy.

Cancers of the nasal sinuses most commonly involve the maxillary sinus or nasal cavity. They usually present with a nasal discharge.

Orbital tumors can be primary (lymphoma, sarcoma) or metastatic (breast, bronchus, thyroid). The typical features are proptosis (forward displacement of the eye), opthalmoplegia (reduced eye movement) and chemosis (red watering eye that can mimic cellulitis).

Treatment — Radiotherapy is often first-line treatment for most head and neck tumors, as it is less mutilating than surgery. Surgery can be reserved for failed radiotherapy.

Radical radiotherapy is the treatment of choice for **laryngeal cancers**, with total laryngectomy the treatment of choice for recurrent disease. Following laryngectomy, patients require vocal rehabilitation by the speech therapist and training in tracheostomy care. (see Tracheostomy Care)

The treatment of choice for **pharyngeal cancers** is radical radiotherapy, usually around 6,000cGy delivered over 6 to 7 weeks. Radiotherapy to the nasopharynx is technically difficult because sensitive structures (spinal cord, cornea, temporal lobe) must be avoided. 5 year survival is less than 50% even for early stage disease and less than 30% if cervical nodes are involved. A significant portion of patients alive at 5 years will still die of recurrence. Surgery can sometimes be offered for recurrent disease, but these operations are complex and require close cooperation between the head and neck surgeon and the plastic surgeon responsible for reconstruction.

Small tumors of the **oral cavity** are usually treated by radioactive implants and have an excellent cure rate. Larger tumors are treated by external beam radiotherapy. Nodes in the neck are usually excised by radical neck dissection. Local recurrence requires wide resection and often results in substantial local damage (for example, recurrent tumor in the floor of the mouth may require excision of the floor of the mouth with hemi-glossectomy and hemi-mandibulectomy). Sophisticated reconstructive surgery is required. The use of free-flap skin grafting with microvascular anastomosis has improved results. Radical resection and repair may still be appropriate (as a palliative procedure) to control the local disease even if small metastases are present.

Cancers of the **salivary glands** are treated with surgery (which attempts to preserve the facial nerve) and post-operative radiotherapy.

Treatment of cancer of the **maxillary sinus** usually involves combined surgery and radiotherapy. Modern prostheses can restore facial appearance despite the large deficit. Advanced tumors cause swelling of the cheek and spread upwards into the orbit (diplopia, opthalmoplegia) or downwards into the oral cavity, distorting the hard palate. Radiotherapy alone is used if the tumor is too advanced for surgery, and about 20% of these patients will survive 5 years.

Radiotherapy techniques for **orbital tumors** attempt to shield sensitive structures (cornea, lens, lachrymal sac). Useful vision is usually retained in the treated eye.

Common problems include:

- Recurrent tumor
- Pain
- Bleeding
- Fistula
- Dysphagia
- Airways obstruction
- Radiation fibrosis

Recurrent tumor, causing tumor bulk with obstruction, bleeding, slough or smell, can be controlled by cryosurgery or lasers. Both can be used in areas previously treated with radiotherapy or surgery.

Pain usually responds to titrated doses of morphine. Escalating pain may be due to infection. (see *Morphine*)

Bleeding due to malignant ulceration may be controlled by topical adrenaline, tranexamic acid or radiotherapy. Hemostatic dressings sometimes help. (see *Bleeding*)

Fistulas in the mouth or pharynx cause leakage of saliva. Surgical repair may be possible. A fistula in a malignant area can shrink after radiotherapy. It is sometimes possible to plug a fistula with a molded occlusive dressing.

Dysphagia may be due to tumor recurrence, radiation damage or candidiasis. A fine-bore nasal feeding tube or a cervical esophagostomy may be necessary. (see *Nutrition*)

Airways obstruction due to malignant tracheal compression will often regress after radiotherapy or laser treatment. Tracheostomy may be necessary if there is inoperable laryngeal obstruction. (see *Tracheostomy Care*)

Radiation fibrosis can cause trismus of the lower jaw and inability to open the mouth, obstruction of the eustachian tube and deafness (sometimes relieved by inserting a grommet in the tympanic membrane) or obstruction of the nasolacrimal duct with watering of one eye (sometimes corrected by probing the duct or inserting a catheter).

Problems in advanced disease — Advanced disease tends to spread to lymph nodes and lungs. Malignant lymph nodes may not become apparent until 2 years after the initial diagnosis. A radical block dissection of the neck to remove malignant lymph nodes is a palliative procedure to prevent pain and disfigurement. Most patients with cervical node metastases will already have internal metastases, so the procedure rarely extends life, although it can occasionally be curative. About 25% of patients will develop local recurrence after block dissection, usually within six months.

HEPATOMA

Background information — Primary liver cancer (hepatoma) is associated with cirrhosis and hepatitis B (although there may be no underlying cause). It is 10 times more common in men. Patients present with abdominal pain or with a lump. Untreated, the mean survival is only 6 months.

Treatment — Surgical resection offers a chance of cure and must be considered particularly in a non-cirrhotic patient, because the liver will regenerate even if three-quarters of the organ is removed. The value of **liver transplantation** is limited because the operative mortality is high and 60% of patients suffer recurrence. **Chemotherapy** can produce tumor regression (as assessed by ultrasound and CT scan) in about 20% of patients. Radiotherapy has no place in treating primary liver cancer.

Problems of advanced disease:

- Pain
- Ascites
- Thrombosis
- Metastases (lung and bone)
- Hypercalcemia
- Rare syndromes (ectopic ACTH, hypoglycemia)

Liver pain responds well to titrated doses of morphine. Embolization or ligation of the hepatic artery is sometimes used to infarct and shrink the tumor and reduce stretching of the liver capsule (but can itself be a very painful procedure). Celiac plexus block should be performed if pain is not well controlled with morphine. Involvement of the porta hepatis nodes can cause biliary distention and episodes of acute pain. (see Liver Pain, Nerve Blocks)

Ascites can occur early, and insertion of a peritoneo-venous shunt should be considered if the patient is in reasonably good condition and the ascites is symptomatic. (see Ascites)

Deep vein thrombosis can occur (made more likely by tumor invasion of the inferior vena cava). Anti-coagulation with warfarin can reduce swelling and pain. Careful monitoring is necessary in view of poor liver function. (see Anti-coagulants)

Metastases to lung and bone occur occasionally. Lung metastases may cause no symptoms. Bone pain is best treated by palliative radiotherapy. (see Bone Pain)

Hypercalcemia may cause thirst, nausea and drowsiness. (see Hypercalcemia)

Rare syndromes include polycythemia, carcinoid syndrome (wheezing, flushing, diarrhea), ectopic ACTH or hypoglycemia (which may be a terminal event).

LEUKEMIAS

Background information — There are four main types of leukemia:

- Acute lymphoblastic (ALL)
- Acute myeloid/acute nonlymphoblastic (AML or ANLL)
- Chronic lymphocytic (CLL)
- Chronic myelocytic (CML)

Many forms of leukemia are treatable. 50% of children and 25% of young adults can be cured.

Leukemia cell proliferation in the bone marrow causes:

- Anemia (lack of red cells)
- Infections (lack of white cells)
- Bleeding (lack of platelets)

Acute leukemias can occur at all ages. Chronic leukemias mainly affect the elderly. Diagnosis is confirmed by identification of leukemia cells in the bone marrow.

Treatment:

Acute lymphoblastic leukemia (ALL) is the most common type in childhood. Initial chemotherapy usually produces a rapid remission. Therapy continues for about 2 years, including cranial irradiation and intrathecal methotrexate, to prevent relapse. If relapse occurs further chemotherapy can induce a remission in most, but cure is then very unlikely without a successful bone marrow transplant. (*see Bone Marrow Transplant*)

Acute myeloid leukemia (ALL), also called **acute non-lymphoblastic leukemia** (ANLL), is much less responsive to treatment. Chemotherapy will produce a remission in around 80% of younger patients but cure is rare. In elderly patients chemotherapy may be considered inappropriate but supportive treatment, particularly blood transfusions, may be beneficial.

Chronic lymphocytic leukemia (CLL) is rare below the age of 40. It causes the gradual enlargement of lymph nodes (usually symmetrically) and in the early stages no treatment is required. The patient is more susceptible to infections (candida, shingles, pulmonary infections) and live vaccines must be avoided. Chlorambucil and steroids may be used if symptoms develop (auto-immune anemia, thrombocyto-penia or symptomatic lymphadenopathy). Splenic radio-therapy is sometimes useful.

Chronic myelocytic leukemia (CML) occurs mostly in adults over 35. There is usually splenomegaly. In 30% of patients it is discovered as an accidental finding on a blood test. Chemotherapy with busulphan or hydroxyurea may produce survival for several years (50% of patients die within 3 years) but cure is not possible except by successful bone marrow transplant. The patient may be able to live a normal life for some years but terminally the disease trans-forms into acute leukemia (blast crisis) when aggressive chemotherapy is only rarely beneficial.

Problems in advanced disease:

1. When to stop chemotherapy
2. Anemia
3. Thrombocytopenic bleeding
4. Infections
5. Pain
6. CNS disease

1. The decision to **stop further chemotherapy** is often a very difficult one. Chemotherapy may have already worked

by inducing a remission. A second remission is a possibility, but at the cost of side-effects (hair loss, nausea and vomiting, many weeks in a hospital). The chance of a third remission is always very poor. Treatment decisions need to be discussed in detail with the patient. (*see Chemotherapy*)

2. **Anemia** should be treated only if it is causing troublesome symptoms (angina, dyspnea, dizziness, tiredness). A trial of blood transfusion may be indicated to see if it improves a patient's condition. (*see Anemia*)

3. Bleeding is usually due to **thrombocytopenia**.

The main problems are:

- Skin purpura (harmless)
- Mucous ulceration (sore mouth)
- Nose bleeds (avoid cautery)
- Retinal bleeds (loss of vision)
- Hematuria
- GI bleeds
- Intracranial bleeds (as a terminal event)

Platelet transfusion produces only a temporary improvement and is rarely indicated. An exception would be a patient with distressing bleeding (perhaps into the eye or heavy nose bleeds).

4. **Bacterial, fungal and viral infections** are all common. Painful urinary tract infections or cellulitis are usually treated. Pneumonia or septicemia are usually regarded as terminal events. Thrush is common, and careful mouth care is essential (long-term prophylaxis may be indicated). Herpes simplex can cause severe peri-oral lesions which can become hemorrhagic. Acyclovir is effective if started early, and ice can be soothing. Shingles is common. If caught early, IV or even oral acyclovir can abort the attack. In corneal involvement the eye should be closed (tarsorrhaphy, or use paper tape temporarily).

5. **Pain is unusual** in leukemia. The gross splenomegaly of CML can be painful and responds to titrated doses of opioids, plus high dose steroids as a co-analgesic if necessary. Bone pain can occur, and steroids can be helpful. (*see Bone Pain, Steroids*)

6. **CNS disease** is potentially very unpleasant — headache, vomiting, cranial nerve palsies and paraplegia. It may be reasonable to continue active treatment against CNS disease (for example, weekly intrathecal methotrexate) after systemic chemotherapy has been stopped.

LUNG CANCER

(see Pancoast's Syndrome)

Background information — The risk of lung cancer is proportional to the number of cigarettes smoked. 15 years after stopping smoking the risk returns to about normal. 15% of lung cancers (usually adenocarcinomas) occur in non-smokers. Smoking plus exposure to asbestos increases the risk by 40 times. Industrial exposure to uranium, chromium and nickel have been linked to lung cancer.

Common presenting symptoms are:

Cough	80%
Hemoptysis	70%
Dyspnea	60%
Chest pain	40%
Wheeze	15%
Stridor	5%

It can also present as a symptomless mass on a routine x-ray.

Diagnosis is based on histology. Biopsy is usually by bronchoscopy (or sometimes needle biopsy or open lung biopsy). Further investigations are needed to assess spread and detect metastases (to see which treatment is appropriate). Lung function tests may be needed to assess fitness for surgery.

There are four types of lung cancer:

Squamous	45%
Adenocarcinoma	20%
Small (oat) cell	20%
Large cell	15%

Squamous cell carcinoma usually causes a large obstructing lesion in a main bronchus. It may cavitate and mimic an abscess.

Adenocarcinomas tend to occur in the periphery of the lung, unrelated to a bronchus. They are slower growing and may reach a large size before causing problems or being detected on a routine chest x-ray.

Small (oat) cell tumors spread rapidly into blood and lymphatics and have an explosive course, disseminating rapidly to bone, lymphatics, liver and brain. Survival time after diagnosis can be as short as a few months.

Large cell carcinomas are undifferentiated and bulky and tend to invade locally and disseminate widely.

Prognosis depends on histology. The average survival from diagnosis to death is approximately:

Squamous	18 months
Adenocarcinoma	36 months
Small (oat) cell	6 months
Large cell	18 months

Treatment — For cancers **other than small (oat) cell**, surgery offers the best hope of cure. About 20% of patients are suitable for surgery.

Surgery is usually not considered if:
- Metastases are present
- Central tumor is large (within 2cm of carina)
- Para-tracheal nodes present
- Pleural effusion present
- Mediastinal involvement (hoarseness)
- Poor lung function
- Age over 70 (high operative mortality)

After surgery 40% of patients survive 5 years. The outcome is best for small squamous carcinomas (less than 3cm). 80% of these patients survive 5 years.

Radiotherapy — Several studies have shown that radiotherapy does not prolong survival (and therefore it is not given routinely). The best palliation occurs when treatment is delayed until the onset of specific symptoms. This often allows 4 to 5 months before treatment is necessary, and for 50% of patients radiotherapy is never necessary.

Palliative radiotherapy is most useful for:
- Hemoptysis
- SVC compression (stridor, dysphagia)
- Bone pain

Hemoptysis is controlled or reduced in 90% of patients.

Palliative radiotherapy is also sometimes given for:
- Dyspnea
- Chest pain
- Cough

Palliative radiotherapy is less effective for these symptoms, and only about 40% of patients respond. The usual dose is 2,000cGy in 5 fractions which can be repeated after a month. Radical radiotherapy (6,000cGy over 6 weeks) is occasionally given to small tumors where surgery is hazardous or refused, and a small number of such tumors may be cured. Side-effects of treatment include dysphagia, pericarditis, skin reaction and (occasionally) damage to the spinal cord.

Combination chemotherapy is disappointing for non-small (oat) cell tumors and only 10% of patients get a complete response.

For patients with **small (oat) cell carcinomas**, surgery and radiotherapy fail to prolong survival. The main treatment is combined chemotherapy, sometimes with local radiotherapy to the primary tumor. With limited disease (limited to one lung and the ipsilateral supraclavicular nodes) 20% will survive 2 years with intensive chemotherapy, but with extensive disease few patients live longer than 1 year (although occasionally patients survive 2 or 3 years). Chemotherapy can help to prevent symptoms (pain, cough, dyspnea, hemoptysis, dysphagia and SVC obstruction), but is rarely helpful once these symptoms develop. 30% of patients will develop cerebral metastases even after chemotherapy.

Intrathoracic spread causes:

- Hilar node enlargement
- Pleural effusion
- Pericarditis (pain, dysrhythmias, effusion)
- Mediastinal node enlargement:
    - SVC obstruction (venous swelling)
    - Laryngeal nerve compression (hoarseness)
    - Sympathetic chain (ptosis)
    - Phrenic nerve (paralyzed diaphragm)

Problems in advanced disease:

- Dyspnea
- Pain (chest, bone, liver, nerve)
- Cough, hemoptysis
- Stridor, dysphagia, SVC compression
- Hoarseness
- Nodal metastases

- Skin nodules
- Brain metastases
- Hypercalcemia
- Hyponatremia
- Rarer non-metastatic features

Dyspnea may be due to obstruction of a large airway (consider radiotherapy) or lymphatic obstruction at the mediastinum, causing lymphangitis carcinomatosa and stiff lungs (consider high dose steroids) or a large effusion. (see *Dyspnea*)

Pain may be from the tumor (visceral pain) or due to rib metastases or rib erosion. Pleuritic pain may be due to underlying infection and responds to antibiotics. Involvement of the brachial plexus causes nerve pain in the arm. Bone pain and liver pain are also common problems. Liver metastases can be painless, or cause liver pain which usually responds to morphine. Ascites can occur. (see *Bone Pain, Liver Pain*)

Hemoptysis can be frightening. It responds rapidly in 90% of cases to palliative radiotherapy.

Productive cough suggests retained secretions and responds to antibiotics. **Dry cough** due to tumor irritation may respond to low dose morphine, radiotherapy, high dose steroids or nebulized local anesthetic. (see *Cough*)

Stridor or dysphagia can occur due to compression by nodal metastases at the thoracic inlet. Radiotherapy, high dose steroids or passage of an esophageal tube may be indicated. (see *Superior Vena Cava Compression*)

Hoarseness is due to recurrent laryngeal nerve damage. It is common. The patient often fears losing his voice altogether and can be reassured that this will not occur. It is possible to inject teflon into the paralyzed vocal cord to fix it medially, allowing the mobile cord to approximate. Consider referral to an ENT specialist.

Nodal metastases in the neck and axillae and skin nodules are distressing mainly because they are a visible reminder of the cancer. Large or painful lumps can be treated with radiotherapy.

Brain metastases are common in lung cancer, and occur in 40% of patients. They occur most commonly with small (oat) cell carcinomas and adenocarcinomas. They may present with personality change, seizures, weakness of an arm or leg, or headache and vomiting due to raised intracranial pressure. Diagnosis can be confirmed by CT scan. Treatment is with high dose steroids. Whole brain irradiation extends median survival from 1 to 5 months, and may be considered in the small group of patients who are relatively fit, have no evidence of metastases elsewhere, and who have had a long interval (1 year or more) from diagnosis to the development of metastases, since this group does best. Occasionally a patient with brain metastases lives for several years. (see *Brain Metastases*)

Hypercalcemia is common with squamous (23%) and large cell (12.7%) carcinomas, less common with adenocarcinoma (2.5%), and rare with small (oat) cell tumors. **Hyponatremia** occurs in about 20% of small (oat) cell tumors. The kidneys retain water. (see *Confusion, Hypercalcemia*)

Other non-metastatic features of lung cancers include:
- Clubbing
- Arthralgia in wrists and ankles (HPO)
- Ectopic hormones (ACTH)
- Neuropathy, myopathy, myasthenia
- Thrombophlebitis
- Endocarditis

LYMPHOMAS

Background information — Lymphomas are malignancies of the lymphoid tissues. **Non-Hodgkin's lymphomas** are more common than **Hodgkin's Disease** and account for about 3% of all cancers.

Hodgkin's Disease is one of the commonest malignancies of young adults. It typically presents with painless enlargement of lymph glands, sometimes with malaise, sweats and weight loss. The disease can spread outside the lymph system to involve skin, lung, bowel, liver, bone marrow, bone and CNS. Diagnosis is by biopsy of an involved node. Investigations (bone marrow, CT scan, lymphangiogram) are performed to stage the spread of the disease.

Diagnosis is based on distinctive histology (Sternberg-Reed cells).

Stage	Spread	Treatment	Approximate % 5-year survival
1	Single node	Radiotherapy	85
2	2 or more nodes same side of diaphragm (may include spleen)	Radiotherapy	80
3	Nodes on both sides of diaphragm	Radiotherapy/ chemotherapy	60-80
4	Liver, bone marrow (or any diffuse organ involvement)	Chemotherapy	50

The criteria for staging are in fact more detailed than given in this simplified table. For example, there can be a place for chemotherapy in Stage 1 and 2 disease if there are systemic symptoms (fever, night sweats, weight loss).

Note that there is a good chance of cure at all stages, even with advanced disease. Even with Stage 4 disease 40% to 50% of patients survive 10 years, although late relapse can occur. Staging is essential, so that all the disease is treated from the start. CT scan is beginning to replace the staging laparotomy.

In **non-Hodgkin's lymphomas**, staging of the disease follows the same scheme, but the great majority of patients present with Stage 3 or 4 disease, and the prognosis is worse than for Hodgkin's Disease.

Prognosis also depends on histology. The follicular lymphomas have a good prognosis, and lymphocytic better than histiocytic or undifferentiated lymphomas.

Most patients present with nodal disease, which tends to be more widespread than for Hodgkin's Disease. Diagnosis can be difficult when the disease presents at extra-nodal sites (bowel, stomach, bone, CNS, pharynx, eye, skin).

Treatment depends on accurate staging of spread of disease. The median survival with low grade non-Hodgkin's lymphomas is about 8 years and treatment is usually with a single agent (chlorambucil). Local radiotherapy may be used. High grade non-Hodgkin's lymphomas can cause death within a few months despite treatment with combination chemotherapy. The cure rate for high grade lymphomas is about 40%.

Problems in advanced disease:

- Lymph node masses
- Bone marrow failure (anemia, thrombocytopenia)
- Infections (thrush, herpes simplex)
- CNS disease
- Itching (see *Itching*)
- Fever and sweats (see *Sweating*)

Lymph node masses may be painful or unsightly, and local radiotherapy may produce shrinkage. Blood transfusion may be indicated for symptomatic anemia. Platelet transfusion may be indicated for distressing bleeding (into the eye or heavy nose bleeds). Prophylactic antifungal therapy may be indicated to prevent thrush recurring.

MELANOMA

Background information — Melanoma is rare and accounts for only 2% of skin cancers, although its incidence appears to be increasing. If diagnosed early it is a curable form of cancer (lesions less than 0.75mm deep on histology have a 95% cure rate). It arises in melanocytes in the skin (or sometimes in the choroid layer of the eye, when enucleation is usually necessary). Only 30% arise in pre-existing moles. It occurs most frequently in people of fair complexion. Incidence correlates with amount of sunlight received (which has a cumulative effect).

Treatment — Primary treatment is excision down to fascia with a wide margin (to remove skin lymphatics) and skin grafting if necessary. Prophylactic dissection of normal lymph nodes is not performed unless the lesion is already advanced (2mm to 3mm deep). An occasional disaster occurs through mis-diagnosis of melanoma as a benign lesion, and mis-treatment by simple curettage which causes dissemination.

Spread to lymph nodes indicates a poor prognosis. Only 10% of patients survive 5 years. Block dissection of lymph nodes is usually performed. Fixed nodes can be treated with radiotherapy but high doses are needed since it is a radio-resistant tumor. Regional limb perfusion with cyto-toxic drugs is sometimes used for advanced unresectable tumors, and the disease may regress for a time with relief of symptoms. Amputation, except of a digit, is seldom advised. Cryotherapy can be used on advanced fungating skin lesions. Extensive skin involvement can be excised and skin grafted, but this is rarely indicated for a disease with such a short prognosis.

When the disease has spread beyond regional lymph nodes, median survival is only 5 months. 20% of patients develop distant metastases without any prior evidence of lymphadenopathy. Melanomas are notorious for produc-ing metastases years after apparently adequate surgery or enucleation.

Metastases occur in liver, brain, bone and lung (and less commonly to spleen and heart). Chemotherapy is disap-pointing — about 20% respond for 3 to 6 months with regression of skin deposits but with no effect on visceral metastases. Spontaneous regression of this tumor has been described but is very rare.

Problems in advanced disease:
- Massive hepatomegaly
- Bone pain
- Brain metastases
- Paraplegia
- Cranial nerve palsies
- Fears about heredity

Hepatomegaly can be massive but often causes re-markably few symptoms. The small stomach syndrome can occur with heartburn, nausea, and the need for small fre-quent meals. These symptoms may be reduced by meto-clopramide 10mg to 20mg 4 times a day. (see *Small Stomach Syndrome*)

Bone metastases can cause pain. These respond to pallia-tive radiotherapy (even though the primary tumor is radio-resistant). Pathological fractures can occur. (see *Bone Pain, Fractures, Spinal Cord Compression*)

Brain metastases are very common in the terminal stages.

Melanoma deposits can sometimes occur within the spi-nal cord. This may cause paraparesis or **paraplegia** without marked sensory loss (unlike total spinal cord compression due to collapse of a vertebra which causes a sensory loss).

Cranial nerve palsies can occur, especially to 3, 4, and 6 (affecting eye movements) and to 7 (causing facial weakness). They are caused by meningeal infiltration.

Some **families** have the dysplastic nevus syndrome, a large number of distinctive large moles which can become malignant. Families have been described in which melanoma occurs with unusual frequency. Carers should know the **standard advice on prevention**: avoid excessive sunlight and observe moles regularly for significant changes (darkening, enlargement or satellites, itch, ulceration or bleeding).

MESOTHELIOMA

Background information — A mesothelioma is a malignant tumor of the pleura. In 90% of patients it is related to asbestos exposure. The association between asbestos exposure and mesothelioma was described in 1960 by Wagner in South Africa. About 5 to 10% of those exposed develop the disease.

Most patients with mesothelioma recite a history of exposure to asbestos, although characteristically there is a delay of 10 to 50 years between exposure and presentation. The histology is sarcomatous or anaplastic.

The typical presentation is with chest pain (which can be severe) or dyspnea due to pleural effusion. Chest x-ray may show typical pleural plaques. Diagnosis is by pleural biopsy which may require open thoracotomy.

The tumor spreads by direct extension to invade ribs and chest wall (and can infiltrate the skin and cause enlarging subcutaneous lumps). It can extend through the diaphragm and spreads to the lymph nodes. It rarely involves the contralateral chest and rarely causes distant metastases.

Treatment is highly unsatisfactory. Surgery is possible in only a small minority of cases with localized involvement. (Prior assessment by CT scan is important.) Recurrence is common. Radiotherapy is of very little value. Many chemotherapeutic drugs have been tried with little success.

Problems in advanced disease:
- Pleural effusions
- Dyspnea
- Pain
- Infections

Recurrent **pleural effusions** may need aspirating. Sometimes the effusion becomes loculated as the tumor extends and the need for aspiration lessens or ceases altogether. After pleural aspiration a tumor nodule often develops at the site of the needle puncture, but these are not usually painful. (see *Pleural Effusion*)

Dyspnea may be due to effusions or to restricted chest wall movements or both. In fact, one lung generally remains healthy and it is usually possible to control dyspnea by a combined approach. (see *Dyspnea*)

Chest pain usually responds well to morphine, but involvement of the ribs and intercostal bundles can cause severe chest wall pain which only partially responds to morphine. A paravertebral nerve block (which can be repeated at different levels) can be very helpful in controlling this pain.

Chest infections can occur as the disease progresses to encase one lung causing restricted expansion and predisposing to pooling of secretions. Infections should be treated promptly.

MYELOMA

Background information — Myeloma (multiple myelomatosis) is a disease of the elderly (rare under the age of 50). It is a malignant disorder of plasma cells in the bone marrow. These produce an excessive amount of immunoglobulin (usually IgG, but sometimes IgA or IgM). Sometimes an excessive production of light chains (part of the IgG molecule) causes heavy proteinuria (Bence-Jones protein).

The clinical features are due to:

- Bone involvement (pains, hypercalcemia)
- Bone marrow replacement (low Hb, WBC, platelets)
- Abnormal proteins (high ESR, renal damage, infections)

The patient usually presents with tiredness (anemia) or bone pains (osteolytic lesions). Recurrent bacterial infections can occur (immune paresis). The abnormal proteins also cause a very high ESR (above 100) and sometimes renal damage (with recurrent infections or renal failure).

Immuno-electrophoresis of plasma or urine may be diagnostic (abnormal immunoglobulins). Bone marrow aspirate is often diagnostic, showing an excess of plasma cells.

Solitary **plasmacytoma** is a single lesion found either in bone or soft tissue (particularly nasal cavity, bowel or bronchus). It is treated with radiotherapy. A proportion of these patients develop myeloma later. Progression is more common with plasmacytoma in bone.

Treatment for myeloma includes radiotherapy to local bone lesions and combination chemotherapy which increases the median survival from 6 to 12 months (untreated) to 2 to 3 years. Patients with early renal failure should be considered for dialysis.

Problems of advanced disease:

- Weakness
- Bone pain
- Hypercalcemia
- Anemia
- Soft tissue deposits
- Renal failure
- Respiratory infection

Increasing **weakness** and **bone pain** are the predominant features. Vertebral crush fractures and spinal cord compression can occur. (see *Bone Pain, Spinal Cord Compression*)

Hypercalcemia in myeloma responds to steroids more frequently than hypercalcemia in solid malignancies. (see *Hypercalcemia*)

It can be a difficult decision to stop repeated blood transfusions for **anemia**. Transfusions should be stopped if they no longer relieve symptoms, and this does not necessarily reduce survival. (see *Anemia*)

Soft tissue deposits (subcutaneous, lymph nodes, liver and spleen) of myeloma occur as a late feature of the disease. Large subcutaneous lumps will shrink with radiotherapy. Skin changes may be noticed with purpura (low platelets) or poor circulation (hyperviscosity syndrome).

Uremic coma or **respiratory infection** is the usual mode of death.

OVARIAN CANCER

Background information — These tumors **present late** (usually with abdominal distention) and therefore the prognosis is poor. Most are adenocarcinomas. Poorly differentiated tumors tend to be more aggressive.

Rare germ cell tumors occur in younger patients (10 to 30 years old) and can be curable with radiotherapy and chemotherapy. Rare cases of spontaneous regression of ovarian tumors are well documented.

Management depends on clinical staging:

Stage	Spread	Treatment	Approximate % 5-year survival
1	Ovary	Surgery	60
2	Pelvis	Debulking and radiotherapy	40
3	Abdomen	Debulking and chemotherapy	5
4	Distant metastases	—	—

Treatment — Laparotomy is essential for diagnosis and assessment.

The most important part of **management** is adequate surgical removal of as much tumor as possible. Only 20% of patients present with Stage 1 disease, and are treated by hysterectomy and bilateral salpingo-oophorectomy. Very careful inspection of the entire abdominal cavity is essential to exclude small peritoneal seedlings (which make it Stage 3 disease requiring chemotherapy).

Debulking large tumors surgically delays the appearance of symptoms but probably has little effect on survival. The size of the post-operative residual tumor is a good indicator of prognosis. The aim is to leave no tumor masses larger than 1cm.

In Stage 2 disease survival is probably improved by post-operative radiotherapy (but there is a high incidence of side-effects). In Stage 3 disease debulking followed by single agent (usually a platinum analog) or combined chemotherapy will result in 40% of patients being free of tumor 1 to 2 years after initial treatment, as judged by laparoscopy or second-look laparotomy. Only a very small number will be cured.

Palliation with single agent chemotherapy (such as chlorambucil) for 14 days a month can be helpful, since there are few side effects. About 30% of patients have a response (reduction in ascites or abdominal masses) which can occasionally last several months. The white cell count should be checked monthly.

Problems in advanced disease:

- Pain
- Ascites
- Intestinal obstruction
- Cachexia
- Metastases (liver, lung, lymph nodes, CNS)

Pain is usually visceral (continuous, deep, aching pain) and responds to opioids. Colicky pain may be due to constipation or intestinal obstruction.

Abdominal distention may be due to **ascites** or enlarging tumor masses or both — test for shifting dullness and consider an ultrasound scan. In a relatively fit patient consider a peritoneovenous shunt for troublesome ascites. Chemotherapy can occasionally be beneficial even in advanced disease. (see *Ascites*)

Intestinal obstruction occurs in 25% of patients. Usually the disease is known to be multi-focal from a previous laparotomy, but it is important to consider the possibility of a single (surgically correctable) block. In advanced disease, intestinal obstruction is best managed medically with a continuous **subcutaneous** infusion of drugs. It is usually possible to avoid intravenous fluids or nasogastric suction. (see *Intestinal Obstruction, Subcutaneous Infusions*)

Cachexia and weight loss can be profound. The usual picture is one of gross abdominal distention with severe wasting of arms and legs.

Metastatic spread is mainly to pelvic and para-aortic nodes (sometimes supraclavicular or inguinal). Symptoms due to metastases to lung, liver or brain are rare. Bone marrow involvement is very rare.

PANCREATIC CANCER

Background information — Most cancers of the pancreas are adenocarcinomas. (Cystadenocarcinomas in elderly women have a better prognosis. Rare acinar cell carcinomas produce lipase and can cause painful skin lumps due to subcutaneous fat necrosis.) The mean age at presentation is 55, and cancer of the pancreas is twice as common in men as in women. It is twice as common in smokers.

70% of cancers occur in the head of the pancreas (when obstruction of the duodenum and bile duct are common). Cancers in the body and tail of the pancreas tend to present with weight loss or pain. 80% of patients already have metastases in regional nodes or liver at diagnosis. Spread to the peritoneum can cause ascites, and is present in 15% of patients at diagnosis.

Cancer of the pancreas is very difficult to diagnose. There are no definitive diagnostic tests, and the pancreas can be difficult to visualize with x-ray or scans. It usually presents with epigastric pain, but this is a very common symptom. Patients commonly have pain for some time before the diagnosis is made, and are often angry at the delay in diagnosis. ("If it had been found earlier, could I have been cured?")

Tissue diagnosis is important because chronic pancreatitis can mimic cancer. Tissue may be obtained at laparotomy, by needle biopsy under CT or ultrasound control, or by cytology of duodenal aspirate or brush biopsy at endoscopic retrograde cholangiopancreatography (ERCP).

Treatment — 90% of patients die within one year of diagnosis (50% within six months). Small tumors are sometimes treated by total pancreatectomy, but the operative mortality is around 20%, and the tumor usually recurs. Only 5% of patients survive five years. After total pancreatectomy insulin is required.

There is little place for radiotherapy or chemotherapy. Radiotherapy needs to be high dose and often causes vomiting. About 20% of patients have a partial response to chemotherapy (usually fluorouracil), but the duration of response is usually short.

The recent discovery of estrogen receptors in tumor tissue suggests tamoxifen may prolong survival.

Problems in advanced disease:

- Pain
- Jaundice
- Obstructive vomiting
- Steatorrhea
- Thrombosis
- Ascites
- GI bleeding
- Metastases (liver, lung, bone, brain)

Pain can be severe. It is typically worse with food, relieved by sitting forward, and radiates into the back. Pain control is achieved with opioids and (if necessary) celiac plexus block (CPB), which should always be considered for pancreatic cancer pain. CPB can be done at the time of laparotomy, or under local anesthetic and x-ray image intensifier. CPB can abolish the pain, but more commonly it reduces the pain so that it can be well controlled with morphine. Longstanding chronic pain can cause depression, and thus some textbooks describe depression as a particular feature of this disease. (see *Celiac Plexus Block, Depression*)

Jaundice is common due to pressure on the bile duct. It can cause severe itching. If the diagnosis of cancer of the head of the pancreas is made at laparotomy, the surgeon usually performs a palliative cholecystojejunostomy to prevent later obstruction. If the diagnosis is made medically (with biopsy of the mass under ultrasound or CT control) bypass can be achieved by placing an endoprosthesis into the common bile duct via endoscopy or via a percutaneous transhepatic approach. This should be considered for jaundice and itching in a relatively fit patient. (see *Jaundice*)

Obstructive vomiting can occur due to direct tumor expansion causing malignant duodenal or pyloric obstruction. The pattern of vomiting is usually large volumes (often with some undigested food). There may be little nausea. A palliative gastrojejunostomy can solve this problem. Palliative surgery does not alter prognosis, but reduces symptoms and can improve quality of life. If surgery is not possible, a trial of high dose steroids (dexamethasone 8mg per day) is worthwhile and effective in about 50% of patients, abolishing obstructive vomiting for several weeks or months. (Until vomiting settles, use IM or IV steroids.) The trial should last at least a week. (see *Steroids*)

Obstruction of the pancreatic ducts is common, and the lack of pancreatic enzymes causes malabsorption of fat, causing **steatorrhea**. (The patient may complain only of "diarrhea".) Bowel movements (4 to 5 a day) are loose, pale or silver in color, very smelly, and difficult to flush away. Steatorrhea responds poorly to standard anti-diarrheal agents, but responds well to pancreatic enzyme replacements. (These are destroyed by gastric acid, and are best taken with food. They are more effective if cimetidine 200mg is taken 30 minutes before eating.) This usually stops the "diarrhea" immediately. If the patient is also taking morphine he will need laxatives once enzyme replacements have stopped the malabsorption. (see *Diarrhea, Morphine*)

Thromboses are common with carcinoma of the pancreas, due to an abnormal thrombotic tendency which can be resistant to anti-coagulants. This may cause deep vein thrombosis or superficial thrombophlebitis. If anti-coagulation is not appropriate the pain and swelling of deep vein thrombosis can be reduced by support hose and a small dose of morphine.

Peritoneal spread can occur (particularly from tumors in the body and tail of the pancreas) and can cause **ascites**. This may be asymptomatic, but if it causes symptoms (painful distention, dyspnea) it should be drained. (see Ascites)

Gastrointestinal (GI) bleeding can occur. Portal vein occlusion can cause esophageal varices (dilated veins) which can bleed on minimal trauma.

Metastases are common to the liver, causing hepatomegaly. Less frequent sites for metastases are lung, bone and brain.

PROSTATE CANCER

Background information — Prostate cancer is the third most common cancer in men (after lung and colon). It becomes increasingly common with age (it is said that 90% of men over 90 have some malignancy in the prostate gland). The majority of tumors are well differentiated adenocarcinomas.

It may present with urinary problems (hesitancy, urgency, poor stream, terminal dribbling) or with metastases (bone pains, anemia). However, it is often asymptomatic and is diagnosed at routine rectal examination, or after trans-urethral resection for benign prostatic hypertrophy.

Diagnosis is strongly suspected if acid phosphatase levels are raised, and is confirmed by biopsy (usually transrectal). Investigations are carried out first by CT scan to exclude spread to the pelvic area, and by bone scan and liver function tests for distant metastases.

Treatment — Localized disease (with no evidence of spread or distant metastases) can be treated by radiotherapy or surgery.

Radical prostatectomy should be considered in younger men, in view of the excellent contemporary results of nerve-sparing total prostatectomy (preserving sexual function), and preservation of the bladder neck, (or its reconstruction with an implantable prosthetic sphincter). While radical prostatectomy has previously had a reputation for complications (impotence, incontinence, rectal injury and urethral stricture), even the incidence of these may have been exaggerated.

Radiotherapy is often the treatment of choice for localized disease, to shrink the tumor, relieve symptoms and hopefully prolong survival (although 30% of patients develop previously undetected metastases within 2 years). 6,000cGy over 6 weeks is a common course of treatment. Side effects occur (dysuria, proctitis and soreness of perineal skin) but they are usually not severe.

In the **elderly patient** a small prostatic cancer can remain asymptomatic for years, and it can be left untreated. The elderly have a higher risk of dying from causes unrelated to the cancer, which is usually managed by trans-urethral resection for symptoms of obstruction, and routine follow-ups to detect metastases.

50% of patients presenting with prostate cancer already have metastases, making cure impossible. The majority of these patients die within 3 years (although 10% live 10 years).

Management options:

- Trans-urethral resection for outflow obstruction
- Hormone therapy (75% respond)
- Bilateral subcapsular orchiectomy
- Palliative radiotherapy for bone pain
- Palliative radiotherapy for prostatic pain

Huggins (1941) showed that the tumor is hormone-dependent. Conventional hormone therapy with estrogens is being replaced by newer **anti-androgens**.

Hormones are usually delayed until symptoms occur because they do not prolong survival, the maximum response occurs early in treatment, and they cause side effects (flushes, impotence). Diethylstilbestrol 1mg 3 times a day causes gynecomastia and thromboses. Bilateral subcapsular **orchiectomy** causes hot flushes (in 25%) and sometimes personality changes — and still leaves adrenal androgens intact.

The modern aim is complete suppression of testosterone using newer agents, such as LHRH analogs (by monthly implant) together with an anti-androgen (flutamide, cyproterone) to prevent the initial flare-up of the disease that can occur. Other drugs are occasionally used (such as aminoglutethimide which suppresses the adrenal hormones). If hormone therapy fails, cytotoxics are sometimes tried, but results are disappointing.

Problems in advanced disease:

1. Obstructive symptoms
2. Bone pain from metastases
3. Perineal pain
4. Lymphedema of the legs
5. Rectal stenosis
6. Anemia
7. Groin nodes (pain, bleeding)
8. Soft-tissue metastases (liver, lung)

1. **Trans-urethral resection** (repeated if necessary) is indicated if the malignant prostate causes urinary obstruction (hesitancy, poor stream).

2. **Bone pain** is the main symptom. Palliative radiotherapy is the treatment of choice, and occasionally hemibody irradiation can be useful for multiple painful secondaries. Pathological fractures can occur, but are less common than in carcinomas of the breast and bronchus (presumably because bone metastases from the prostate tend to be sclerotic rather than lytic). (see *Bone Pain*)

3. **Perineal pain** usually responds well to carefully titrated doses of oral morphine (with laxative and anti-emetic started simultaneously). Radiotherapy to the prostate can reduce perineal pain due to advanced local disease (but takes time to take effect). (see *Morphine*)

4. **Lymphedema** can occur as a late feature due to involvement of pelvic lymphatics. Treatment with radiotherapy, high dose steroids or diuretics is usually of little help. A firm elastic stocking plus the use of a compression sleeve can reduce swelling. (see *Lymphedema*)

5. **Rectal narrowing** can occur as the enlarging prostate encroaches on the anterior wall of the rectum. This rarely causes complete obstruction provided the bowel movements are kept soft and regular.

6. **Anemia** is common, and transfusion may be indicated if it is symptomatic (Hb usually below 7g/dl). (see *Anemia*)

7. The tumor spreads to pelvic **nodes**, then inguinal nodes, and para-aortic (and even supra-clavicular) nodes. Inguinal nodes occasionally ulcerate with pain and bleeding. Radiotherapy can be helpful to shrink the nodes. (see *Bleeding*)

8. **Metastases** to visceral organs (liver, lung) can occur, but are very late features of the disease.

RECTAL CANCER

Background information — The disease is rare under the age of 40; average age at presentation is 60. Like colon cancer, no definite cause is known. It is rare in developing countries, and low fiber diet has been suggested as a possible cause (because of longer fecal transit time allowing more contact with possible toxins in feces). Most rectal cancers are adenocarcinomas.

Typical symptoms at **presentation** are altered bowel habits, rectal bleeding and tenesmus. The majority of patients present with advanced lesions. About 50% are palpable on rectal examination.

Small lesions of the rectum may be missed on barium enema (obscured by large volume of barium), therefore sigmoidoscopy is important to diagnose lesions in the upper rectum.

Prognosis relates to the Dukes classification (1932) of degree of infiltration through the bowel wall:

Stage	Spread	Approximate % 5-year survival
A	Limited to mucosa	90
B	Penetrating mucosa	60
C	Spread to lymph nodes	25
D	Metastases	—

Treatment — About 60% of rectal tumors are operable at presentation.(operative mortality is around 5%, rising with age).

There are two main operations:

- Anterior resection (upper rectum)
- Abdomino-perineal resection (lower rectum)

Anterior resection and anastomosis is preferred since the anal sphincter is maintained. (Sphincter-saving operations are now possible even for quite low-lying lesions because of surgical stapling devices which allow anastomosis deep in the pelvis.)

Tumors very low down in the rectum require abdomino-perineal (A-P) resection and a permanent colostomy. A-P resection often causes nerve damage leaving male patients impotent.

After surgery about 40% of patients will survive 5 years.

The place of adjuvant radiotherapy (either preoperative or post-operative) is being assessed at some cancer centers. There is some evidence that it reduces local recurrence rates (currently around 40%). Endocavity radiation has been used as a primary treatment for patients in poor general condition, with good results.

Prognosis is poor (usually less than 1 year) if the tumor recurs within 2 years of surgery. After anterior resection, patients with recurrent disease usually present with rectal discharge and bleeding. After A-P resection recurrence usually causes a residual mass of tumor on the anterior sacrum (visible on CT scan) causing sacral root pain, urinary symptoms and vaginal bleeding. Perineal nodules suggest a sacral recurrence. Radiotherapy (for example, 2,000cGy over 4 days) can shrink the tumor mass and can reduce pain and discharge, but the response is usually partial and short-lived, and local disease returns. Occasionally, if there is a long interval between surgery and recurrence, it is worthwhile giving aggressive radiotherapy (for example, 5,000cGy over 4 weeks) since some of these patients can survive a number of years.

If the tumor is inoperable radiotherapy is unlikely to reduce tumor volumes enough to make it operable. A palliative colostomy should be considered if there is fecal incontinence or obstruction (but this will not improve local symptoms of pain and discharge).

If metastases are present most patients die within a year (although survival for 5 years is recorded). Solitary metastases in liver and lung can be resected with occasionally good survival.

Problems in advanced disease:

- Pain
- Discharge (mucus, blood, feces)
- Obstruction
- Urinary incontinence
- Perineal cavity
- Metastases (liver, lung, bone, brain)

Pain occurs in three main patterns, sometimes combined:

- Tenesmus (see Tenesmus)
- Perineal pain (sacral nerve involvement)
- Radiating sciatic pain (see Nerve Pain, Pelvic Pain)

The patient may have had increasing pain for several months and (characteristically) difficulty in sitting down. Often the correctly titrated dose of morphine reduces but fails to abolish the pain (because of the component of nerve pain), and adjuvant maneuvers are necessary. Any patient who has had chronic pain for weeks or months may become depressed, and may benefit from a tricyclic in full doses, which can raise the pain threshold. (see Depression)

Rectal discharge is very distressing. Incontinence of foul-smelling materials requires the wearing of incontinence pads, and oral metronidazole 250mg to 500mg 3 times a day to reduce odor.

Local symptoms other than pain (discharge, bleeding, tenesmus) can sometimes be reduced by local palliative techniques:

- Interstitial radiation
- Electrocoagulation
- Transanal resection
- Endoscopic laser therapy

Interstitial radiation is a technique sometimes used to reduce small tumors when the patient is not fit for general anesthetic and radical resection.

Electrocoagulation (under general anesthetic) is a rather crude technique which can debulk tumors and reduce bleeding.

Transanal resection (under general or spinal anesthetic) is performed via an enlarged rectoscope with a cutting loop and diathermy (somewhat similar to trans-urethral resection techniques). In-patient admission for several days is required because of the risk of secondary hemorrhage. In one series, 20 out of 24 patients had good symptomatic relief.

Endoscopic laser therapy can be performed without general anesthesia. It can reach higher tumors than other techniques. It coagulates as it burns so the risk of hemorrhage is reduced. Laser therapy gives good symptom relief, and it is becoming more widely available. (see Lasers)

A perineal recurrence can break down into a fungating, painful, foul-smelling **perineal cavity**. This may be packed with an alginate dressing soaked in metronidazole solution, or sometimes a sialastic foam dressing can be made to plug the cavity. **Explanation is particularly important.** Far too often a patient suffering with a perineal cavity has been offered virtually no explanation about what is happening, how big the cavity is, the rationale behind management, and the likely outcome. Fears abound. Explanation alone can raise morale. "Out of sight" does not mean "out of mind" with this problem. (see *Pressure Sores*)

RENAL CANCER

Background information — Renal cell adenocarcinoma (hypernephroma) arises in the renal tubular epithelium. It occurs in men three times more frequently than in women, and is associated with smoking. Nephroblastoma (Wilm's tumor) is one of the most common childhood malignancies.

Renal cancer presents typically as painless hematuria which is present in 50% of patients. Anemia may develop. It can also present as pain, a lump in the loin, or with symptoms due to metastases (in bone, lung or brain). Rare features are fever, hypertension, polycythemia or hypercalcemia.

Prognosis depends on stage:

Stage	Spread	Approximate % 5-year survival
1	Small tumor	70
2	Large tumor	50
3	Nodes, renal vein involvement	30
4	Diaphragm, abdominal wall involvement	—

Prognosis also depends on degree of differentiation. (Poorly differentiated tumors have a worse prognosis.)

Diagnosis may require intravenous urography, ultrasound and sometimes CT scan and retrograde pyelography (or cyst-puncture and aspiration cytology). About 7% of renal cancers occur in the renal pelvis, and these are urothelial tumors associated with carcinomas of the ureter and bladder.

Treatment — Surgery is the most important treatment. Radical nephrectomy (with lymph nodes excision) may include removal of ureter and a part of the bladder (for tumors of the renal pelvis), since urothelium lines the renal pelvis, ureter and bladder. Before surgery metastases must be excluded (chest x-ray, CT scans, liver scan, bone scans, etc.). Radiotherapy can be given post-operatively if there is evidence of extra-renal spread.

25% of cases are technically inoperable. In inoperable cases radiotherapy can be given (usually 3,500cGy to 5,000cGy over 3 to 5 weeks) but only delays the onset of local progression of disease.

Patients with advanced (Stage 4) disease rarely survive more than 18 months. If the local disease is still operable, palliative surgery can offer the best means of controlling local disease and controlling or preventing symptoms of renal pain and hematuria. In a reasonably fit patient, resection of a solitary metastasis (lung, skin, bone, brain) can occasionally produce a long tumor-free interval. Rarely (in about 1% of patients) metastases can regress after nephrectomy, but the operation itself has a 5% mortality.

If surgery is unwise, an alternative treatment is renal artery embolization (using an injection of material to occlude the artery) which causes infarction of the tumor and temporary control of the tumor, which may prevent or delay local symptoms.

An occasional response (in about 5% of patients) to hormone therapy can occur, and medroxyprogesterone acetate 100mg 3 times a day is sometimes given. Only about 20% of patients show some response to chemotherapy.

Problems in advanced disease:

- Pain
- Hematuria
- Bone metastases
- Thromboses
- Hypercalcemia

Local disease can cause **visceral pain** (which is morphine-responsive) or hematuria.

Hematuria is usually not heavy. It may be controlled by radiotherapy or oral anti-fibrinolytics. (see *Bleeding*)

Symptoms in advanced disease can be mainly due to **metastases**. 40% of patients develop bone metastases. Other common sites for metastases are lung, mediastinum, liver, skin and brain). (see *Bone Pain*)

The tumor characteristically grows into the inferior vena cava causing venous **thrombosis**. This can cause bilateral leg edema and can also obstruct the hepatic veins causing jaundice and ascites (Budd Chiari syndrome). Anti-coagulation may be necessary. (see *Anti-coagulants*)

Hypercalcemia occurs in around 5%. (see *Hypercalcemia*)

Rarely the tumor may cause heart failure due to an arteriovenous shunt within the tumor. Hypertension, polycythemia and fever can also occur.

SARCOMA

Background information — Sarcomas are malignant tumors of the soft tissues. They can arise deep in the tissues, and may present with few signs other than painful enlargement of the area, commonly the buttock, calf or thigh. Most are liposarcomas (fat) or leiomyosarcomas (muscle). Untreated, the tumor can reach a massive size. CT scan will define the extent of the tumor, but diagnosis must be confirmed by biopsy.

Treatment is by radical excision including a 2.5cm cuff of normal tissue (attempts to simply "shell out" the tumor lead to local recurrence). After a wide radical excision only 10% get local recurrence. Amputation may be performed if wide excision is not possible.

Sarcomas are resistant to radiotherapy and chemotherapy. Radiotherapy is sometimes given post-operatively but has little potential for improving survival.

Problems in advanced disease — Spread to lymph nodes is unusual but metastases commonly occur to lung and liver, with median survival around 12 months. A single pulmonary metastasis can be excised which extends the prognosis to 5 year survival for 25% of patients.

Recurrent disease and distant metastases are more malignant than the initial primary tumor and grow rapidly.

STOMACH CANCER

Background information — Almost all stomach cancers are adenocarcinomas. Patients often present late with a long history of dysepsia.

A family history of gastric cancer, pernicious anemia or a partial gastrectomy more than 10 years before (causing hypo-acidity) all increase the risk. Signs (mass, nodes, ascites) suggest advanced inoperable disease but most patients require a laparotomy in order to assess operability. Lymphatic spread increases with the depth of gastric wall invasion but can be present even in the most superficial tumors.

Treatment — Curative surgery is attempted in about 40% of patients, but only 10% are cured. Attempted surgical cure usually involves radical subtotal gastrectomy (leaving the fundus) with gastrojejunostomy (Billroth II operation). Lesions in the upper third of the stomach require a total gastrectomy with roux-en-Y esophagojejunostomy. After total gastrectomy long-term survivors require iron supplements and monthly B12 injections. Patients have to adapt to having frequent small meals.

In about 60% of patients the cancer is incurable and survival is measured in months. **Resection** of the primary tumor by subtotal gastrectomy with gastrojejunostomy (to drain the stomach) offers the best palliation by reducing the problems of pain, hemorrhage or obstruction. Intubation can be offered for dysphagia due to obstructing proximal tumors. Neither the size of the lesion nor extension to neighboring structures need prevent resection, but such palliative surgery has a high mortality.

Radiotherapy has no place in management (treatment causes anorexia and nausea and survival is rarely improved).

Chemotherapy with fluorouracil has about a 20% response rate but does not prolong survival. It is rarely if ever useful for control of symptoms. Trials of combination chemotherapy are continuing.

Problems in advanced disease:

- Dyspepsia
- Visceral pain
- Nausea
- Obstructive vomiting
- Metastases (liver, lung, peritoneum)
- Ascites
- Pancreatic invasion
- Acanthosis nigricans

Antacids and H2-receptor antagonists will relieve the **dyspepsia** of an ulcerated cancer, and may promote temporary healing. They do not reduce blood loss.

Visceral pains may be from the gastric carcinoma itself, or from involved lymph nodes, or due to liver metastases. All respond well to titrated doses of morphine. Occasionally severe pain occurs that is not well controlled by a full dose of morphine (i.e., a dose that begins to cause drowsiness for the patient) and a celiac plexus nerve block should then be considered. (see *Celiac Plexus Block*)

Nausea is a common problem and usually controllable with anti-emetics (by suppository, injection or continuous subcutaneous infusion until nausea is controlled). Remember to exclude constipation. For persistent nausea consider ranitidine or a trial of steroids in addition to anti-emetics.

Most patients are able to continue eating right up to a few days before death. (see *Nausea & Vomiting*)

Malignant **pyloric stenosis** causes a typical pattern of obstructive vomiting (large volumes of undigested food with little nausea). Anti-emetics are of little help (since nausea is not the problem). About 50% of patients respond within 2 to 3 days to high dose steroids (dexamethasone 8mg per day), by injection until the vomiting settles. (see *Nausea & Vomiting*)

Metastases to the peritoneum can cause ascites. Invasion of the pancreas can cause steatorrhea. (see *Ascites, Diarrhea*)

Acanthosis nigricans is a rare skin condition sometimes associated with stomach cancer. Brown or black benign eruptions, which have a velvety surface and multiple small papillary outgrowths, occur in the armpits and groin. There is no treatment.

UNKNOWN PRIMARY CANCER

Definition — Histologically confirmed metastatic tumor with no evidence of a primary site (despite routine tests). It occurs in about 7% of cancer patients.

Background information — The patient is clinically ill, with weight loss and weakness. Further investigations to find the primary are not helpful if they will not alter the outcome. It is important to obtain a tissue diagnosis whenever possible and not to accept a diagnosis of carcinomatosis based upon tests such as scans or x-rays.

The prognosis is poor. Median survival is only 3 to 5 months and only 10% of patients are alive at two years. This is presumably because the tumor is usually aggressive, with a tendency to early metastasis when it is still small (and difficult to detect).

In the majority of patients the primary site will be pancreas, lung, stomach or colon. Intensive investigations will identify the primary tumor in only 10% of patients.

Histology usually shows adenocarcinoma or poorly differentiated carcinoma. A review of the histology is important. Special staining techniques may show that a tumor thought to be anaplastic carcinoma is in fact a treatable lymphoma or germ cell tumor.

The likely primary depends on the site of the metastases:

Site of Metastasis	Likely Primary Tumor
Cervical nodes	Nasopharynx, thyroid, breast, lung
Supraclavicular nodes	Lung, intra-abdominal
Axillary nodes	Breast, lung
Inguinal nodes	Vulval, anorectal, prostate, ovary
Brain	Lung, breast, prostate, melanoma
Skin	Breast, lung, melanoma
Intra-abdominal, with ascites or hepatomegaly	Ovary, stomach, pancreas, colon

The aim of further investigations is to exclude cancers which it may be possible to treat:

- Lymphoma
- Germ cell tumors
- Well-differentiated thyroid cancer

or to palliate:

- Ovary - chemotherapy
- Bronchus (small (oat) cell) - chemotherapy
- Breast - chemotherapy or hormone therapy
- Prostate - hormone therapy

Other tests that may be useful include:

- Acid phosphatase (prostate)
- Human chorionic gonadotropin (germ cell tumor)
- Alpha-fetoprotein (hepatoma)
- Urine microscopy for red blood cells (renal carcinoma)
- Bone marrow examination (lymphoma)
- Mammogram

Treatment — Combination chemotherapy can sometimes induce a regression, but treatment is usually disappointing. In young men with undifferentiated tumors a trial of germ cell tumor chemotherapy may be worthwhile. In women with adenocarcinoma a trial of tamoxifen is worthwhile, even with no evidence that the breast is the primary site. If prostate cancer is suspected but unproven (for example, a man with bone metastases from an unknown primary) a trial of anti-androgen therapy may be warranted, although prostate cancer with a normal acid phosphatase level and negative biopsy is rare.

Management can be very difficult. Having no proven primary site of origin can increase the difficulty of coping with a diagnosis of cancer. Uncertainty is the hardest emotion of all to bear. Explanation (about possible sites and the reason for limited investigations) is very important, and can protect a patient from spending the last few months of life having extensive (and expensive) investigations which have no chance of altering the outcome. If treatment is given its purpose and rationale need to be explained in detail.

VULVAL CANCER

Background information — The majority of vulval tumors are squamous carcinomas affecting older age groups. Dystrophic changes predispose to carcinoma. It is said to be associated with diabetes.

Most patients present with pruritus vulvae, pain, ulceration or discharge. Vulval cancers are usually visible. Diagnosis is by biopsy. Assessment of lymphatic spread may involve lymphography, node aspiration or CT scan.

If nodes are not involved 5-year survival is over 75%. This falls to 40% if femoral or inguinal nodes are involved, and to 20% if pelvic nodes are involved.

Treatment of choice is radical excision of the carcinomas and lymphatics. Primary skin closure without the need of skin grafting is usually possible because of the laxity of the skin in this area. In patients unfit for surgery, palliative radiotherapy can reduce pain and ulceration.

Problems in advanced disease — The disease spreads locally (to vagina, urethra and anus), to superficial nodes bilaterally (femoral and inguinal), and to pelvic nodes (via urethral lymphatics). Bloodborne spread is rare until very late in the disease.

The main problems are local:

- Ulceration (soreness, discharge, smell)
- Lymphedema (legs, vulva)
- Nodes (pain, bleeding)

The preceding summaries provide brief background information only, and are not intended as definitive statements.

NOTES

NOTES

HOSPICE
INFORMATION & REFERRAL

HOSPICELINK® is a nationwide toll-free telephone service offering referral to over 1,700 local hospices and palliative care services in the United States, general information about hospice principles and practices, and limited informal support to callers who wish to discuss personal problems relating to terminal illness and bereavement. HOSPICELINK® is a service of the Hospice Education Institute, and is available to both health professionals and members of the public.

800-331-1620
(Alaska & Connecticut: 203-767-1620)

CANCER
INFORMATION & REFERRAL

The American Cancer Society's nationwide toll-free telephone service offers information about currently accepted cancer treatments for all types of cancer. Local chapters of the American Cancer Society maintain lists of specialist physicians in their areas, and offer many services and support groups to cancer patients and their families.

The Cancer Information Service of the National Cancer Institute offers information about both conventional cancer treatment and experimental trials and protocols currently in progress at designated medical centers, and will assist both health professionals and patients seeking referral to specialist cancer centers.

Other reputable non-profit organizations offer assistance and advice to cancer patients in a particular state or region, or to patients suffering from a particular type of cancer. Additional information about many such organizations is listed in "Health Hotlines," a publication of the U.S. Department of Health and Human Services.

American Cancer Society
800-227-2345

Cancer Information Service
800-422-6237
(Alaska: 800-638-6070   Hawaii: 800-524-1234)

AIDS
INFORMATION & REFERRAL

The Centers for Disease Control AIDS Information Hotline offers general information about AIDS, maintains a directory of local AIDS treatment and support organizations nationwide, and offers advice and support to persons with AIDS, to HIV-positive persons, and to those who fear possible exposure to HIV.

800-342-2437

ALS INFORMATION

The Amyotrophic Lateral Sclerosis Association offers general information about ALS, patient and family educational publications, and referrals to ALS specialty clinics.

800-782-4747

ALZHEIMER'S DISEASE
INFORMATION

The Alzheimer's Disease and Related Disorders Association offers general information about Alzheimer's Disease, and makes referrals to local and state chapters of the association and community support services.

800-621-0379
(Illinois: 800-572-6037)

INDEX OF DRUGS

Tables of Drugs (Generic/Proprietary and Proprietary/Generic) appear at the front of the book

Index of Drugs

Index of Drugs

Index of Drugs

USEFUL REFERENCES

Acworth A, Bruggen P. *Family Therapy when One Member is on the Death Bed.* Journal of Family Therapy (UK) 1985; 7:379-385.

Amiel SA, et al. *Intravenous Infusion of Frusemide as Treatment for Ascites in Malignant Disease.* British Medical Journal 1984; 7 April:1041.

Baines M. *Pain Relief in Active Patients with Cancer: Analgesic Drugs are the Foundation of Management.* British Medical Journal 1989; 7 January:36-38.

Baines M, et al. *Medical Management of Intestinal Obstruction in Patients with Advanced Disease.* Lancet 1985; II:990-993.

Barr H, Krasner N. *Interstitial Laser Photocoagulation for Treating Bleeding Gastric Cancer.* British Medical Journal 1989; 9 September:659-660.

Bulkin W, Lukashok H. *Rx for Dying: The Case for Hospice.* New England Journal of Medicine 1988; 318:376-378.

Carlisle DW, et al. *Intraventricular Morphine Administered by Hospice Nurses to a Patient with Intractable Pain.* The American Journal of Hospice Care 1989; 4:36-39.

Dixon JA. *Current Laser Applications in General Surgery.* Annals of Surgery 1988; 4:355-372.

Filshie J, Morrison PJ. *Acupuncture for Chronic Pain: A Review.* Palliative Medicine 1988; 2:1-14.

Fowlie M, et al. *Quality of Life in Advanced Cancer: The Benefits of Asking the Patient.* Palliative Medicine 1989; 3:55-59.

Hanks GW, et al. *Corticosteroids in Terminal Cancer — A Prospective Analysis of Current Practice.* Postgraduate Medical Journal 1983; 59:702-706.

Hinton J. *Whom do Dying Patients Tell.* British Medical Journal 1980; 15 November:1328-1330.

Jenkins H. *The Family and Loss: A Systems Framework.* Palliative Medicine 1989; 2:97-104.

Kaye PM, Oliver DJ. *Hypercalcemia in Advanced Malignancy.* Lancet 1985; I:512.

Lapin J, et al. *Cancer Pain Management with a Controlled-Release Oral Morphine Preparation.* Journal of Pain and Symptom Management 1989; 4:146-151.

Levy M. (Guest Editor) *Palliative Care.* Seminars in Oncology 1985; 12:No. 4.

Librach SL. *The Use of TENS for the Relief of Pain in Palliative Care.* Palliative Medicine 1988; 2:15-20.

Lipman AG. *Opioid Analgesics in the Management of Cancer Pain.* The American Journal of Hospice Care 1989; 1:13-23.

Lloyd JW, et al. *Cryoanalgesia: A New Approach to Pain Relief.* Lancet 1976; II:932-934.

MacAdam DB. *An Initial Assessment of Suffering in Terminal Illness.* Palliative Medicine 1987; 1:37-47.

Maloney CM, et al. *The Rectal Administration of MS-Contin: Clinical Implications of Use in End Stage Cancer.* The American Journal of Hospice Care 1989; 4:34-35.

Price P, et al. *Prospective Randomized Trial of Single and Multifraction Radiotherapy Schedules in the Treatment of Painful Bony Metastases.* Radiotherapy and Oncology 1986; 6:247-255.

Schell HW. *The Role of Adrenal Corticosteroid Therapy in Far Advanced Cancer.* American Journal of the Medical Sciences 1966; December:641-649.

Scofield GR. *Terminal Care and the Continuing Need for Professional Education.* Journal of Palliative Care 1989; 3:32-36.

Valleri RM, et al. *Palliative Gastrointestinal Endoscopy.* Palliative Medicine 1988; 2:101-106.

Walsh TD. *Oral Morphine in Chronic Cancer Pain.* Pain 1984; 18:1-11.

Walsh TD. *Opiates and Respiratory Function in Advanced Cancer.* Recent Results in Cancer Research 1984; 89: 115-117.

Wanzer SH, et al. *The Physician's Responsibility toward Hopelessly Ill Patients: A Second Look.* New England Journal of Medicine 1989; 320:844-849.

USEFUL BOOKS

Ainsworth-Smith, I & Speck, P
Letting Go: Caring For The Dying And Bereaved
SPCK, 1982
(U.S. Distributor: Abingdon Press)

Amenta, MO & Bohnet, ML
Nursing Care Of The Terminally Ill
Little, Brown and Company, 1986

Bates, TD (Editor)
Contemporary Palliation Of Difficult Symptoms
Clinical Oncology Series, Vol. 1, No. 2
Balliere Tindall (London), 1987

Billings, JA
Outpatient Management Of Advanced Cancer
J. B. Lippincott Company, 1985

Bluebond-Langner, M
The Private World Of Dying Children
Princeton University Press, 1978

Bowlby, J
Attachment And Loss
   Volume I: *Attachment*
   Volume II: *Separation: Anxiety And Anger*
   Volume III: *Loss, Sadness And Depression*
Basic Books, 1984

Corr, CA & DM (Editors)
Hospice Care: Principles And Practice
Springer Publishing Company, 1983

Cousins, N
Anatomy Of An Illness As Perceived By The Patient
W. W. Norton, 1979

Jolly, J
Missed Beginnings: Death Before Life Has Been Established
(The Lisa Sainsbury Foundation Series)
Austen Cornish, 1987
(U.S. Distributor: Hospice Education Institute)

Kübler-Ross, E
On Death And Dying
Macmillan, 1969

Latham, J
Pain Control
(The Lisa Sainsbury Foundation Series)
Austen Cornish, 1987
(U.S. Distributor: Hospice Education Institute)

Useful Books

Lugton, J
Communicating With Dying People And Their Relatives
(The Lisa Sainsbury Foundation Series)
Austen Cornish, 1987
(U.S. Distributor: Hospice Education Institute)

McCaffery, M
Nursing Management Of The Patient With Pain
J. B. Lippincott Company, 1979

Neuberger, J
Caring For Dying People Of Different Faiths
(The Lisa Sainsbury Foundation Series)
Austen Cornish, 1987
(U.S. Distributor: Hospice Education Institute)

Parkes, CM
Bereavement: Studies Of Grief In Adult Life
(New Edition)
International Universities Press, 1986

Pincus, L
Death And The Family
Random House, 1974

Saunders, C (Editor)
The Management Of Terminal Malignant Disease
Edward Arnold (Publishers) Ltd., 1984
(U.S. Distributor: Williams & Wilkins)

Saunders, C Summers, DH & Teller, N (Editors)
Hospice: The Living Idea
Edward Arnold (Publishers) Ltd., 1981
(U.S. Distributor: Williams & Wilkins)

Speck, P
Being There: Pastoral Care In Time Of Illness
SPCK, 1988
(U.S. Distributor: Abingdon Press)

Spilling, R (Editor)
Terminal Care At Home
Oxford University Press, 1986

Stedeford, A
Facing Death: Parents, Families, Professionals
Heinemann, 1984
(U.S. Distributor: Butterworth & Co.)

Stoddard, S
The Hospice Movement
Random House, 1978

Twycross, RG & Lack, SA
Therapeutics In Terminal Cancer
Pitman, 1984
(U.S. Distributor: Urban & Schwarzenberg)

Wall, PD & Melzack, R (Editors)
Textbook Of Pain (2nd Edition)
Churchill Livingstone, 1989

Wilson-Barnett, J & Raiman, J (Editors)
Nursing Issues And Research In Terminal Care
John Wiley & Sons, 1988

Worcester, A
The Care Of The Aged, The Dying, And The Dead
Thomas, 1935

Worden, JW
Grief Counseling And Grief Therapy
Springer Publishing Company, 1982

Zimmerman, JM
Hospice: Complete Care For The Terminally Ill
(2nd Edition)
Urban & Schwarzenberg, 1986

Zorza, R & V
A Way To Die
Knopf, 1980

USEFUL JOURNALS

Palliative Medicine
Doyle D, Editor-in-Chief

Cambridge University Press
(North American Distributor)
110 Midland Avenue
Port Chester, New York 10573

The American Journal of Hospice Care
Lescohier D, Managing Editor

Prime National Publishing Corporation
470 Boston Post Road
Weston, Massachusetts 02193

The Journal of Palliative Care
Roy DJ, Editor-in-Chief

110 Pine Avenue West
Montreal, Quebec H2W 1R7
Canada

ABOUT THE AUTHOR

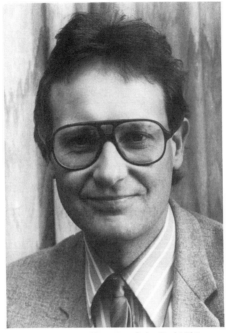

Photograph by Yoshi Shimazu

Dr. Peter Kaye is Consultant in Palliative Medicine to the Oxford Regional Health Authority, and Medical Director of Cynthia Spencer House, a hospice in Northampton, England. Educated at Cambridge University and Westminster Hospital Medical College, Dr. Kaye practiced as a family physician before completing his residency in hospice medicine at St. Christopher's Hospice in London. Dr. Kaye is a Member of the Royal College of Physicians and the Royal College of General Practitioners, and is a Diplomate of the Royal College of Obstetricians & Gynecologists. He is the author of a medical textbook on obstetrics and gynecology. Dr. Kaye lectures frequently on hospice topics in Great Britain, has broadcast on BBC radio and television, and has lectured throughout the United States.